BIPOLAR DISORDER

FRANCIS MARK MONDIMORE, M.D.

Bipolar Disorder

A Guide for Patients and Families

Third Edition

JOHNS HOPKINS UNIVERSITY PRESS   BALTIMORE

NOTE TO THE READER. This book is not meant to substitute for medical care of people with bipolar disorder or depression, and treatment should not be based solely on its contents. Nor is it meant to offer legal advice, which must be obtained from a practicing attorney.

Johns Hopkins University Press
2715 North Charles Street
Baltimore, Maryland 21218-4363
www.press.jhu.edu

LIBRARY OF CONGRESS CATALOGING-IN-PUBLICATION DATA

Mondimore, Francis Mark, 1953–
   Bipolar disorder : a guide for patients and families / Francis Mark Mondimore, M.D. — Third edition.
       pages cm. — (A Johns Hopkins press health book)
   Includes bibliographical references and index.
   ISBN 978-1-4214-1205-4 (hardcover : alk. paper) — ISBN 978-1-4214-1206-1 (pbk. : alk. paper) — ISBN 978-1-4214-1207-8 (electronic) — ISBN 1-4214-1205-5 (hardcover : alk. paper) — ISBN 1-4214-1206-3 (pbk. : alk. paper) — ISBN 1-4214-1207-1 (electronic)
       1. Manic-depressive illness—Popular works. 2. Affective disorders—Popular works. I. Title.
RC516.M64 2014
616.89′5—dc23   2013015236

A catalog record for this book is available from the British Library.

Figures 2-1, 2-4, 2-5, 5-1, 6-1, 15-1, and 16-1 by Jacqueline Schaffer.

Special discounts are available for bulk purchases of this book. For more information, please contact Special Sales at 410-516-6936 or specialsales@press.jhu.edu.

Johns Hopkins University Press uses environmentally friendly book materials, including recycled text paper that is composed of at least 30 percent post-consumer waste, whenever possible.

To the memory of Sallie Mink, R.N.
Caring nurse, tireless educator, and
passionate advocate for those
with bipolar disorder and their families.
You are sorely missed, my friend.

Contents

Preface

About 2 percent of the population suffers from some form of bipolar disorder. Winston Churchill, George Frideric Handel, Lord Byron, Virginia Woolf, Edgar Allan Poe, Napoleon Bonaparte, and Vincent van Gogh are only a few of the politicians, writers, artists, and musicians who, despite having bipolar disorder, left a mark of greatness upon the world.[1] Most persons who are affected by this illness, however, are ordinary people who want nothing more than to get back to their everyday lives after they or their family members have been diagnosed with it. This book is written for them.

We psychiatrists have at times become a little complacent about this disease. When lithium became widely available in the United States in the mid-1970s, many psychiatrists thought the battle to control the illness had been won. Indeed, lithium was—and still is—a miracle drug for many people who suffer from what was then known as manic-depression. More recent studies indicate that a substantial proportion of patients—according to some studies, as many as half—have a relapse of their illness despite taking lithium.[2] But even as we become more aware of the sobering facts about the difficulty of successfully treating bipolar disorder, an explosion of developments in science and medicine holds great promise for those affected by the disease. In this book I shall relate this good news.

Clinical research has shown again and again that many relapses of bipolar disorder occur not because of medication failure, but rather because patients stop taking medication and drop out of treatment. Perhaps patients don't understand that relapse and repetition of illness episodes are the hallmark of the illness, that *abruptly* stopping medication has been shown to be especially risky, that medication side effects can often be treated or controlled, and that new medications are becoming available all the time. I hope this book helps those who face difficult treatment decisions to make well-informed and intelligent choices.

A survey of patients with bipolar disorder and other mood disorders, carried out by the National Depressive and Manic-Depressive Association (now, the Depression and Bipolar Support Alliance) in the early 1990s, found that 36 percent of those who responded to the questionnaire had not sought professional treatment until more than *ten years* after their symptoms had begun.[3] Of the bipolar patients in this study, 73 percent had received at least one incorrect diagnosis before being identified as having bipolar disorder—often many years after first seeking help. The average respondent had seen 3.3 physicians before being correctly diagnosed. Why is this illness so difficult to identify correctly? One reason is that full-blown manic-depressive illness is only one of the several forms this chameleon disorder can take—and manic-depressive illness may in fact be less common than the milder forms (the so-called soft bipolar disorders), in which symptoms of mild depression and subtle "mood swings" may be the only manifestations of bipolar disorder. We are realizing that many patients with these milder forms of the disorder benefit from treatment with mood-stabilizing medications, too. But they can do so only if they seek treatment and are correctly diagnosed. We shall see why many patients who have a bipolar disorder are told they have "only depression" or a "personality disorder" and shall also see the consequences of these and other diagnostic errors.

Like any other serious illness, bipolar disorder affects not only the person who suffers from the disease but family, friends, and colleagues as well. Family support is crucial to the effective management of symptoms. The disrupted relationships and interpersonal conflicts that the symptoms of the illness can cause make bipolar disorder all the more difficult and complicated to treat. Information and understanding are definitely part of the treatment for this disease, and this book was written not only for the patient but for the patient's family and friends as well.

Bipolar disorder can be a fatal disease. Although the figures vary among studies, about 15 percent of persons with bipolar disorder commit suicide;[4] many more make suicide attempts. These are preventable deaths, because very effective treatments for this illness exist. I hope that the information this book provides about the treatment of bipolar disorder addresses some of the reasons why individuals are reluctant to enter treatment and dissuades some from stopping treatment against medical advice. Yes, it is my hope that this book will save lives.

PART I

SYMPTOMS, SYNDROMES, AND DIAGNOSIS

A professor of mine once told me, "When you can't figure out *what* the patient has, he or she probably has bipolar disorder." I remember thinking at the time that this was one of the most foolish things I had ever heard a Johns Hopkins faculty member say. But over the years I have come to realize that he was right.

Bipolar disorder is the chameleon of psychiatric disorders, changing its symptoms from one patient to the next and from one episode of illness to the next even in the same patient. It is a phantom that can sneak up on its victim cloaked in the darkness of melancholy but then disappear for years at a time—only to return in the resplendent but fiery robes of mania. Although both depression and mania had been described over two millennia previously by Greek and Persian physicians—several of whom thought the conditions were linked in some way—it wasn't until the early part of the twentieth century that a German psychiatrist, Emil Kraepelin, convincingly presented the idea that these opposite conditions were two sides of one pathological coin, the two profiles of a Janus-faced disease that he called manic-depressive insanity.

Why did it take more than two thousand years for someone to solve a puzzle having only two pieces? Because, as my professor knew, there are so many more than two pieces to this mysterious disorder. The depressed phase can be merely gloomy or profoundly despairing; torpid and lethargic, or agitated and churning. The manic phase can be no more than an enthusiastic glow, or it can be an exultant, transcendental fervor, frenzied panic, or delirious, crashing, raving psychosis. Sometimes opposite moods seem to be combined, as inseparable as smoke and fire, mood states that have been given names like *depressive mania, manic stupor, agitated depression,* and more recently and more simply, *mixed states.* The tendency of the illness to hibernate—for symptoms to spontaneously disappear for years, even decades at a time—adds to the confusion, perplexing the diagnostician and lulling the patient into dangerous complacency regarding the need for treatment.

In this first part of the book, there are four chapters examining the symptoms, the syndromes, and the diagnosis of bipolar disorder. In chapter 1, "Normal and Abnormal Mood," we review the many symptoms of bipolar disorder, collected into three main clusters: *mania, depression,* and the *mixed mood states.* I have not minimized the severity of the symptoms in this chapter; I present all the possible symptoms of the illness, many of them frightening and terrible. But it is important to remember, first, that not every person with bipolar disorder develops all the possible symptoms, and second, that modern treatments usually prevent the development of the worst of them, many of which are now rarely seen even by psychiatrists.

The different forms the disorder can take is the subject of chapter 2, "The Diagnosis of Bipolar Disorder." The diagnosis of bipolar disorder is complex, and there is still some disagreement about how the different symptom clusters are related to one another. Are there several different diseases of mood with different causes? Is there a group of disorders that share common features *and* common causes? Are these illness forms essentially the *same* disorder differing only in details of expression? Do these different forms remain the same over time in each patient, or can one form develop into another? The answers to some of these questions remain unknown. Nevertheless, there are several forms of the illness that can be reliably identified and separated from one another. Identifying one or another of these forms allows for predictions about the course of the illness over time and about the type of treatment that has the best chance of being effective.

Chapter 3, "Bipolar Disorder and the *DSM-5*," reviews the official classification system for the illness that is currently used by the American Psychiatric Association (and by many psychiatrists throughout the world). This chapter might be considered optional reading and will probably be of more interest to students and professionals concerned with the details of illness classification and diagnostic categories.

In chapter 4, "The Mood Disease," I show how psychiatrists came to realize that bipolar disorder is indeed a disease. For decades, persons afflicted with mood disorders were often given the covert message by their physicians that they themselves were to blame for their symptoms. Depression and other mood symptoms were blamed on emotional immaturity or "maladjustment" rather than being recognized as expressions of disordered functioning of the brain. It was only with the discovery of effective pharmaceuticals that psychiatry realized that bipolar disorder is indeed a disease—as real as diabetes or hyperthyroidism.

CHAPTER 1

Normal and Abnormal Mood

BIPOLAR DISORDER IS A *MOOD* DISORDER, ONE OF SEVERAL EMOTIONAL disorders whose main symptom is an abnormality of mood. The first step in understanding the illness, then, is to understand what we mean by the word *mood*. Perhaps more to the point, I want to talk about what *psychiatrists* mean by the word. The dictionary isn't much help here; it defines *mood* simply as "a conscious state of mind or predominant feeling."[1] The "predominant feeling" part of this definition begins to capture the psychiatric concept, but mood is much more than just a feeling.

Our mood includes our happiness or sadness, our state of optimism or pessimism, our feelings of contentedness or dissatisfaction with our situation, and even physical feelings such as how fatigued or robust we feel. Mood is like our emotional temperature, a set of feelings that expresses our sense of emotional comfort or discomfort.

When individuals are in a good mood, they are confident and optimistic, relaxed and friendly, patient, interested, content. The word *happy* captures part of it, but good mood includes a lot more. People in a good mood usually feel energetic and have a sense of physical well-being; they sleep soundly and eat heartily. It's easy for them to be sociable and affectionate. The future looks bright and the moment ripe for starting new projects. When we're in a good mood, the world seems a wonderful place to live in; it feels good to be alive.

When we're in a low mood, an opposite set of feelings takes over. We tend to turn inward and may seem preoccupied or distracted by our thoughts. The word *sad* captures some of the experience, but low mood is a bit more complicated. There may be a sense of emptiness and loss. It's difficult to think about the future very much, and when one does, it's hard not to be pessimistic or even intimidated by it. We may lose our temper more easily and then feel guilty about having done so. It's difficult to be affectionate or sociable, so we avoid others and prefer to be alone. Energy is low. Self-doubt takes over; we become preoccupied, worrying about how other people see us.

Abnormal Mood

Some of life's more common stresses and the normal human reactions to them are such common experiences that common terms have been coined for some mood changes—and most people recognize these mood changes as quite normal. Moving to a new community where we don't know anyone often leads to a sense of dislocation and loneliness that we know as homesickness, an unpleasant experience that may last for days or even weeks and that everyone has probably experienced at one time or another. When someone close to us dies, a profound sense of sadness and loss—the deep sorrow that we call bereavement or mourning—occurs, and it can become temporarily incapacitating. When we come to various milestones of personal achievement, we experience changes of mood in the other direction. A graduation or wedding or the birth of a child can fill a person with joy and pride and a sense of limitless optimism that are nearly overwhelming. We wouldn't call any of these moods "abnormal," even though they may be extreme.

Like many other things we can measure in human beings—body temperature, blood pressure, and hormone levels, for example—a person's mood state normally varies within a certain range. People are not in the same mood state all the time; it is quite normal to have ups and downs of mood. Do persons with bipolar disorder simply have higher ups and deeper downs? Well, it's certainly true that the bipolar patient's ups and downs are sometimes so far outside the range of normal that it doesn't take a psychiatrist to know that something is very wrong. The abnormal mood states of bipolar disorder are accompanied by changes in thinking and bodily functions, changes that further demarcate them from normal mood. Examples include sleeplessness, changes in appetite, impaired concentration and memory, and problems with motivation and energy level. To say that persons with bipolar disorder simply have more extreme ups and downs of mood isn't even nearly right. The symptoms of bipolar disorder, which seem to be caused by a defect in the brain's *regulation* of mood, also spill over to other areas of functioning.

Laura is a forty-year-old vice president of one of the largest banks in the country.[2] When I walked out into the waiting room to call her for our first appointment, she was sitting with a laptop computer balanced on her knees and a cell phone held up to her ear. "No, Steve, that's not good enough," she was saying into the phone as she nodded to me. "No, that won't work either, we need the last quarter's *real* numbers, not an estimate. Listen, I'm . . . ah . . . in the doctor's office. I'll call you in an hour." I raised my eyebrows and shook my head. "Make that two hours. Bye." Click, click, snap, phone and computer were shut, and in a moment we were sitting in an interviewing room.

"I made this appointment as soon as I could after I read this." Laura handed me a pamphlet that the local chapter of the Depression and Bipolar Support Alliance had been handing out at a local shopping mall during a health fair recently. "I've known for years that something was wrong, but I didn't know what. Reading this has made me think medication might help."

"What have you noticed that's 'wrong'?" I asked.

"I go into these, these *things*," she started. "I get this wired, can't-slow-down feeling. I've always called it 'the crazies,' and I usually crash after it's over. Sometimes I can't get out of bed for days."

"You seem to have a very high stress job," I offered. "Maybe that's part of the problem."

"You sound like my mother. 'You don't have to take *every* promotion they offer you,' she says. But this isn't just stress, there's something else going on. The worst part is, I think these things are getting worse."

Laura's use of phrases like "the crazies" and "these things" seemed to indicate that she felt that these feelings were foreign, not like her normal feelings.

"Are you saying that sometimes your feelings and moods are controlling you rather than the other way around?" I asked.

Laura sat up straight in her chair. "That's the best way I could possibly describe it," she said decisively. "I can *feel* them coming on; it's almost physical. But I know they're . . . well, *mental,* I guess, is the best way to put it." Her face suddenly clouded over. "Does this mean I'm mentally ill?"

"Well," I said, "we know that there are illnesses that affect mood, and mood is certainly a mental state. But we have a lot more to talk about before I'll be able to say just what explains what you're going through."

Laura looked slightly relieved and said, "Well, that's why I'm here, for an explanation." She picked the brochure up from the edge of the desk. "This is the best explanation I've come across yet," she said thoughtfully. "And that means I can get rid of them, right? There's a treatment that will get rid of them?"

"There are many treatments for mood disorders. It may just take some time to find the one that works best."

"Then I came to the right place," she said as she sat back in her chair again. "'You're not crazy,' my mother said. 'You don't need to see a psychiatrist.'"

"Well, I think your mother was at least half right," I said.

Laura smiled for the first time. "OK, then let's—" Suddenly a beep-beep-beep sounded from her jacket pocket. She took out her cell phone again. "If that's, um, confidential," I offered, "I can—"

Laura pushed a button, and the beeping stopped. She put the phone back in her pocket. "No, that can't possibly be as important as this. It can wait. I want to give you my undivided attention."

"Excellent!" I thought to myself. "This is a woman who understands priorities."

Imagine a person whose temperature regulation system doesn't work correctly—a person who suddenly starts shivering on a warm sunny day or breaks out into a sweat in a room in which everyone else is chilly. This person's reactions to warm and cold are abnormal; her body "thinks" it is cold when it isn't and she feels hot when the temperature is cool. We can think of mood disorders as problems with *emotional* temperature regulation.

In mood disorders, the mood becomes disconnected from the individual's environment, and "happy" and "sad" feelings take on rhythms and fluctuations of their own. Sometimes the fluctuations are mild, and the affected person only seems to have *more* ups and downs than other people have and to have mood fluctuations that are more difficult to understand. But because such individuals don't get profoundly depressed or irrationally "high," their problems are dismissed as being due to a difficult personality or to "immaturity." Sometimes, though, the mood states are so extremely abnormal that a person's ability to judge reality is shattered; his behavior can be bizarre and frightening. (It is in some of these cases that a diagnosis of schizophrenia can be mistakenly made, with the result that proper treatment goes wanting.) If the mood-disorder patient and his situation are examined with enough care, however, the basic underlying problem, the regulation of mood, will be found.

It is because the basic problem is *regulation* of mood that the disorder can present different symptoms at different times. Persons afflicted with the classic form of the illness have periods of severe *depression* as well as periods of *mania* (a mood state that is in some ways the opposite of depression). The observation that both of these mood states occur at various times during the course of the illness gave rise to the older name for the disorder: manic-depressive illness. These opposite moods occur in affected persons because the brain mechanisms that normally regulate mood don't work properly. This observation—that the mood states of affected persons move to either of the two polar opposite extremes of mood—gives the disorder its modern name, bipolar disorder. In the following sections we'll take a closer look at these opposites, or poles, of bipolar disorder, as well as an abnormal mood state in which the two opposites seem to be combined, a condition simply called a *mixed mood state.* Then, in chapter 2, we will see how the various combinations of these mood syndromes define the different forms of bipolar disorder.

A word you will frequently come across in discussions of mood disorders is *affect* (pronounced with the accent on the first syllable). To be precise, *affect* refers to the appearance of a person's mood state. *Mood* refers to the patient's inner experience, while *affect* refers to what others observe about a person's mood, the external signs of mood. (Psychiatrists talk of a patient's affect being depressed or irritable, and so forth.)

Mania

The manic state, or more simply *mania,* is the most extreme and dramatic of the symptom clusters of bipolar disorder.[3] Many persons who have bipolar disorder never have a full-blown manic episode. But since mania is the most unmistakable and probably the most dangerous of the abnormal mood states associated with mood disorders, it is a good place to start.

In the manic state, the mood regulator switches into "high." Mania usually starts gradually and may take weeks to develop fully. Although the symptoms may be almost imperceptible at first, they gradually become more extreme, more unpleasant, and more unmistakably pathological (table 1-1).

In the early stages of mania, the mood state of affected persons begins gradually to move "upward," and they find themselves filled with pleasant feelings of exuberance—what a physician writing over a hundred years ago called "a welling up of a sense of well being and an overflowing of the spirits."[4] This heightened sense of well-being and confidence grows and expands and gradually evolves into euphoria. One bipolar patient described it this way:

> The world was filled with pleasure and promise; I felt great. Not just great, I felt *really* great. I felt I could do anything, that no task was too

TABLE 1-1 Symptoms of mania

Mood symptoms	Bodily symptoms
Elated, euphoric mood	Increased energy level
Irritable mood	Decreased need for sleep
Grandiosity	Erratic appetite
	Increased libido
Cognitive (thinking) symptoms	
Feelings of heightened concentration	*Symptoms of psychosis*
Accelerated thinking ("racing thoughts")	Grandiose delusions
	Hallucinations

difficult. My mind seemed clear, fabulously focused, and able to make intuitive mathematical leaps that had up to that point entirely eluded me. . . . Not only did everything make perfect sense, but it all began to fit into a marvelous kind of cosmic relatedness.[5]

And here we confront one of the many ironies of this illness: at the onset of an episode of the disorder, it is not uncommon to feel *better* than usual. One manic patient said, "If I'm ill, this is the most wonderful illness I've ever had."[6]

Changes in thinking accompany the changes in mood. The feeling that one is thinking more clearly and more rationally than usual is especially common in the early stages of mania. This is an especially troublesome symptom, since such a mental state is not likely to make a person suspect that something is wrong. Not only does thinking seem clearer than usual to the manic patient, but a feeling that mental processes are moving *faster* than usual also develops. At first there may be only a pleasant sense of nimbleness of thinking. Invariably, however, thinking processes accelerate: "quick" becomes "fast" and finally "racing." This vivid description of such an acceleration of thinking—illustrating what psychiatrists call *flight of ideas*—comes from a collection of patient accounts written early in the twentieth century:

My thoughts ran with lightning-like rapidity from one subject to another. All the problems of the universe came crowding into my mind, demanding instant discussion and solution—mental telepathy, hypnotism, wireless, telegraphy, Christian science, women's rights, and all the problems of medical science, religion and politics.

Thoughts chased one another through my mind with lightning rapidity. I felt like a person driving a wild horse at a weak rein, who dares not use force but run[s] his course, following the line of least resistance, mad impulses rush through my brain carrying me first in one direction then in another.[7]

Racing thoughts are a symptom so typical of mania that the diagnosis becomes doubtful if this symptom is absent. This tumbling, jumbled jumping from one thought to another becomes progressively worse and more unpleasant as the episode develops.

As the manic individual's thinking speeds up, her speech does as well. Rapid or *pressured* speech (the term normally used by psychiatrists) is nearly always seen in mania. Manic individuals speak more and more quickly as the episode develops, attempting to express the ideas that are whirling through their consciousness at ever-faster speeds. A psychiatric text from the beginning of the twentieth century mentions one early researcher who actually counted the number of syllables per minute spoken by manic patients. He found that manic patients spoke 180 to 200 syllables per minute, compared with 122 to 150 in nonmanic persons.[8]

Sometimes the racing thoughts and pressured speech lead to an outpouring of frenzied writing:

> I made notes of everything that happened, day and night. I made symbolic scrapbooks whose meaning only I could decipher. I wrote a fairy tale. . . . I noted down cryptically all that was said or done around me at the time, with special reference to relevant news bulletins and to jokes which were broadcast in radio programs. The time, correct to the nearest minute, was written in the margin. It was all vitally important. [I was convinced that] the major work [that] would be based on this material would be accurate, original, provocative and of profound significance.[9]

The feelings of exuberance and overconfidence that characterize mania can lead to several patterns of behavior typical of the manic state: spending sprees, sexual promiscuity, and overuse of alcohol and other intoxicating substances.

Spending sprees can be extravagant and financially catastrophic, because the manic person has no concern for where the money will come from to pay the bills. The increased sexual feelings of this stage of mania may lead to infatuations and even betrothals. One early psychiatric expert noted that "incomprehensible engagements, also pregnancies, are not rare in these states. I know cases in which the commencement of [mania] was repeatedly announced by a sudden engagement."[10] The loss of inhibitions typical in mania may also lead to promiscuity as well as to uncharacteristic bisexual or homosexual behaviors in some persons.

We shall explore the complex relationship between bipolar disorder and substance abuse in chapter 15. Suffice it to say here that increased and uncharacteristic use of intoxicating substances is frequently seen in mania.

One way to understand this hedonistic triad of mania—spending sprees, sexual overactivity, and increased substance abuse—is to group these behaviors together as expressions of an increase in "motivated behaviors" seen in mania,[11] an exaggeration of the normal drives toward pleasurable goals.

There are almost always changes in sleeping and eating habits in mania. A decreased need for sleep is in fact one of the first symptoms to develop in mania—often a clue for individuals who have been manic before that another episode may be starting. Food intake is usually reduced because manic individuals simply don't have time to eat. Constantly distracted by new thoughts and ideas, they feel pressed to continue to act; they just can't sit still long enough to finish a meal. The ensuing weight loss can be dramatic.

As the combination of euphoric mood and mental quickness develops, the manic individual begins to feel tremendously self-confident, even fearless. This is the so-called *grandiosity* of the manic state. Fears of unpleasant consequences disappear altogether, and reckless enthusiasm takes over. The affected person may seek out new adventures and experiences with no regard for the possible adverse repercussions. This is one of the points at which the manic person can begin to lose touch with reality—when the grandiose thinking leads the individual to start *believing* the great things he feels capable of.

In a landmark work on bipolar disorder that we'll discuss in detail in chapter 4, the German psychiatrist Emil Kraepelin recorded the symptoms and course of the illness he called *manic-depressive insanity*. (I also quote Kraepelin extensively here and in chapter 2. Not only did Kraepelin write some of the most vivid and enduring descriptions of the symptoms of bipolar disorder, but his insights into the different forms and the course of the illness have proved to be correct again and again.) Kraepelin's description of the grandiose delusions of mania, written in 1896, is classic:

> The patient asserts that he is descended from a noble family. That he is a gentleman; he calls himself a genius, the Emperor William, the Emperor of Russia, Christ, he can drive out the devil. A patient suddenly cried out on the street that he was the Lord God, the devil had left him. Female patients possess eighty genuine diamonds, are leading singers, leading violinists, Queen of Bavaria, Maid of Orleans, a fairy; they are pregnant, are going to be engaged to St. Francis, are to give birth to the redeemer . . . the Messiah.[12]

Modern patients are more likely to become convinced that they are president or prime minister rather than king or queen, a rock star rather than a great violinist, but the feelings that lead to such beliefs are the same: a fantastic, indescribable feeling of mental power and significance. Feelings of religious inspiration are very common. Patients may feel that they are a modern prophet, the founder of a new religion, a reincarnation of Christ, even a new god.

The "feeling good" stage of mania is sometimes very short-lived, and the elated mood and grandiosity can be quickly replaced by an angry, irritable mood. Quoting Kraepelin again:

> The patient is dissatisfied, intolerant, faultfinding . . . even rough. Trifling external occasions may bring about extremely violent outbursts of rage. In his fury, he thrashes his wife and children, threatens to smash everything to smithereens . . .
>
> . . . At the most trifling affront it may come to outbursts of rage of extraordinary violence . . . clamorous abuse and bellowing, to dangerous threats with shooting and stabbing, to blind destruction and actual attacks.[13]

Sometimes the manic individual alternates between elation and irritability for a time, but usually the irritable, unpleasant mood becomes predominant. It is often this irritability that brings the patient to medical attention.

As the manic state continues to develop, pressured, racing thoughts, an increased energy level, and loss of inhibitions lead to more grossly disorganized and disturbed thinking and behavior. A psychiatric textbook written in the 1950s described this stage as follows:

> Driven by greater pressure of activity, terror and excitement, [the manic person] becomes violent, attacks his neighbor, begins to shout all kinds of accusations against his alleged persecutors. . . . Distortions [and] misinterpretations . . . are now elaborated into delusions of persecution accompanied by violence and panic, the patient runs down the street nude, sets fire to the house, starts an argument with the police, shoots a gun on the street or starts suddenly to preach the gospel in a frenzied manner. . . . If crossed or interfered with in any way he becomes abusive, destructive, homicidal.[14]

Thinking patterns not only spin faster and faster but also become more bizarre. Hallucinations can develop, and beliefs called *delusions* can occur. The very best modern written descriptions of the symptoms of severe mania are those of Kay Redfield Jamison. Dr. Jamison's nearly unique qualification to set them down is that she is an internationally recognized medical expert on bipolar disorder who suffers from it herself. This passage by Dr. Jamison is what I give medical students to read so that they can learn about the symptoms of severe mania:

> Although I had been building up to this for weeks and certainly knew something was seriously wrong, there was still a definite point when

I knew I was insane. My thoughts were so fast that I couldn't remember the beginning of a sentence halfway through. Fragments of ideas, images, sentences, raced around and around in my mind like the tigers in a children's story. Finally, like those tigers, they became meaningless melted pools. Nothing familiar to me was familiar. I wanted desperately to slow down but could not.[15]

These passages vividly make the point that the manic state is not pleasant—even if it may sometimes start out that way. Those unfamiliar with the illness sometimes think that persons with bipolar disorder simply experience swings of mood between "happy" and "sad." As the foregoing illustrates, this is usually not true. The full-blown manic state is not only intensely unpleasant but also very dangerous. The danger arises not only from the increased risk of violence toward others (or toward the patient himself) but also from the physical stress the syndrome causes.

The combination of severe manic symptoms and the physical stress from such frenzied hyperactivity can lead to what Kraepelin called *delirious mania,* in which there is "profound clouding of consciousness and extraordinary and confused hallucinations. . . . The patients become stupefied, confused, bewildered and completely lose orientation for time and place."[16] Fortunately, it is now rare for a psychiatrist to see patients suffering from this severest form of the manic state, but in Kraepelin's time and even more recently, mania had a significant mortality rate. Persons with mania died "in a state of progressive exhaustion,"[17] suffering dehydration and cardiovascular collapse.

In 1973, just as lithium, the first effective treatment for bipolar disorder, was becoming available, a study from the National Institutes of Health attempted to describe a typical manic episode from beginning to end. Patients who had been admitted to a research unit that was trying to figure out how to use lithium safely and effectively for the treatment of bipolar disorder were carefully observed. The course of their symptoms was meticulously documented and described. The authors concluded that three stages could be described in a manic episode:

[Stage I]: Increased psychomotor activity which included increased . . . rate of speech and increased physical activity. . . . Euphoria predominated, although irritability became obvious when the patients' many demands were not instantly satisfied. . . . Expansiveness, grandiosity and overconfidence [were observed]. Thoughts were coherent though sometimes [disconnected]. Also frequently observed during this stage were increased sexuality or sexual preoccupations, increased interest in religion, increased and inappropriate spending of money, increased smoking, telephone use and letter writing. Some of the patients were aware of the mood change on some level and described the feeling of "going high," having racing thoughts and feeling like they were in an airplane. At this stage the patients were not out of control.

[Stage II]: Pressure of speech and . . . activity increased still further. Mood, although euphoric at times, was now more prominently characterized by increasing [unpleasantness]. . . . The irritability observed initially had progressed to open hostility and anger, and the accompanying behavior was frequently assaultive. Racing thoughts progressed to . . . increasing disorganization. Preoccupations that were present earlier became more intense with earlier . . . grandiose trends now apparent as frank delusions.

[Stage III]: A desperate, panic stricken, hopeless state experienced by the patient as clearly [unpleasant], accompanied by frenzied and frequently even more bizarre . . . activity. Thought processes that earlier had been only difficult to follow now became incoherent. . . . Delusions were bizarre. . . . Hallucinations were present [in about one-third of the patients].[18]

More recently some researchers have questioned whether typical manic episodes include all of these stages. Specifically, some researchers believe that Stage III mania (or *dysphoric mania,* as it has come to be called) occurs only in a subgroup of patients with bipolar disorder. There is some evidence that these patients have a variant of the disorder and may need medications different from what others with a more typical bipolar disorder would need. (More on this in "Mixed States," later in this chapter.) Nevertheless, this study on the "stages of mania" was important because its investigators used modern clinical methods to document how sick patients with mania can get. Even more important, it made the researchers realize that it would be easy to misdiagnose a very disorganized patient in Stage III mania as having schizophrenia, a psychiatric illness that requires a very different treatment approach and has a different prognosis from bipolar disorder.

Hypomania

In 1881 a German psychiatrist named Mendel published a book about the manic state called *Die Manie* and in it proposed that another term be used for states of milder euphoria and hyperactivity that did not progress to full-blown mania. He called this condition *hypomania,* "similar to the state of exultation in typical mania [but] with a certain lesser grade of development."[19] (The prefix *hypo-* comes from a Greek word meaning "under.") Hypomania can be thought of as having only the symptoms present at the beginning of a manic episode (Stage I in the study described above): the elated mood, the increased energy level, the rapid thinking and speaking, and sometimes a bit of the irritability. Norman Endler, another psychologist who himself suffered from a mood disorder and wrote of his experiences with the illness, described hypomania this way: "Most of the time I was busy, busy, busy; taping records, playing tennis, skiing, writing manuscripts, talking . . . reading, going to movies, staying up at night, waking up early in the morning, always on the go—busy, busy, busy. Furthermore, I was boasting about all the energy I had that enabled me to keep up this fast pace. . . . Instead of occasionally 'idling' in neutral I was always in overdrive."[20]

Although persons in the hypomanic stage do not have the severe mental disorganization of mania and are by definition not agitated and frenzied to the point of violence toward themselves or others, hypomania can nevertheless have unpleasant consequences. Feelings of increased confidence can lead to foolish investments in real estate or the stock market, and patients can squander personal resources on grandiose and risky business ventures. Increased sexual feelings can lead to extramarital affairs or promiscuity—actions that can be life-threatening in the age of HIV disease. The irritability of hypomania can lead to arguments and disagreements with family, colleagues, or neighbors that can sour relationships, sometimes irreparably. Dr. Endler described it this way:

> As a hypomanic, I didn't stop to analyze my thoughts, feelings, or behavior. I was much too busy and didn't always stop to think about what I was doing. . . . I was critical of others and occasionally told some people off publicly. I was not so concerned about . . . the effect my behavior had on [others]. I was aggressive, talked incessantly, and interrupted others while they were speaking. Whenever I had a thought I felt compelled to utter it, and I didn't always censor my thoughts and feelings. At times I seemed to have lost my sense of judgment. I was having a good time, I was narcissistically preoccupied with myself, but (without being aware of it) I was making my wife miserable.[21]

Persons with even mild hypomania can quit a good job in a burst of overconfidence or irritability, withdraw their life savings for a get-rich-quick scheme, or simply begin to drive their car too fast—all behaviors with potentially devastating consequences.

Words like *seductive* and *addictive* are frequently applied to the hypomanic syndrome. Because individuals in a hypomanic state feel so good, they seldom seek treatment. Even for persons who have a history of previous manic or depressive episodes of bipolar disorder and perhaps should know that trouble is brewing, the giddy delight of being hypomanic often seems

TABLE 1-2 Length of time before hospitalization for mania in ninety-four manic patients

Time	Percentage of patients	
	Male	Female
14–30 days	69	62
3 months	11	11
6 months	11	10
1 year or more	6	15

Source: Data from George Winoker, *Mania and Depression: A Classification of Syndrome and Disease* (Baltimore: Johns Hopkins University Press, 1991), 13.

Note: Notice that some patients have symptoms for many months before receiving needed treatment. During this time, hypomanic symptoms can wreak havoc on their lives.

too delicious to interrupt. Persons whose abnormal mood states are successfully controlled with medication sometimes stop treatment to recapture the wonderful feelings that accompany hypomania.

Because hypomanic individuals are *not* psychotic, they often cannot be involuntarily treated for their illness, because criteria for involuntary treatment insist upon "dangerous" behaviors. (We shall discuss involuntary treatment in chapter 22.) Hypomanic persons can avoid treatment for weeks, even months (table 1-2), consequently ruining their financial status, credit rating, employment history, relationships, and health.

As we shall see in a later section, many patients go through episodes of hypomania only and never become completely manic. Others have both hypomanic and manic episodes. Observations about the frequency and intensity of hypomanic versus manic episodes in different individuals are beginning to suggest that the classic "manic-depressive disorder" with episodes of full-blown mania and depression may be only one of many forms of the illness. (We shall discuss this new way of thinking about bipolar disorder in chapter 2, in the section "Bipolar Spectrum Disorders.")

The Syndrome of Depression

The depression of bipolar disorder is both easier and more difficult to describe and discuss than mania or hypomania. It is easier to discuss because depression is a more familiar set of feelings: everyone, whether suffering from bipolar disorder or not, has gone through periods of depressed mood. But the depressive syndrome of bipolar disorder is more difficult to discuss for that very reason: it is a very different experience from "normal"

TABLE 1-3 Symptoms of depression

Mood symptoms	*Bodily symptoms*
Depressed mood	Sleep disturbance:
Dysphoric mood	insomnia
Diurnal variation of mood (early-morning	hypersomnia
depression, mood improving as day	Appetite disturbance:
goes on)	weight loss
Guilty feelings	weight gain
Loss of ability to feel pleasure (anhedonia)	Loss of interest in sex
Social withdrawal	Fatigue
Suicidal thoughts	Constipation
	Headaches
Cognitive (thinking) symptoms	Worsening of painful conditions
Poor concentration	
Poor memory	*Symptoms of psychosis*
Indecision	Delusional thinking
Slowed thinking	Hallucinations
	Catatonic states

depression. In modern psychiatric terminology, this abnormal depressed mood state is called *major depression* or sometimes *clinical depression* (table 1-3).

When persons who do not suffer from a mood disorder go through a period of low mood, such as after a romantic disappointment, the loss of a job, or a period of homesickness, not only is their depressed mood temporary, but they retain the normal *reactivity* of mood. Anyone who has attended a funeral and then returned to the home of the bereaved afterward has probably observed this normal reactivity of mood, perhaps even in herself. Mourners who might have been grief-stricken during the funeral service or at the grave site can afterward often relax, reminisce about good memories of the person who has died, and enjoy catching up with friends and relatives whom they may not have seen for a long time. The reactivity of mood is also retained in the lonely or homesick person who goes to the movies and loses himself in a good film. We are able to dispel the feelings of bereavement, isolation, or disappointment—even if it's only for a few hours—if the depressed mood is a "normal" one.

The most significant feature of the depressed mood in the syndrome of depression is that instead of being reactive, the mood is *constricted*. Years ago AM radio stations used to give away free radios, gifts that came with only one catch: they couldn't be tuned to any of the sponsoring station's competitors. These radios were built to receive only the signal of the station that gave them away. The mood state of the person who is suffering through a depressed episode of bipolar disorder is like one of those radios, "set" to receive only one mood signal: depression. The mood of the syndrome of depression is a relentless, pervasive gloom that continues from one day to the next and from which the afflicted person cannot rouse herself. As Pulitzer Prize–winning novelist William Styron said of his own depression, "The weather of depression is unmodulated, its light a brownout."[22]

In these constricted-mood states, depressed individuals find their thinking dominated by thoughts of sadness and loss, regret and hopelessness. Guilty ruminations are especially characteristic of the syndrome of depression, and psychiatrists often make a special point to ask about guilty feelings when they examine a person being evaluated for depression. Ruminations on themes of guilt, shame, and regret are common in the depressed states of the mood disorders, but they are uncommon in the "normal" depressed mood. Persons experiencing the normal depressed mood that comes after a personal loss attribute their bad feelings to the fact that a loss has occurred; only in unusual circumstances will they feel that they are to blame for their problem and be preoccupied by guilty feelings or feelings of shame. The individual with a depressive syndrome, however, frequently feels to blame for his troubles, and sometimes for other people's troubles as well. The presence of guilty preoccupations is very significant for making a diagnosis of the syndrome of depression.

Feelings of inadequacy and worthlessness are similarly significant and especially common in the syndrome of major depression. Psychologist Norman Endler described how depression caused him to be tormented by feelings of incompetence even at the height of a successful academic career:

> [When I became depressed] I was positive I was a fraud and a phony and that I didn't deserve my Ph.D. I didn't deserve to have tenure; I didn't deserve to be a Full Professor; I didn't deserve to be a Fellow of the American Psychological Association and the Canadian Psychological Association; I didn't deserve the research grants I had been awarded; I couldn't understand how I had written the books and journal articles that I had and how they had been accepted for publication. I must have conned a lot of people.[23]

Another typical symptom of major depression is the loss of interest in usually pleasurable activities. This can be understood as another aspect of the loss of normal reactivity of mood. The depressed person is unable to derive any pleasure from listening to music, going to a movie, engaging in the sports or hobbies that usually provide enjoyment. This loss of the ability to feel pleasure has come to be called *anhedonia* (derived from the Greek word for "pleasure"). In Johann Wolfgang von Goethe's novel *The Sorrows of*

Young Werther, the main character expresses a loss of responsiveness to the joys and beauty of nature: "Nature lies before me as immobile as in a little lacquered painting, and all this beauty cannot pump one drop of happiness from my heart to my brain."[24] Patients say that food has lost its taste, the colors have drained away from sunrises and landscapes, and flowers have lost their textures and perfumes—everything has become bland, dull, and lifeless.

For some, the bright and beautiful things of the world are a source of anguish rather than pleasure. The nineteenth-century Austrian composer Hugo Wolf described a terrible sense of sorrowful isolation during his depressions, a feeling of separation from the world of ordinary pleasures—all the more painful when it occurred in springtime:

> What I suffer from . . . I am quite unable to describe. This wonderful spring with its secret life and movement troubles me unspeakably. These eternal blue skies, lasting for weeks, this continuous sprouting and budding in nature, these coaxing breezes impregnated with spring sunlight and fragrance of flowers . . . make me frantic. Everywhere this bewildering urge for life, fruitfulness, creation—and only I . . . may not take part in this festival of resurrection, at any rate not except as a spectator with grief and envy.[25]

Just as the manic syndrome infuses the affected person with feelings of inexpressible joy, the syndrome of depression brings indescribable anguish. Many individuals who have suffered from depression have struggled to describe the feelings, and even great writers seem to falter in the attempt. William Styron said, "If the pain were readily describable most of the countless sufferers from this ancient affliction would have been able to confidently depict . . . their torment. Healthy people [cannot] imagine a form of torment so alien to everyday experience. For myself, the pain is most closely connected to drowning or suffocation—but even these images are off the mark."[26]

Sometimes the "indescribable" mental discomfort seen in major depression is a feeling that seems different from the sad, pessimistic mood people usually mean by the word *depression.* Instead, people with major depression may have a tense, irritable, miserable sort of mood called *dysphoria.* (Remember that the term *dysphoric mania* is used to describe a tense, unpleasant, irritable mood that can be seen along with the agitation and hyperactivity of the manic state.)

The changes in thinking and physical well-being caused by the syndrome of depression are perhaps easier to describe. One's energy level and thinking as well as mood are affected—in an opposite direction of polarity from that seen in mania. The depressed person experiences slowing and inefficiency in thinking and a feebleness of memory and concentration. Information-processing and reasoning falter, and simple decisions can become overwhelming dilemmas. Endler expressed it this way: "My indecisiveness was the worst of all. I couldn't decide what to eat or what to wear. I couldn't decide whether to get out of bed or to stay. I couldn't decide whether to shower or not to shower. I could never decide what to do because I didn't know myself."[27]

These *cognitive* functions (from the Latin *cognoscere*, meaning "to know") become progressively debilitated as the depression deepens, but even in milder depressions, ordinary mental tasks seem to require extraordinary effort. Kraepelin described the severe cognitive slowing he observed in his severely depressed patients: "[The patient's] thoughts are as if paralysed . . . immobile. He is no longer able to perceive or to follow the train of thought of a book or conversation. . . . He has no memory, he has no longer command of knowledge formerly familiar to him [and] must consider a long time about simple things."[28] In the elderly, these sorts of thinking problems can be so severe that depression is misdiagnosed as Alzheimer's disease.

Severe depression almost always causes a change in the person's sleeping pattern. Depressed persons frequently suffer from insomnia—but also from its opposite, sleeping too much (*hypersomnia* is the technical term). In the depression associated with bipolar disorder, hypersomnia seems especially common, perhaps more common than in other types of clinical depression, where insomnia predominates.

Sometimes depressed persons have a peculiar rhythmic pattern of sleep disturbance and mood changes throughout the day, called *diurnal variation of mood* (*diurnal* is a word used in biology to refer to a twenty-four-hour cycle). It causes persons to fall asleep at the usual time and without much difficulty but wake up very early in the morning after only a few hours of sleep. Lying awake hours before sunrise, they experience their lowest mood of the day, and minor problems and regrets seem magnified and overwhelming during this early-morning period. I recall one patient who told me that during those early-morning hours, "I lie awake thinking about every stupid thing I've ever done in my life." American author F. Scott Fitzgerald, who described his struggles with depression in the 1936 autobiographical work *The Crackup*, gave a vivid account of this mood pattern. He experienced the worst of his moods during the predawn hours, recalling that "at three o'clock in the morning, a forgotten package has the same tragic importance as a death sentence." For Fitzgerald, these nocturnal agonies were the nadir of his depressions, which he called "the dark night of the soul."[29] Individuals notice a gradual lifting of their mood as sunrise approaches, and when the morning dawns, they can often rouse themselves and start their daily activities. As the day goes on, their mood continues to improve little by little, until by day's end they feel nearly back to normal. They go to bed and usually fall asleep normally, but several hours later, it's "three o'clock in the morning" again: they awaken depressed, and the cycle repeats itself.

Novelist William Styron experienced a very striking diurnal variation in his mood during his depression, but with a reversal of the usual pattern: "While I was able to rise and function almost normally during the earlier part of the day, I began to sense the onset of the symptoms at mid-afternoon or a little later—gloom crowding in on me, a sense of dread and alienation and . . . stifling anxiety."[30]

The disruptions of various bodily rhythms that occur in depression and mania have convinced many scientists that some persons with mood disorders have a disturbance of their *chronobiology* (from *chronos,* the Greek word for "time"). Persons with mood disorders have been observed to have disturbances in the normal rhythmic pulsing of various hormone levels, in body temperature fluctuations, in the sleep-wake cycle, and in other natural rhythms. Later in this book we shall examine connections between these natural rhythms and mood and also look at other cycles: the monthly cycles of mood in women with premenstrual mood symptoms (chapter 14) and the twelve-month cycles of persons with seasonal affective disorder (chapter 16).

Appetite is also usually disturbed in depressed individuals. As with sleep problems, changes occur in both directions, and patients may eat too much or too little. They may lose or gain a significant amount of weight during periods of depression. As might be expected, the depressed person loses interest in sex; this symptom is perhaps best understood as part of the person's inability to experience pleasurable activities of any kind, the "anhedonia" of depression.

Of the other bodily symptoms that occur in depression, one of the most striking is a sense of fatigue with prominent low energy and listlessness. As Endler put it: "[My] fatigue [was] extreme to the point of exhaustion. I was too tired to make decisions and felt as if I had a huge weight on my back that wouldn't allow me to achieve anything. . . . No matter how long I stayed in bed and slept I never felt rested and refreshed. . . . When I did get out of bed I was lethargic. I was slow as molasses."[31] Headaches, constipation, and a feeling of heaviness in the chest are common, as are other more difficult-to-describe sensations of physical discomfort. Styron said: "I felt a kind of numbness, an enervation . . . an odd fragility—as if my body had actually become frail, hypersensitive and somehow disjointed and clumsy. Nothing felt quite right. . . . There were twitches and pains, sometimes intermittent, often seemingly constant, that seemed to presage all sorts of dire infirmities."[32]

It is not clear whether these symptoms are caused by depression itself or arise from the lack of restful sleep, the lack of exercise, and the poor eating habits that depression brings on. Persons who have preexisting painful medical conditions such as arthritis or inflammatory bowel disease are usually more bothered by the physical symptoms of these illnesses when they are depressed. The connections between depression and problems with fatigue seen in chronic fatigue immunodeficiency syndrome and the painful joint and muscle disease fibromyalgia are well known but poorly understood. Depression seems to lower the pain threshold: depressed individuals are more sensitive to pain and are more distressed by it.

Some persons may be willing to seek treatment for these physical symptoms but reluctant to mention their mood problems. So sometimes patients with depression end up getting all kinds of tests and treatments for physical illnesses from their physicians, when their real problem is depression.

Just as in the syndrome of mania, persons suffering through an episode of the depression of bipolar disorder can experience the distortions of thinking that psychiatrists call *delusions*. As their view of the world and of themselves becomes increasingly colored by their pervasive mood changes, depressed individuals can come to believe that terrible things are happening all around them: "I was positive that I was going to be fired from the university because of incompetence and that [my family] would become destitute—that we would go broke," wrote Endler. "I felt guilty at the prospect of not being able to support my family."[33] In addition to such *delusions of poverty*, delusions can arise from the uncomfortable physical sensations of depression. Patients believe they have cancer, AIDS, or some other terrible illness.

Kraepelin described the increasingly bizarre *hypochondriacal delusions* he sometimes observed in his patients: "[The patient believes he is] incurably ill, half-dead, no longer a right human being, has lung disease, a tapeworm, cancer in his throat, cannot swallow, does not retain his food. . . . Face and figure have changed; there is no longer blood in his brain, he does not see any longer, must become crazy, remain his whole lifetime in an institution, die, has already died." Patients with such beliefs may refuse to eat or drink, convinced that their body cannot absorb the food. *Paranoid delusions,* beliefs that one is in danger or the victim of evil people and forces, can also occur.

> Everywhere danger threatens the patient. . . . Strange people are in the house; a suspicious motorcar drives past. People mock him, are going to thrash him, to chase him from his post in a shameful way, incarcerate him, bring him to justice, expose him publicly, deport him, throw him into the fire, drown him. The people are already standing outside; the bill of indictment is already written; the scaffold is being put up; he must wander about naked and miserable. . . . His relatives also are

being tortured. . . . His family is imprisoned, his wife has drowned herself; his parents are murdered; his daughter wanders about in the snow without any clothes on.[34]

It's easy to understand why suicidal thinking and behavior are so common in the syndrome of major depression: compared with the horrors of such delusional imaginings, death may seem a welcome alternative. It's also possible to understand why delusionally depressed persons can occasionally be dangerous to others as well as to themselves: they can come to believe that those close to them are in similar danger of gruesome persecution and would be better off dead.

Hallucinations occur in severe depression, but not as frequently as in mania (table 1-4). The hallucinations are consistent with the mood and are frightening, even horrifying: "The patients see evil spirits, death, heads of animals . . . crowds of monsters . . . dead relatives. . . . The patient hears his tortured relatives screaming and lamenting. . . . His food tastes of soapy water or excrement, of corpses and mildew."[35]

Some seriously ill patients sink into a state of lethargy and despair that is called *depressive stupor*. Styron's description of this horrible condition is the best I have ever read:

> I had now reached that phase of the disorder where all sense of hope had vanished, along with the idea of a futurity; my brain . . . had become less an organ of thought than an instrument registering, minute by minute, varying degrees of its own suffering. . . . I'd feel the horror, like some poisonous fog bank, roll in upon my mind, forcing me to bed. There I would lie for as long as six hours, stuporous and virtually paralyzed, gazing at the ceiling.[36]

TABLE 1-4 Delusions and hallucinations in bipolar disorder: Mania versus depression

Category of symptoms	Percentage of patients
Delusions	
Mania	44
Depression	12
Hallucinations	
Mania	14
Depression	8

Source: Data from D. W. Black and A. Nasrallah, "Hallucinations and Delusions in 1,715 Patients with Unipolar and Bipolar Affective Disorders," *Psychopathology* 22 (1989): 28–34.

Just as few modern psychiatrists have ever seen the most extreme stage of mania, so-called *delirious mania,* it is also fortunately rare today to see a patient depressed to the point of unresponsiveness and immobility that psychiatrists call *catatonia.* Kraepelin, describing patients in an era when virtually no treatment was available for this terrible condition, starkly describes this deepest abyss of depression: "The patients lie in bed taking no interest in anything. They betray no pronounced emotion; they are mute, inaccessible; they pass their [bowel movements] under them; they stare straight in front of them with [a] vacant expression of countenance like a mask and with wide open eyes."[37]

Electroconvulsive therapy (ECT), discussed in more detail in chapter 10, is a very effective treatment for these extreme states of the depressive syndrome. Although there have been misguided attempts to ban this safe and effective treatment technique in the United States, and equally misguided activists still occasionally appear in the media to disparage it, ECT fortunately remains available to treat this most extreme stage of depression, rescuing these individuals from a kind of living hell.

Mixed States

Another type of abnormal mood can be seen in bipolar disorder. This mood, a strange combination of both the frenzied intensity of mania and the horrors of deep depression, has been called a *mixed state* (sometimes it's termed *mixed affective state*). Kay Jamison described it as the most terrible expression of the illness for her: "On occasion, these periods of total despair would be made even worse by terrible agitation. My mind would race from subject to subject, but instead of being filled with . . . exuberance and cosmic thoughts . . . it would be drenched in awful sounds and images of decay and dying; dead bodies on the beach, charred remains of animals, toe-tagged corpses in morgues."[38]

Although psychiatrists do not yet agree on the defining characteristics for this mood state, they have long recognized that symptoms of depression and mania seem to exist almost simultaneously in some patients (table 1-5). This state represents a distinct variety of abnormal mood that is separate from depression and typical mania yet combines features of both. The accelerated thinking and hyperactivity typical of the manic state remain its most striking features, but instead of a euphoric mood, these changes become combined with a depressed, despairing, desperate mood. Kraepelin described patients with "flight of ideas, excitement and anxiety" who were at the same time "anxiously despairing."[39] Other labels used for the mixed state are "mixed mania" and "dysphoric mania."[40] As we shall see in chapter

TABLE 1-5 Symptoms in ten patients with mixed mania (dysphoric mania)

Symptoms	Percentage of patients
Depressed mood	100
Irritable mood	100
Increased activity	100
Insomnia	93
Pressured speech	93
Hostility	79
Flight of ideas	43
Anxiety attacks	43
Delusions (depressive)	36
Delusions (nondepressive)	21

Source: Data from Frederick K. Goodwin and Kay Redfield Jamison, *Manic-Depressive Illness* (New York: Oxford University Press, 1990), 49.

2, there is some evidence that this mood state does not occur in all patients with bipolar disorder and that, when it does occur, a different treatment approach is necessary.

Just as full-blown mania is unmistakable, so is a full-blown mixed state. But in the same way that a state of mild hypomania can be difficult to distinguish from an elevated but normal mood, milder mixed states can be difficult to recognize. A mild mixed state sometimes lasts only a few hours. Whenever a patient tells me about being troubled by uncomfortable angry "rages," I suspect that he may be having mild mixed states. "Anxiety" is another word that persons experiencing this mood state use to describe it, although it is not the fearful fretfulness of ordinary anxiety; this state is more like a pressure cooker full of depressed emotions ready to explode.

The mixed state is very dangerous because the patient has negative, depressing thought patterns together with excess energy, restlessness, and an inner sense of pressure and tension. This negative energy puts patients in mixed states at high risk for hurting themselves with suicidal behaviors. And it is often while in a mixed state that an individual is propelled into a variety of self-destructive behaviors that are not immediately life-threatening. They may cut or burn themselves. Patients have told me that desperate behaviors like these help them shift a terrible inner pain and tension to "the outside" and that the physical pain is somehow easier to deal with than the painful agitation of a mixed state.

Another type of mood "mixture" occurs when, rather than a true mixture of simultaneous mania and depression, there is rapid alternation between the two states. Kraepelin described "transition periods from one state to another, which often [extended] over weeks," during which his patients seemed depressed one moment and manic nearly the next:

> Manic patients may transitorily appear not only sad and despairing, but also quiet and inhibited. A patient goes to bed moody and inhibited, suddenly wakes up with the feeling as if a veil had been drawn away from his brain, passes the day in manic delight in work, and the next morning, exhausted and with a heavy head, he again finds in himself the whole misery of his state. Or the hypomanic exultant patient quite unexpectedly makes a serious attempt at suicide.[41]

Recently the term *ultra-rapid cycling* has been proposed for such alternations in mood.

Now that you have some familiarity with the symptoms of bipolar disorder, I can talk about diagnosis. As I have already said, most people with bipolar disorder never develop all the possible symptoms of the illness. It is the presence or absence of certain symptoms as well as the pattern of mood symptoms that allows a diagnosis of a particular type of bipolar disorder. And once a diagnosis has been made, a treatment plan can be developed. In the next chapter you'll see how the diagnostic process works.

CHAPTER 2

The Diagnosis of Bipolar Disorder

WHEN LITHIUM BECAME AVAILABLE IN THE 1970S AS A TREATMENT for bipolar disorder, psychiatrists started to realize that not all cases of the disorder were the same. For some patients, lithium was indeed a miracle; their symptoms were completely controlled by it, and their illness seemed simply to end. But other patients—often those with less severe symptoms or more frequent episodes of abnormal mood—didn't respond as well to the medication. Did these people have bipolar disorder, or something else? Patients who had been thought to have "cyclothymic personality disorder"—a diagnostic category in an old edition of the diagnostic manual of the American Psychiatric Association—also saw their troublesome and unpredictable mood variations stop when they took lithium; did these people have bipolar disorder, and not a personality problem after all? Was this a milder form of "manic-depressive" illness, or a different disorder altogether? Did it matter? What difference does diagnosis make, anyway?

Diagnostic classification has two purposes in medicine: to make predictions about the course of an illness, and to aid the clinician in selecting the treatment most likely to be effective. In the practice of psychiatry, since the physical basis for most psychiatric illnesses has yet to be discovered, classification systems are largely derived from studying groups of patients with different combinations of symptoms and seeing how the different groups vary in the course of their illness or in their response to medications.

As more and more medications have become available to treat mood disorders, the classification system for bipolar mood disorders has continued to evolve. In this chapter, various subtypes of bipolar disorder are described. These are the subtypes that currently seem to make sense to clinicians because they serve one of the two purposes of diagnosis: they allow for a better prediction of the course of the illness, and they allow for a more rapid selection of effective therapy—saving the patient time that would be wasted on trying an ineffective medication.

Psychiatric Diagnosis

At least once a month, it seems, I see a patient who asks to be "tested for bipolar disorder." It's not an unreasonable request. Unfortunately, it's not a request that can be satisfied—not just yet. There's no blood test or x-ray or biopsy that can diagnose bipolar disorder (and, for that matter, there is none that can be used to confirm the diagnosis of most of the problems psychiatrists treat).

The reason for this sorry state of affairs is that the biological and chemical basis of bipolar disorder remains a nearly complete mystery; no one knows what to test for. Despite literally hundreds of years of examining the bodily fluids and brain tissues of individuals with mood disorders—first with the naked eye, then with microscopes, later with x-rays and scanning devices, and more recently with incredibly sophisticated biochemical probes—no one has been able to find in patients with this illness any abnormalities that can be accurately and reliably measured as an aid in diagnosing the disorder. Although work in the genetics of bipolar disorder holds the promise that genetic markers for the illness may be discovered in the not-too-distant future—suggesting that a blood test might be possible that will identify at least some cases of the illness—and although some individuals with bipolar disorder have been identified as having subtle brain-scan abnormalities (see "Picturing Bipolar Disorder in the Brain" in chapter 18), again suggesting a possible diagnostic tool, the clinical applications of these findings are still in the future. Modern psychiatrists are left with the same diagnostic tools that Emil Kraepelin and other nineteenth-century psychiatrists had: their eyes and ears.

We psychiatrists listen to what the patient and her family members say when they describe symptoms—their onset, course, fluctuation, and impact upon the patient. Whether other members of the family suffer from a mood disorder is an important piece of information. We observe the patient for the signs of bipolar disorder described in chapter 1 by performing a *mental status examination,* the psychiatrist's equivalent of the physical examination. This examination consists of observing speech patterns and behavior, asking questions about mood and thinking processes, and evaluating other aspects of mental functioning such as concentration and memory. After this process of history-taking and examination, a picture emerges of the person and of her symptoms, and the course of her illness becomes clear. A particular diagnostic category that seems to be a good fit with the clinical information is identified. Once the diagnostic category of the illness is determined, we can make predictions about the future course of the symptoms and, perhaps more important, can select a treatment that has a good chance of relieving them. In the sections that follow, you can learn about the different forms of bipolar disorder the same way young physicians training to be psychiatrists do: by hearing from patients.

Bipolar I

It had been several years since I had seen Richard in the mood-disorders clinic. He looked great. Although he was only in his late thirties, some silver tones in his hair made him look older and quite distinguished. I remembered that he had always dressed well, but today, in an obviously finely tailored suit, a crisp white shirt, and a beautiful silk tie, he looked—well, like a million. I knew that this could be a very good sign—or a very bad sign.

"That's a handsome suit you've got on, Richard. Is it new?" I asked.

"I got it about a month ago," he said proudly, "in London. A terrific shop on Savile Row, the same one Prince Charles goes to." He smiled a little mischievously. "And I know what you're thinking: no, I wasn't manic when I bought it!"

Rich certainly knew what mania was, as did several members of his family. His wealthy parents had taken control of his financial affairs in a legal-guardianship proceeding; for years he hadn't even been able to write a check at the supermarket. Rich first developed manic symptoms during law school; he made down payments on not just one Porsche but three before a check bounced. He angrily stormed into the bank's branch office to protest, created quite a scene, and ended up in jail, where an astute nurse fortunately arranged an immediate psychiatric evaluation. Richard was admitted to a local psychiatric hospital and had taken his first dose of lithium before his parents even knew what had happened.

He stopped taking his lithium within a month after leaving the hospital and started having manic symptoms almost immediately. This time his manic enthusiasm turned to travel rather than cars, and he used a credit card to buy an airline ticket to Fiji. He made it as far as Los Angeles before his mania turned dysphoric and irritable again. He started yelling at and shoving a security guard who wanted to examine his luggage and wound up in jail again—this time with federal charges. After a talk with a good lawyer, another hospitalization, more lithium, a leave from law school, and a move back home, he came for treatment at the university outpatient clinic where I was training.

Richard's father also suffered from bipolar disorder and knew, from his own turbulent experiences with the illness, just how to handle the situation. A pair of scissors to the credit cards, a power of attorney, and a trip with Richard to the psychiatrist's appointments made the difference—as did the fact that Richard was an intelligent fellow who (eventually) learned from experience as well. Moreover, he learned from his father that a paternal uncle who had been killed in a car accident when Rich was a child had also actually probably died from the disease; the single-passenger accident had most likely been a suicide. Rich made the decision to take control of the illness rather than let it control him. And as with most things, once he made the decision, he stuck to it. Rich applied himself to staying well with energy and determination.

There was a time after he broke up with a girlfriend when severe depressive symptoms almost necessitated another hospitalization for Rich; he spent fourteen to sixteen hours in bed every day for nearly three weeks and put on almost fifty pounds. Fortunately, family support, an excellent clinical psychologist who saw him for therapy, and a higher lithium dose for several months got him through. After about a year of maintaining a stable mood, he got into a local law school to finish his studies and eventually graduated at the top of his class. He took a job in New York but now had returned home. "I couldn't pass up the opportunity to open my firm's new branch office in my hometown, could I?" he beamed.

Rich brought me up to date. A little hypomania had occasionally emerged during the summers while he was working in New York, especially if he was working too hard and didn't watch his sleep habits. But Rich had obviously remained serious about his mental health; he monitored his moods and saw his psychiatrist regularly. Most important, he was making career decisions that reflected his knowledge of his illness. "I think the pace will be slower here than in New York. I may not become a millionaire quite as quickly," he said mischievously, "but there will also be less risk of getting sick, blowing it all, and having to start over again. So . . . I had my last lithium level done three months ago, and it was 0.8. When do you want me to get another?"

It looked as if the suit had been a very *good* sign.

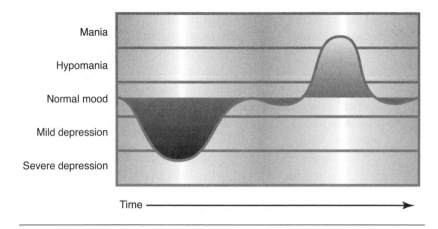

FIGURE 2-1 Mood changes in bipolar I.

Bipolar I is the designation for the classic variety of bipolar disorder, characterized by full-blown manic attacks and deep, paralyzing depressions. A schematic representation of the moods of bipolar I appears in figure 2-1. The pattern of abnormal mood episodes seems to vary widely, and the rhythm of the illness is almost as individual as the patient who has it. Symptoms of bipolar I usually begin in the late teens or early twenties (figure 2-2), although onset at later ages is not uncommon.[1]

Bipolar I is what physicians refer to as a relapsing and remitting illness; during the course of the illness, its symptoms come and go. This feature of bipolar I—it is actually a feature of *all* mood disorders—makes it difficult to diagnose, difficult to treat, and fiendishly difficult to study. This deserves a closer look.

THE DISEASE THAT SLEEPS

When we think about illnesses of the body, we usually think of diseases that have a beginning, a middle, and an end. Take, for example, pneumonia, an infection of the lungs caused by bacteria. The disease begins when fever, cough, chest pains, and breathing problems appear. These symptoms build and worsen over a period of hours or sometimes days. Before the antibiotic era, patients reached what was called a *crisis* point, when their bodies' natural defenses had mounted their best effort against the bacterial invaders, and the patient either started getting better or died. Either the patient killed off the bacteria or vice versa, but in any case the disease process came to an end. (Fortunately we can now administer antibiotics that usually give the patient's defenses the crucial edge against a bacterial invader.)

How about a disease not caused by a foreign invader like bacteria but instead one in which the body seems to turn on itself: a disease like cancer—

say, leukemia? In this case a white blood cell in the body develops an abnormality that causes it to start reproducing uncontrollably. Most of the cells in the body reproduce from time to time, replacing those that wear out. It is thought that most cancers are caused by an error during cell duplication that results in an abnormality in the control center of one of the new cells. This abnormality causes the cell to start reproducing continuously. More and more abnormal cells are produced, and in the case of leukemia they fill the bloodstream and lymph nodes such that the normal cells cannot do their job properly, the immune system fails, and the patient dies. Many types of leukemia are now curable. The cures basically involve using ingenious methods to eradicate every single cancer cell, eliminating the abnormally reproducing cells altogether; when the abnormality is eliminated from the body, things return to normal. Again, the illness begins when something goes wrong in the body, and it ends (is cured) when the abnormality is corrected and eliminated. The illness is finished for good.

Bipolar disorder is very different from these diseases, because it does not simply have a beginning, a middle, and an end. Or perhaps it is more

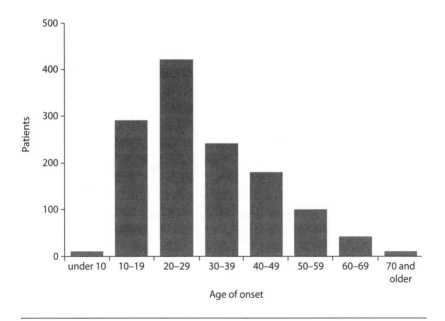

FIGURE 2-2 Age of onset of bipolar disorder in 1,304 patients. These data were compiled from ten different studies carried out between 1969 and 1984. Notice that early adulthood is the peak time for the onset of the disorder.

Source: Frederick K. Goodwin and Kay Redfield Jamison, *Manic-Depressive Illness* (New York: Oxford University Press, 1990), 132. Copyright © 1990 by Oxford University Press, Inc. Used by permission of Oxford University Press, Inc.

accurate to say that the illness seems to have many beginnings and endings: the symptoms of bipolar disorder can develop in an individual, and then *without any treatment at all* the symptoms may go away for years at a time— a pattern that is nearly unique among the diseases that afflict humankind.

Since most people are more familiar with diseases that end when their symptoms go away, it is often very difficult for patients and their families to understand that although the symptoms of bipolar disorder can go into *remission* after treatment (or even spontaneously), they almost inevitably will come back if treatment to prevent their return is not in place. The hallmark of bipolar illness—especially bipolar I—is the tendency of the illness to *relapse*. No matter how well the symptoms of any one episode are treated, the illness does not end but instead seems merely to hibernate—and *symptoms can come back at any time.*

THE NATURAL HISTORY OF BIPOLAR I

Now, back to a description of the characteristics of bipolar I. Fortunately, many excellent clinical studies about the course of bipolar disorder were done in the years before effective treatments for it were available; these studies document and illustrate the pattern of bipolar-disorder symptoms that occurs if the illness is not treated—what physicians call the *natural history* of the illness.[2]

How many episodes of illness did patients have in the days before treatment was available? How long did their episodes last? What was the length of time between episodes?

In a 1942 study, the records of sixty-six patients with "manic-depressive psychosis" were studied; some of these individuals had been followed for up to twenty-six years. Although a few patients seemed to have had only one episode of illness in the period of study, about one-third had two to three episodes, about one-third had four to six episodes, and about one-third had

TABLE 2-1 Number of episodes of illness in sixty-six patients with bipolar disorder

Number of episodes	Percentage of patients
1	8
2–3	29
4–6	26
More than 7	37

Source: Data from Thomas A. C. Rennie, "Prognosis in Manic-Depressive Psychosis," *American Journal of Psychiatry* 98 (1942): 801–14.

Note: This study was done before any treatments were available for bipolar disorder.

more than seven (table 2-1). A few had twenty or more episodes.[3] Unfortunately, when a diagnosis of bipolar I is made, there is no way to know whether the individual will have another two or three episodes during his lifetime or more than twenty.

How long did episodes of mania or major depression last before effective treatments were available? In the 1942 study, the average duration was about six and a half months. But we also know that depressions and manias were sometimes shorter and sometimes lasted much longer. Kraepelin, writing at a time when there were essentially no effective treatments, noted:

> The duration of individual attacks is extremely varied. There are some which last only eight to fourteen days, indeed we sometimes see that states of moodiness or excitement . . . do not continue in these patients longer than one or two days or even only a few hours. For the most part, however, a simple attack usually lasts six to eight months. On the other hand, the cases are not at all rare, in which an attack continues for two, three or four years, and a double attack [can] double that time. I have seen manias, which even after seven years, indeed after more than ten years, recovered, and a state of depression which after fourteen years recovered.[4]

Modern psychiatrists no longer see patients who are manic for years at a time. Effective modern treatments bring these episodes to a close, and the patient is usually better in a few days—weeks at the most. Modern psychiatrists do, however, see patients who seem to become manic again and again, month after month, year after year—often every time they stop taking medication. Do these patients have many episodes, or do they have many relapses of a single episode of several years' duration? I tend to think it's the latter, but the rhythm of the illness makes research very difficult.

How about the time between attacks? For many persons with bipolar disorder, modern treatments are quite effective at keeping the episodes from recurring. But how long did remissions last in the days before these treatments were available? Kraepelin noted that the time between episodes could be years, even decades. Among 703 "intervals" that he studied in his patients, Kraepelin found one case in which there were forty-four years between one episode of illness and the next.[5] However, subsequent studies have shown that, if untreated, episodes of bipolar disorder often occur more and more frequently in individual patients (figure 2-3). The illness seems to accelerate if untreated, and in the days before treatment was available, mood episodes tended to recur more and more frequently as patients aged. This acceleration has profound implications for treatment and prognosis, as we shall see in chapter 20.

Another finding in these older studies is that some patients tend to "switch" from a depression to a manic episode with no interval of normal mood. In a 1969 study, the course of one hundred manic episodes was described.[6] Many individuals had a period of depression lasting several weeks or months and then switched into a manic episode, again of several months' duration. In a few of these patients, there followed another switch and a third phase of the episode set in: a long period of depression. In this study, about half of the patients' manic episodes showed at least one switch—a depression either before or after a manic episode. Several studies suggest that patients who "switch" from depression to mania have a more difficult-to-treat form of illness than those who switch from mania to depression.[7]

Bipolar I is the classic manic-depressive illness, with fully developed manic episodes and episodes of severe depression, and it is also characterized by long periods of "hibernation" in which the symptoms temporarily

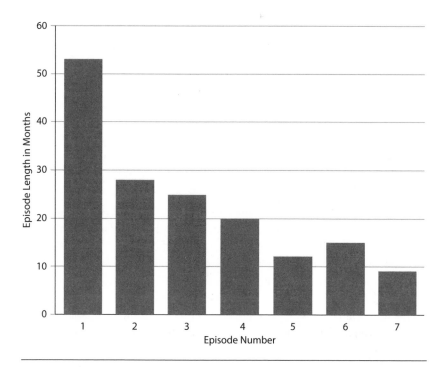

FIGURE 2-3 Acceleration of illness in one hundred patients. This graph shows that the cycle length of episodes of bipolar disorder (the time from the onset of one episode to the onset of the next) becomes shorter and shorter in patients whose symptoms are not well controlled and who continue to have episodes of the illness.

Source: Data from P. P. Roy-Burne, R. M. Post, T. W. Uhde, T. Porcu, and D. Davis, "The Longitudinal Course of Recurrent Affective Illness: Life Chart Data from Patients at the NIMH," *Acta Psychiatrica Scandinavia* 71, suppl. 317 (1985): 1–34.

TABLE 2-2 Features of bipolar I

Mood
Fully developed manic episodes
Fully developed depressive episodes

Other features
Untreated episodes average six months
Hallucinations and delusions frequently seen
Three-phased episodes (depression, mania, depression)
Relapses more frequent as patient ages

---

disappear (table 2-2). The number of episodes varies enormously, but patients who have only one or two episodes seem to be the exception rather than the rule. Before effective treatments became available, the average length of each episode if untreated was about six months—but episodes that lasted years were not at all uncommon.

Bipolar II

Robert was a thirty-nine-year-old accountant who had been seeing a psychologist for treatment of depression for about three months. Both he and his therapist were frustrated because, despite the best efforts of both, Robert's depression seemed to be getting worse.

"I can usually pull myself out of these things—or at least I can usually slog through them until they finish," he told me at our first appointment. Right away, his description of his depressions as "these things" made me feel pretty certain that this fellow had a mood disorder. Robert's moods had an alien, external quality to him; they came upon him like a fog bank rolling in, lasted for a few weeks, and then slowly dissipated. Where they came from and where they went was a complete mystery to Robert. He would sleep away the weekends, put on weight, fall behind in his work. "This has been happening to me since college," he said, "and I really want it to stop." In fact, this was not the worst his depressions had ever gotten. Shortly after graduation, Robert had had such a severe depression that he had spent most of the summer at home in his room. At one point he seriously contemplated suicide. The only reason he didn't get into treatment then was because he felt he was no worse off than his mother.

Robert's mother was a closet alcoholic. "There was always one of those huge bottles of wine in the refrigerator," he told me. "It always seemed either full or half full, and when I was in high school I realized that this was because she drank about a half a gallon every day." Robert's mother had never had any treatment for either her drinking problem or depression, but his description of the long "naps" she took most afternoons and the "sick headaches" that put her in bed for weeks sounded like more than alcoholism—more like a smoldering depression complicated by alcohol addiction. Another red flag for a mood-disorder diagnosis: a positive family history.

Robert had always blamed his melancholic moods on his childhood. The memories of his shame and worry about his mother seeped back into his consciousness during these times, as did guilty feelings that he had put hundreds of miles between himself and his mother now, hadn't seen her in over two years, and could bring himself to call her only on holidays. Here was more evidence pointing to a mood disorder: guilty feelings and painful preoccupations with the past that seemed really to bother him only when his mood changed. Although I wasn't quite finished taking his history, I was already thinking about which antidepressant to recommend to him, when Robert gave me another piece of information that changed everything.

"I even feel like my thinking is slower than usual. I'll never get through tax season unless I do something to get some help—or unless one of my highs kicks in."

"One of your . . . ?"

"I call it a high. But it's not like I'm manic-depressive or anything. It's just that sometimes when things get back to normal I'm so relieved and happy that—oh, I don't know, it just feels so good not to be depressed."

"Do you find that you're especially productive during these times?" I asked.

"Oh, definitely. One year I came out of a depression just in time for tax season. I didn't feel overwhelmed like I usually do. It was spring, and I wasn't depressed for a change, and I had just met the girl I was going to marry—in fact we got married that summer, and so of course things settled back down. But that was a great year."

"Do other people notice?"

"Um, yes, especially at the office. 'Slow down, Rob.' 'Take it easy, Rob.' Sometimes I get irritated by that."

I had a few more questions to ask, but I was beginning to think about how to tell this fellow that he probably had "manic-depression" after all.

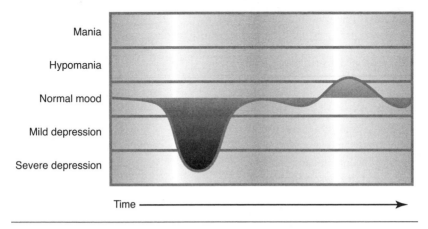

Mania

Hypomania

Normal mood

Mild depression

Severe depression

Time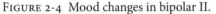

FIGURE 2-4 Mood changes in bipolar II.

Bipolar II is characterized by fully developed depressive episodes and episodes of *hypomania*. A schematic representation of the moods of bipolar II appears in figure 2-4.

When lithium became available in the United States in the 1970s and researchers were trying to find better diagnostic criteria for bipolar disorder, several of them noticed that there was a large group of patients who didn't have a history of fully developed manic episodes but who seemed to be bipolar nonetheless. They had severe depressions, but their "highs" never developed into mania. Were these patients "manic-depressives" who were still early in the course of their illness and simply hadn't had time to have a fully developed manic episode? Several studies attempting to answer this question concluded that these patients did *not* usually go on to fully developed mania. In one study, fewer than 5 percent of the patients with recurrent depressions and hypomania ever became manic.[8]

It is fairly clear from the research literature that bipolar II is not merely a prelude to "full-blown" manic-depressive illness—that is, bipolar II patients are not in the early stages of bipolar I.

Bipolar II is sometimes erroneously characterized as a milder form of bipolar I. But although patients with bipolar II do not develop the most severe symptoms of full-blown mania, they tend to be symptomatic more of the time, and their long periods of depression can be even more debilitating than the dramatic, but shorter-lived, episodes of bipolar I illness.

Bipolar II disorder is more common, more genetically complex, and more challenging to treat than bipolar I. Depending on the criteria used to make the diagnosis, this form of the illness has been estimated to afflict about 5 percent of the general population, meaning that it may be five times more common than bipolar I disorder.[9] Several studies show that bipolar

TABLE 2-3 Features of bipolar II

Mood
Fully developed depressive episodes
Hypomanic episodes

Other features
Increased sleep and appetite during depressions
Depressions sometimes more chronic
Bipolar II history in family members
Later age at first hospitalization
Fewer hospitalizations
Possible increased risk for alcoholism

II patients often have relatives who also suffer from a bipolar mood disorder characterized by major depressions and hypomanias, but they also often have family members who have bipolar I as well as unipolar depressive disorders (that is, symptoms of depression but without either mania or hypomania).[10] In one study of bipolar I and II volunteers, 26 percent of bipolar II patients had a relative with some kind of psychiatric illness (especially anxiety disorders and addiction), as compared to only 15 percent of bipolar I patients.[11] This genetic information is not of academic interest alone. As you will see in a later chapter, we can think of the brain's mood-control system as a very complex and finely tuned clock with a myriad of intricate moving parts, each of which is fabricated using instructions coded in our DNA (genes). We can think of bipolar I as being caused by defects in a few of the bigger parts, caused by glitches in the instructions (the genes); then bipolar II is caused by many more defects in many more of the smaller parts. Because more parts need fixing, there are more complicated symptoms and a need for more complicated treatments.

And indeed, studies indicate that the symptoms and course of illness of bipolar II are different from those of bipolar I (table 2-3). Bipolar II patients have more problems with depression—in fact, the depression is sometimes so prominent that many receive a diagnosis of depressive disorder and don't get treatment for bipolar disorder at all. In a study from the National Institutes of Health published in 1995, 559 patients diagnosed with a depressive disorder were followed over time, some for up to eleven years. It was reported that almost 9 percent of them developed symptoms of bipolar II.[12] The first hypomanic episode could usually be documented within several months of the onset of severe depression, but sometimes it took up to nine years for the correct diagnosis to become clear. Some of these 559 "depression" patients also developed a manic episode—that is, they turned out to have bipolar I—

but this was far less common (only 3.9 percent). The study also found that bipolar II patients had longer depressive episodes (52.2 weeks) than bipolar I patients (24.3 weeks) and that, if untreated, their symptom-free intervals were shorter. This means that they had symptoms over longer stretches of time; they had what doctors call a *chronic* course of illness.

Persons with bipolar II are more likely to have a seasonal variation in their symptoms (they tend to get depressed in the fall and winter and feel better—or even develop hypomania—in the spring and summer), and they have more rapid cycling (see below). Whereas patients with bipolar I frequently have irritable manic symptoms, the hypomanic periods of bipolar II patients are characterized by an elated mood—irritability is less common. With regard to depressive symptoms, psychomotor agitation, guilty feelings, and thoughts of suicide were more frequently observed in bipolar II. Bipolar II patients also have a higher incidence of phobias and eating disorders.[13]

Cyclothymic Disorder

Cyclothymic disorder (-*thymia*, from the Greek word for "mind," is used in psychiatry to refer to mood) is characterized by frequent short periods (days to weeks) of depressive symptoms and of hypomania separated by periods (which also tend to be short, on the order of days to weeks) of fairly normal mood. By definition, the patient does not have either fully developed major depressive episodes or fully developed manic episodes. A schematic representation of the moods of cyclothymia appears in figure 2-5.

Emil Kraepelin believed that there were "certain temperaments which [could] be regarded as rudiments of manic-depressive insanity" that might continue "throughout the whole of life as peculiar forms of psychic person-

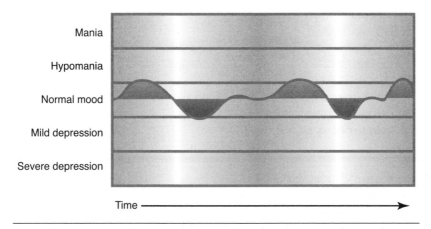

FIGURE 2-5 Mood changes in cyclothymia.

ality without further development." He described the "cyclothymic temperament" as "characterized by frequent, more or less regular fluctuations of the psychic state to the manic or to the depressive side."[14] He reported that 3 to 4 percent of his patients had the cyclothymic temperament but speculated that many more persons might have similar illnesses that "run their course outside of institutions." Modern research on community populations has proved Kraepelin (as usual) quite correct. Several studies have shown that cyclothymic disorder probably affects 3 to 6 percent of the population.[15] Clearly, most of these individuals are neither diagnosed nor treated for these mood problems (fewer than 6 percent of the general population ever receive treatment for any psychiatric problem).

Kraepelin's descriptions of the symptoms of cyclothymia are lively and vivid: "These are the people who constantly oscillate hither and thither between the two opposite poles of mood, sometimes 'rejoicing to the skies,' sometimes 'sad as death.' Today lively, sparkling, beaming, full of the joy of life, the pleasure of enterprise, and the pressure of activity, after some time they meet us depressed, enervated, ill-humored, in need of rest, and again a few months later they display the old freshness and elasticity."[16]

For many years American psychiatric classification systems regarded cyclothymia as a personality problem. The concept of "temperament," which can be thought of as a person's usual manner of thinking, behaving, or reacting, captures the same idea. Cyclothymia was thought to be better understood as an expression of a person's personality than as an illness caused by an abnormality of brain chemistry. In early editions of the *Diagnostic and Statistical Manual* of the American Psychiatric Association (the *DSM*), the disorder was called *cyclothymic personality disorder*. In 1980 *cyclothymic disorder* moved over to the mood-disorder section of the manual—where it remains today.

Individuals with cyclothymic disorder have very frequent ups and downs

TABLE 2-4 Features of cyclothymic disorder

Mood
Frequent alternation between mild depression and mild hypomania
Short, irregular cycles (days)
Only short periods of normal mood

Other features
Patients often wake up with mood changes
Pattern appears in late teens, early twenties
Frequently mistaken for problem with "personality"
Sometimes develops into bipolar I or II

TABLE 2-5 Mood, thinking, and behavior patterns in forty-six cyclothymic patients

Mood	Percentage of patients
Irritable periods lasting a few days	50
Explosive, aggressive outbursts	50
Thinking	
Shaky self-esteem alternating between lack of self-confidence and overconfidence	75
Periods of mental confusion alternating with periods of sharpened, creative thinking	50
Activity and behavior	
Increased sleep alternating with decreased need for sleep	75
Unevenness in quantity and quality of work	75
Buying sprees, extravagance, or financial disasters	75
Repeated shifts in work, study, interest, or future plans	50
Drug or alcohol abuse	50
Extroversion alternating with introversion	50
Unexplained promiscuity or extramarital affairs	40
Joining new movement with enthusiasm, rapidly changing to disillusionment	25

Source: Data from H. Akiskal, M. K. Khani, and A. Scott-Strauss, "Cyclothymic Temperamental Disorders," *Psychiatric Clinics of North America* 2 (1979): 527–54, quoted in Frederick K. Goodwin and Kay Redfield Jamison, *Manic-Depressive Illness* (New York: Oxford University Press, 1990), 54.

of mood, with only comparatively few periods of "normal" mood (table 2-4). As Kraepelin noted, they seem to "constantly oscillate . . . between the two opposite poles of mood." (This almost constant instability perhaps explains why psychiatrists thought of this as a "personality" characteristic for so long.) As might be expected, constant mood instability causes instability in many areas of the patient's life. In a 1977 study of forty-six patients with cyclothymia, the patients demonstrated a whole variety of oscillations of emotions and behavior—from sleep patterns to work habits to group affiliations (table 2-5).[17]

Cyclothymic disorder begins early in life—in the late teens or early twenties.[18] Although many persons with cyclothymic disorder never develop more severe mood symptoms, a significant number of them eventually experience a fully developed depression or manic episode—that is, they develop bipolar disorder. In one study, about 6 percent of patients with cyclothymic disorder eventually had a manic episode, putting them in the bipolar I category, but a higher number (25 percent) developed severe depression—that is, they turned out to have bipolar II.[19] However, perhaps half of patients with the cyclothymic pattern never develop symptoms of full-blown bipolar disorder—a finding that makes cyclothymic disorder a true diagnosis in its own right.

Family-history studies indicate some relationship between cyclothymia and other bipolar disorders. Patients with cyclothymia often have relatives with bipolar disorder but rarely have relatives suffering from depressions only.[20] Treatment experiences seem to confirm this relationship: the mood swings of cyclothymic disorder often respond to many of the same treatment approaches as the bipolar disorders. This finding also confirms that cyclothymia is just as much a "chemical" problem as the other bipolar disorders and shows that thinking of the mood swings of cyclothymia as arising from personality problems is not helpful in making treatment decisions.

Bipolar Spectrum Disorders

If you look at the end of the section on bipolar disorders in the fifth edition of the *Diagnostic and Statistical Manual* of the American Psychiatric Association, you will see the category "bipolar disorder not elsewhere classified" (also, simply, "bipolar NEC"). This odd category exists because the developers of the *DSM* recognized that there are patients who seem to have some kind of bipolar disorder but who don't meet the diagnostic criteria for bipolar I or II or cyclothymia.

Maria is a violinist in the local symphony orchestra. She is nearly seventy but looks much younger. Born in what is now the Czech Republic, she defected to the United States during a tour of a chamber music group in the 1980s. Maria found herself in New York with only a small suitcase of clothes, her violin, and a charming European accent. She credits the latter two with her success in finding good work with several American orchestras over the years.

"I must tell you, Doctor, that my son has started taking Lamictal, just like me. His psychiatrist asked him about my medications and put my son on the same one. It's so good to know he's being treated by a psychiatrist as brilliant as you."

"Now, now, it was hardly brilliant of me to—"

"Oh, yes, so humble, so modest you are, just like all geniuses."

This was a little game we had played for years, ever since I had put her on a mood stabilizer instead of an antidepressant; the new medication had controlled her mood symptoms for the first time in many years.

Because she had moved to a new city every five years or so, Maria had seen many different professionals for her mood problems—mostly depression. For many of those years she received no treatment at all but simply slogged through her periods of depression on her own. During the 1970s, a physician gave her a prescription for the tranquilizer Valium, and although it didn't treat her depression very well, it numbed Maria's feelings enough to keep her going. When she moved to a new community, she would be able to get more prescriptions for Valium by reporting to her new doctor that it helped her—which, after a fashion, it did. During the really bad times, Maria used alcohol to augment the Valium's effect. By the time she was in her mid-forties, she was well on her way to chemical dependency. One terrible year, she lost a job because of missing several rehearsals and an important concert while in a week-long alcohol- and Valium-induced fog during a period of depression. Her husband left her, and a month later she got word that her son, also a talented musician, had dropped out of the prestigious conservatory he had been attending and had disappeared.

Maria's depression worsened to the point that she took a nearly fatal overdose of Valium and alcohol. It was only because the manager of the apartment building where she was living happened to go into her apartment that particular day that she ended up in a hospital rather than in the city morgue.

It was in the psychiatric hospital that she started taking an antidepressant for the first time, but the Lexapro that she started taking made things worse rather than better. Within three days of starting the antidepressant, Maria started to have hypomanic symptoms. She felt "wired" and agitated and couldn't sleep. She started staying up late at night writing music, becoming convinced that she had discovered new musical forms and new harmonies that would make her famous. Her antidepressant medication was immediately stopped, and she was started on lamotrigine. Within days the agitation had stopped. It took much longer for her depression to lift completely, but it eventually did.

"You were the first doctor to understand that I needed a mood stabilizer for depression, and that makes you truly brilliant," Maria continued, a raised eyebrow emphasizing her slightly teasing tone.

I was the lucky recipient of a lot of gratitude—gratitude she sometimes archly exaggerated to keep me from taking myself too seriously—because her moods were stable for the first time in years on a mood stabilizer.

Starting a patient with a history of manic symptoms on an antidepressant is something psychiatric textbooks warn against—but Maria had had manic symptoms only once in her life, at age sixty-six, while taking an antidepressant. Did this really make her bipolar? She didn't have the history of manic or even hypomanic episodes that would make her fit the bipolar I or II diagnosis—yet she clearly had some type of bipolar disorder.

Psychiatrists have long recognized that there are many forms of bipolar disorder. Kraepelin noted that "it is fundamentally and practically impossible to keep apart in any way" the various forms of bipolar disorder and that "everywhere there are transitions."[21] For many years various clinicians have described various types of "soft" bipolar disorder (table 2-6), mostly in patients who had come to them to be treated for depression but whose illness seemed related to bipolar disorder.[22] Terms like *pseudo-unipolar depression* and *bipolar III* have been coined to describe various types of severe depressions that have some features of bipolar disorder but do not fall into traditional categories for bipolar diagnoses. Often these patients have had a long history of depressive-like or manic-like features in their usual mood state, or "temperament," which are punctuated by the more severe mood symptoms that cause them to seek treatment.

As more treatments for bipolar disorder become available and as more research on the mood disorders is done, it is becoming clear that many patients who suffer from mostly depressive symptoms can benefit from treatment with medications for bipolar disorders and may in fact have a type of bipolar disorder.

Nathan is the fifty-five-year-old executive director of a philanthropic foundation. He describes himself as a "workaholic" who for years has worked sixteen- to eighteen-hour days and slept only four to six hours a night. Nathan is famous around town for his buoyant optimism and the boundless energy that he says comes from "making a living giving away other people's money," but his staff knows that he can be impatient and driven when deadlines approach or personnel problems distract him from devoting himself 110 percent to his mission. He came to me for treatment of miserable, irritable, restless feelings that had bothered him for several years but had become much worse in the previous few months.

Nathan had had problems with depression before but had never received any treatment with medication. When he was twenty-five, he became depressed after a friend died in a freak accident while both of them were skiing. Nathan was a graduate student at the time and nearly dropped out of school. When he was in his forties, he went through several months of depressed mood, trouble concentrating on his work, and appetite and weight loss that he and his psychiatrist at the time labeled a "midlife crisis" exacerbated by some unpleasant changes in his job. He was in therapy for about three months, and he started feeling better after he embarked on the job search that eventually led to his current position with a prestigious foundation.

"Or maybe it was the other way around," he mused.

"What do you mean?" I asked.

"Maybe I was able to look for a new job because I was feeling better."

"Do you know if other people in your family have had trouble with depression?"

"My father left us when I was three, and they say he was in and out of psychiatric hospitals his whole life. Both his sisters were alcoholics. One committed suicide."

Nathan was proud that despite his childhood in a broken, impoverished home, he now headed a foundation, signed checks for millions of dollars every year, and was courted by presidents of hospitals and universities every day of the week. "So why do I feel this way?" he asked. "It can't just be stress; I thrive on stress. These hopeless feelings come over me, these 'what's the point?' feelings. Why now?"

Nathan suffers from one of the "soft" bipolar disorders that some researchers call *bipolar III*.[23] These patients have a baseline mood that is a bit "higher" than that of most people, a personality characteristic that has been called *hyperthymic temperament* (table 2-7). Their usual energy level is high; they are cheerful, talkative, confident, and sociable. The down side of their personality style is that they tend to become irritated easily and can be impulsive, even reckless at times. They usually have a family history of bipolar disorder and are bothered by recurrent depressions. Antidepressant

TABLE 2-6 Indicators of "soft" bipolar disorders

Family history of bipolar disorder
History of mania or hypomania caused by treatment with antidepressants
History of "mixed" mood states
Depressive, "hyper," or cycling temperament
Recurrent depressions

TABLE 2-7 Features of bipolar III

Family history of bipolar disorder
Hyperthymic temperament:
    Habitual short sleeper—less than six hours per day
    Cheerful, optimistic personality style
    Tendency to become irritable easily
    Extroverted and sociable
Recurrent depressions

medication alone can make them more irritable and miserable or provoke a manic or hypomanic episode, but mood stabilizers can be very helpful.

For about a half century, psychiatry divided mood disorders into cases of unipolar depression, an illness characterized by only depressive symptoms, and bipolar disorders, in which patients suffer depressive episodes but also manic, hypomanic, or mixed states as well. Bipolar spectrum disorders seem to challenge this way of thinking; many of these patients have an illness that is dominated by depressive symptoms and shows only the slightest colorings of mania. They may have periods of elevated mood that they don't feel are particularly abnormal but that, when examined more closely, bear the hallmarks of hypomania: decreased need for sleep, increased energy, uncharacteristic overconfidence, and loss of inhibitions. As mentioned previously, periods of agitation and irritability that last only a few hours may represent mild mixed states. I have seen many patients who have been unsuccessfully treated with one antidepressant after another for what they have been told is "unipolar depression." For many of these patients, there are bipolar features in their illness that haven't been recognized as such. When one of the medications more typically used to treat bipolar disorder is prescribed, these patients frequently have a significant improvement in their depressive symptoms.

Some patients with this kind of problem become upset when I try to explain that a better treatment approach for their depression might be to treat it as a form of bipolar disorder; they worry that a diagnosis of bipolar disorder means that they have a more serious problem than "just depression" or that they are "really crazy." This reaction overlooks a couple of facts: first, depression is always a serious illness, and second, many people with bipolar disorder never develop full-blown mania or psychotic symptoms (which is what most people are thinking of when they use the pejorative term *crazy*). I sometimes use the term *complicated depression* to talk about these illnesses.

The important point to remember is that, despite what you might gather from reading short newspaper or magazine articles about depression and bipolar disorder, we haven't yet figured out how to classify these illnesses. It is becoming clear that many cases that seem to be "just depression" are related in some way to bipolar disorder. Many depressed patients who don't seem to have classic "manic-depressive illness" will nevertheless benefit from medications used to treat bipolar disorder.

Rapid-Cycling Bipolar Disorder

Soon after lithium became available for the treatment of bipolar disorder, psychiatrists noticed that some of the sickest bipolar patients didn't seem to derive much benefit from it. These patients clearly suffered from a bipolar mood disorder—they had severe manias and depressions—but they were set apart from other bipolar patients by the frequency of their episodes. Currently, rapid-cycling bipolar disorder is diagnosed if the patient has four or more episodes (mania, hypomania, depression, or mixed state) in one year.

Early impressions and case reports seemed to indicate that there were features other than frequency of episodes that set rapid-cycling bipolar disorder apart from other bipolar disorders. It seemed to occur more often in females, usually began with a depressive episode, and was less responsive to lithium therapy. There also seemed to be some indication that patients with this pattern of illness were more likely to have a history of thyroid gland problems and to have been treated with antidepressant medications.[24] There were suggestions from some researchers that these last two factors—thyroid disease and treatment with antidepressants—might cause "normal" bipolar illness to switch into rapid-cycling illness.[25]

Of these two factors, the most interest has been focused on the possibility that treatment with antidepressant medications can cause the switch from "normal" bipolar disorder into a rapid-cycling form. One study examined the case records of 118 patients who were rapid cyclers (had had four or more episodes of abnormal mood in one year).[26] The researchers found that 86 of these patients seemed to have had a change in the course of their illness—that is, they had "switched" into a rapid-cycling pattern. The authors stated that "the majority" of these switched after they were treated with an antidepressant medication. The role of antidepressants in the treatment of bipolar disorder—whether persons with bipolar disorder should even take antidepressants—remains a matter of debate among experts, one that I will return to in later chapters.

A more recent study casts some doubt on the usefulness of talking about rapid cycling as a specific type of bipolar disorder.[27] In this study, 919 patients were followed over a five-year period, and any who met the criteria for rapid cycling (having had at least one episode of mania or hypomania and three additional episodes of any type during one year) were studied closely.

Forty-five patients turned out to meet the rapid-cycling criteria, and their family history, treatment course, and course of illness were compared with those of the "normal" bipolar patients.

The picture that emerged from these patients suggested that rapid cycling is a temporary phase of bipolar illness that some patients are prone to—not a particular type of bipolar illness. The rapid cycling stopped after a period of several months in forty-four of the forty-five patients who were studied. These patients did not have rapid cyclers in their family, although they did have family members with "normal" bipolar illness. As time went on, their rapid cycling gradually stopped. The only finding from the earlier reports that was confirmed was that more women than men had rapid cycling; nearly three-quarters of the patients with rapid cycling were women (bipolar disorder usually affects both sexes about equally).

Some bipolar patients (18.5 percent in this study) seem to go through a period of rapid cycling for some months, during which their symptoms are more difficult to control—more women than men (I discuss this in more depth in chapter 14). Although there continues to be suspicion among many clinicians that antidepressant medications can cause some patients to start rapid cycling, the exact causes of rapid cycling remain a mystery, as do, unfortunately, the treatment steps that will prevent it.

Schizoaffective Disorder

Some patients have an illness with features both of mood disorders and of a very different psychiatric illness: schizophrenia. In addition to mood-disorder symptoms such as depression, hypomania, or mania, these patients have the hallucinations, delusions, and other bizarre mental experiences typical of schizophrenia; they often receive the diagnosis of schizoaffective disorder.

As we have seen in chapter 1, many patients with bipolar disorder develop delusional beliefs or hallucinations. But in the mood disorders, these symptoms can be understood as arising out of the mood state. For example, in a severe depression a patient might have the delusional belief that she has a terrible illness like AIDS or has lost all of her money, or that family members are being tortured by kidnappers, beliefs that are, well, depressing. Manic patients may hear the singing of angels or the voice of God—again, hallucinations that can be understood as coming out of the expansive, grandiose mood of mania. Delusions (false beliefs and ideas) and hallucinations (false sensory perceptions such as the hearing of voices) are said to be *mood congruent* when they can be understood as being part of the abnormal mood.

Persons with schizophrenia have bizarre delusions and hallucinations too, but they don't usually seem to bear any relation to a change in mood.

Examples of schizophrenic delusions would be the belief that one's next-door neighbors are pumping poisonous gas into one's house, or that one's real spouse and children have been replaced by exact replicas, or that the FBI has implanted a transmitter in one's brain. Patients with schizophrenia sometimes believe that other people are reading their minds or putting into their heads thoughts that are not theirs. They might hear their own thoughts repeated to them aloud or hear the voices of unseen commentators describing their actions to other unseen persons. None of these symptoms have much relationship to mood changes. More importantly, persons with schizophrenia do not experience episodes of sustained abnormal changes in mood. When a person has bizarre delusions or hallucinations like these or has these kinds of symptoms during times when they do not seem to be in an episode of abnormal mood, the diagnosis of schizoaffective disorder is often made.

What is this disorder, and where does it belong in the classification of psychiatric disease? These are questions that have plagued psychiatry for many years; we still don't have very good answers to them.

Is schizoaffective disorder truly a separate disorder, an illness that shares symptoms with mood disorders and schizophrenia but is neither? If it is, it has been very difficult for researchers to agree on its defining symptoms. In an earlier version of the *DSM,* the American Psychiatric Association's classification manual for mental illnesses, the diagnostic category of schizoaffective disorder was included without *any* listing of the symptoms that defined it.

I have seen patients who have been diagnosed with schizoaffective disorder who seem to me instead to have a severe case of a mood disorder that has been difficult to treat. Patients can be delusional and have hallucinations when they are very depressed or very manic, and if they are in a phase of ultra-rapid cycling, these symptoms can change rapidly and do not seem to make much sense in relation to their moods. I have seen patients diagnosed with schizoaffective disorder because they have prominent paranoid symptoms—that is, they believe they are being watched or followed or talked about. Although paranoid symptoms are very common in some types of schizophrenia and not as common in the mood disorders, close questioning often reveals the mood component in these patients. In a book written during the twentieth century called *A Mind That Found Itself,* Clifford Beers described his battle with a mental illness that was almost certainly bipolar disorder. In one scene he describes a train ride to the psychiatric hospital. As the train passed through the stations along the way, Beers noticed people standing on the station platforms reading the newspaper. He became convinced that they were reading about him. At first glance, this symptom doesn't seem to have any mood component, and in fact it is a rather typical symptom of schizophrenia called an *idea of reference*. Fortunately, however, Beers describes this symptom in great detail in his book and writes that he thought the people on the train platforms were reading about his long history of mental illness and about what a failure he had been. With this added detail—the themes of shame and failure in the symptom—the mood component becomes obvious and the real diagnosis clear: a mood disorder.

Another possible explanation for the mingling of symptoms of a mood disorder and of schizophrenia in one patient is that the patient may suffer from *both* illnesses. If one considers that bipolar I affects about 1 percent of the population and that about 1 percent of the population suffers from schizophrenia, then obviously, if there are no other factors operating to prevent the illnesses from occurring together, as many as 0.01 percent of the population will suffer from both disorders—that is, one in ten thousand. If one adds in other mood disorders such as bipolar II, cyclothymia, and the "soft" bipolar disorders, the numbers of persons with schizophrenia who also have a mood disorder will be even greater. Treatment experience would seem to support this idea: patients with a diagnosis of schizoaffective disorder seem to be most effectively treated with medications for mood disorders used in combination with medications for schizophrenia.

Indeed, some patients' illness definitely seems to combine two disorders: they have the kind of bizarre delusions common in schizophrenia, which seem to have nothing to do with an abnormal mood, but also have clear-cut episodes of depression and mania. This seems to be a rare occurrence, but it is important not to miss it. I have occasionally seen patients whose psychiatrist seemed reluctant to make the diagnosis of schizoaffective disorder, perhaps not wanting to frighten patients and families with the diagnosis of an illness that is usually more impairing and difficult to treat than a bipolar disorder. This reluctance to diagnose, however, can result in not treating the illness aggressively enough.

I once saw a patient whose psychiatrist had referred him for consultation because what had been diagnosed as severe bipolar depression with psychotic symptoms had responded poorly to many different treatments for mood disorders. This patient was certainly depressed, but his illness—which had required multiple hospitalizations and had become so disabling that he could no longer work or even live in his own apartment—had other features consistent with schizophrenia. For this patient, treatment for depression was helpful only up to a point. Only when he was also prescribed clozapine (Clozaril), a medication usually reserved for patients with severe schizophrenia who have failed to benefit from other medications, did he have a substantial recovery. Making a change in diagnosis and recommending a very different treatment approach was upsetting for this patient and his family at first—for just the reasons mentioned above. But the patient's parents also admitted that they had long suspected that their son had "more than just bipolar disorder," and after more careful explanation of my reasoning and further discussions with the patient and his family, we shifted the course of the treatment plan, ultimately with positive results. This is a lesson in the importance of making the correct diagnosis in mood disorders.

A diagnosis of schizoaffective disorder is in many ways more serious than that of bipolar disorder, since this illness shares some of the features of schizophrenia and some of the treatment challenges of that illness. Delusions and hallucinations may respond incompletely to medication treatment, and more severe (and sometimes progressive) social and occupational impairment is not uncommon. For this very reason, however, it is even more important, if a diagnosis of schizoaffective disorder is being considered, to be extra careful in reviewing the symptoms and course of illness and to use information from as many sources as possible.

CHAPTER 3

Bipolar Disorder and the *DSM-5*

INDIVIDUALS WHO ARE BEING TREATED BY A MENTAL-HEALTH PRO-
fessional and who read their diagnosis in their medical records or insurance
statements often have questions about the diagnostic categories and terms
that are used. Psychiatry is one of the few medical specialties that has a more
or less official list of disorders and diagnoses, and in this chapter we'll take
a closer look at the latest version of this list, the fifth edition of the *Diagnostic and Statistical Manual of Mental Disorders* (the *DSM-5*), developed
and published by the American Psychiatric Association. I'll present a brief
overview of the *DSM* and explain some of the diagnostic terminology for
bipolar disorder.

What Is the *DSM*?

The roots of the *DSM-5* go back at least as far as the U.S. Census of 1840,
which included the category of "idiocy/insanity" in its system for classifying
American citizens. By 1880 there were seven categories into which persons
with mental illness could be placed: mania, melancholia, monomania, paresis, dementia, dipsomania, and epilepsy.[1] In 1917 the American Medico-
Psychological Association—the forerunner of the American Psychiatric Association—developed a statistical manual for use in mental hospitals that
included various categories of diagnoses. As time went on, other organizations interested in the statistics of mental illness, such as the Veterans Administration and the U.S. Army, developed their own statistical manuals.

After World War II, the World Health Organization included a long section on mental disorders in the sixth edition of its *International Classification of Diseases* (the *ICD 6*).

In 1952 the American Psychiatric Association published the *Diagnostic and Statistical Manual: Mental Disorders* (the *DSM I*), which differed from previous statistical manuals in that it contained a glossary describing the symptoms of the different disorders. Thus, in addition to an official list of categories of mental illness, the *DSM I* provided guidance to the clinician in making psychiatric diagnoses. By the time the third edition of the manual appeared in 1980, each category of psychiatric disorders had a list of *diagnostic criteria*—the symptoms and other characteristics of each disorder that were thought to define it and set it apart from other psychiatric disorders.

Perhaps the most valuable use of the *DSM* is in research into the causes and treatment of mental illnesses. Use of the *DSM* in research means that when you find a study of some particular psychiatric disorder in a professional journal and read that "the patients met the *DSM* diagnostic criteria" for that disorder, you can be sure that the patients all had a certain well-defined collection of symptoms and other characteristics in common, that the researchers were not mixing, as it were, psychiatric apples and oranges in their study.

There are problems with the *DSM,* however, and many experts have been extremely critical of it. The *DSM* is essentially a collection of checklists of *symptoms* for each diagnostic category and is not based on an understanding of the *causes* of emotional problems. This might seem like a quibbling academic question at first, but it's not. As an example, a *DSM*-type classification system for physical illnesses might classify diseases based on the severity and location of symptoms such as pain or fever. A moment's thought reveals how useless such a system would be. Patients coming to an emergency department with symptoms of abdominal pain and a fever might be diagnosed with "Hot Painful Belly Disorder." But since these same symptoms can be caused by a myriad of different problems, ranging from appendicitis to gall stones to porphyria, to make a diagnosis of "Hot Painful Belly Disorder" is completely useless for deciding how to treat the patient. Switching back to psychiatric diagnosis, good clinicians know that two patients might have nearly identical symptoms of depression from many different causes that range from normal bereavement, to reactions to long-term depressing life circumstances such as poverty or ongoing physical abuse, to biologically and genetically caused mood disorders. Cataloging the *symptoms* is only a first step in deciding what to do for the patient. A list of symptoms doesn't help decide whether the patient needs grief counseling, social work intervention to alleviate consequences of poverty, protection from an abusive partner, or a prescription for an antidepressant.

Because the *DSM* contains a list of psychiatric diagnoses followed by succinct and clearly written "criteria" for making those diagnoses, it also has the unfortunate effect of making psychiatric diagnosis look deceptively easy. It is tempting for individuals who have no psychiatric training to use this series of symptom checklists to diagnose mental illness. Well, why not?

First of all, it is only with an enormous amount of training and experience that one can gain an appreciation for the very wide range of *normal* emotions and behaviors and have a sense of what falls outside this normal range. Significant clinical experience and judgment are needed to decide what constitutes an "expansive mood" or an "increase in energy" that is clinically significant. I have been called to see "manic" patients referred by their counselors or their family members and found that the patients, though a bit more intense in manner than most people, have a mood state perfectly within the normal range. The *DSM* is full of diagnostic criteria that use qualifiers like "clinically significant," "marked impairment," and "excessive involvement in . . . ," all of which require judgment based on experience to make a determination. Even some counseling and therapy professionals, if they have not trained in a setting where they have had the opportunity to see very sick patients, may not have an appreciation for what constitutes "severe"—simply because they have never seen and worked with "severely" depressed or manic patients. Nonprofessionals will, of course, usually have even less experience with the range of normal and abnormal moods. Without the experience of seeing many patients with severe mental illnesses and treating them, it is impossible to accurately separate normal from abnormal mental experiences or "clinically significant" mood changes from those that are within the range of the normal. In psychiatry as perhaps in no other field, the dictum "A little learning is a dangerous thing" holds quite true.

Moreover, as we shall see in chapter 18, many *medical* conditions can mimic abnormal mood states, dozens of pharmaceuticals can cause depression or euphoric states in some persons, and drugs of abuse can cause all kinds of mood states and psychoses in almost anyone. Almost all the *DSM* diagnoses contain "exclusion criteria" for medical conditions, such as "the symptoms are not due to a general medical condition." A physician will probably notice the abnormalities in the facial appearance of a patient with Graves' disease or Cushing's syndrome as soon as the patient walks into the room; the nonphysician probably has never heard of these illnesses and doesn't know that they can cause psychiatric symptoms practically identical to those of a major depression episode. The physician knows well the typical walk of the patient with Parkinson's disease and the subtle language problems of the patient who has had a silent stroke—both neurological conditions that can cause mood symptoms. Obviously, only a clinician trained in the diagnosis and treatment of physical illness will be able to pick up these sorts of problems.

Finally, just as the range of normal experiences and behaviors is enormous, so is the range (and complexity) of abnormal mental experiences and behaviors; they cannot be contained in any one book and certainly cannot all be described in a few dozen diagnostic categories. Alfred Kinsey, a great student of human behavior and the pioneering researcher on sexuality, once said, "The world is not divided into sheep and goats. . . . Nature rarely deals with discrete categories. Only the human mind invents categories and tries to force facts into separated pigeonholes."[2] To paraphrase Kinsey, bipolar disorder is probably not divided simply into bipolar I and bipolar II, either—and patients often don't fit into *DSM* pigeonholes. There is also the fact that many patients with one psychiatric disorder also suffer from another—patients with mood disorders often have addiction problems, patients with developmental disorders such as autism frequently get depressed or anxious—not to mention that symptoms of one disorder are often seen in another: the "criteria" for attention-deficit hyperactivity disorder (ADHD) are nearly identical to those of hypomania, for example. Many patients with bipolar disorder also have panic attacks, but to say that these patients suffer from a mood disorder *and* an anxiety disorder simply isn't accurate. In fact, treating anxious and depressed patients with anti-anxiety medications such as clonazepam (Klonopin) and other sedatives often makes things worse rather than better.

For all these reasons, I am not going to list here the *DSM* diagnostic criteria for the bipolar disorders. I don't want to tempt nonclinicians to engage in self-diagnosis or diagnosis of family members. The *DSM* is easily available in libraries, but it should be considered a reference book for researchers and clinicians, not a textbook of psychiatry.

Bipolar Categories in the *DSM-5*

Only two subtypes of bipolar disorder have been characterized well enough to have been assigned their own *DSM* categories: bipolar I and bipolar II. As we saw in chapter 2, in the section on bipolar spectrum disorders, there are probably other forms of the illness that will eventually be described and understood well enough to be demarcated with their own labels as well, but for now a patient having one of these "soft" bipolar disorders would be diagnosed with "bipolar disorder not elsewhere classified (bipolar disorder NEC)," according to the *DSM.* Cyclothymic disorder is included in the *DSM-5* as a diagnosis as well.

CHAPTER 4

The Mood Disease

HAVING REVIEWED THE MANY SYMPTOMS OF BIPOLAR DISORDER and the many forms the illness can take, I want to take a moment to review just how far we've come in our understanding of this illness—and where we've come *from*. I think the understanding of any subject is incomplete unless you know a little about its history; and the history of thinking about bipolar disorder not only is a fascinating story in its own right but also will provide valuable insights into how psychiatrists view the diagnostic process and approach the treatment of psychiatric disorders. (This is a chapter that may be of more interest to students and mental health professionals than to patients and their families. You can skip it without any loss of continuity.)

Before "Bipolar"

The ancient Greeks believed that all maladies of mind and body were caused by imbalances among four vital bodily fluids, or "humors." One of the terms we still use to describe depression, *melancholia,* is derived from the Greek word for one of these humors: black bile. According to humoral theory, depression was thought to be caused by an excess of black bile and mania by an excess of yellow bile.

Although they were incorrect about the causes of the two opposite mood states of bipolar disorder, several ancient physicians had remarkable insight into the connection between them. Aretaius of Cappadocia (ca. 150) described the syndrome of depression in which patients became "peevish, dispirited, sleepless" and "complain[ed] of life and desire[d] to die." In other patients he described manic symptoms: "At the height of [their] disease [they] have impure dreams, and irresistible desire[s]. . . . If roused to anger by admonition or restraint, they become wholly mad." But most remarkably, he stated, "In my opinion, melancholia is without any doubt the beginning and even part of the disorder called mania."[1] Paul of Aegina (625–690) made a similar connection between the two syndromes, basing his thinking on humoral theory. Like other Greeks, Paul assumed that melancholia was caused by too much ordinary black bile, but he postulated that mania was caused by an excess of "yellow bile which, by too much heat," had become burned black bile.[2]

Considerations of possible physical causes for the symptoms of bipolar disorder more or less ceased after the fall of the Roman Empire, and the symptoms and behaviors that we now recognize as arising from psychiatric conditions were usually attributed to witchcraft or demonic possession rather than to disruptions of a person's physiology. When medieval times gave way to the Renaissance and the Enlightenment, mental illness again became the purview of physicians rather than priests, and modern attempts to understand and classify diseases began. Melancholia and mania were often considered to be two separate disorders by these early physicians. However, a few insightful clinicians, such as the English physician Robert James (1705–1776), connected the two syndromes: "There is an absolute Necessity for reducing Melancholy and Madness [mania] to one Species of Disorder, and consequently considering them in one joint View. . . . We find, that they both arise from the same common Cause and Origin, that is, an excessive Congestion of the Blood in the Brain. . . . We find that melancholic Patients . . . easily fall into Madness, which, when removed, the Melancholy again discovers itself."[3] Melancholia and "madness" were thought by most early physicians who wrote about mental disease to predispose to each other but nevertheless to be entirely different conditions.

Not until the middle of the nineteenth century was the idea that depression and mania might be expressions of a single mental illness first proposed. It was suggested by two French *alienists* (a term—from *aliéné*, the French word for "insane"—that was used in France and in English-speaking countries at one time to denote physicians specializing in mental disorders). Jules Baillarger (1809–1890) published a paper in 1854 describing an illness he called *la folie à double forme,* and two weeks later Jean-Pierre Falret (1794–1870) rushed a paper into print in the same journal in which he insisted that he had been teaching his students about *la folie circulaire* at the Salpetrière hospital for ten years. (This was, incidentally, the same hospital where several years later the young Sigmund Freud began to formulate his own theories about mental phenomena.) Both men described a mental illness characterized by alternating periods of melancholia and mania that were often separated by periods of normal mood. After the appearance of their original papers, Baillarger and Falret wrote several "me first!" "no, *me* first!" letters to the *Bulletin* of the Imperial Academy of Medicine, each claiming to be the originator of this idea. Which of them deserves credit as the first to describe bipolar disorder is a matter upon which scholars still disagree.[4] But medical historians do *not* disagree about the identity of the psychiatrist who published the first comprehensive description of the mood disorders and established the basis of the classification system for mental illnesses that we still use today.

Dr. Kraepelin and "Manic-Depressive Insanity"

It was the German psychiatrist Emil Kraepelin (1856–1926) who, in 1899, solidified the modern concept of bipolar disorder in the sixth edition of his enormously influential textbook on mental illnesses, *Psychiatrie: Ein Lehrbuch für Studirende und Ärzte*. Kraepelin had been working for several years to develop a logical and comprehensive classification system for major mental illnesses, and successive editions of his *Textbook of Psychiatry* document the development of his thinking.

In the fifth edition, he divided severe forms of mental illness into two broad categories: those that had a deteriorating course of illness and those that were "periodic." These two groups are still recognizable in modern classifications of psychiatric disorders, the "deteriorating" group containing the various forms of schizophrenia and related disorders and the "periodic" group containing the mood disorders. Although he was not the first to suggest that mania and depression were both expressions of one disorder, Kraepelin was the first to articulate, clearly and convincingly, the idea that *all* disorders of mood were related to one another: "Manic-depressive insanity . . . includes on the one hand the whole domain of so-called periodic and circular insanity, on the other hand simple mania, [and] the greater part of the morbid states termed melancholia. . . . In the course of the years I have become more and more convinced that all the above-mentioned states only represent manifestations of a single morbid process."[5] Kraepelin's "manic-depressive synthesis" was a major breakthrough in the understanding and classification of major mental illnesses.[6]

But Kraepelin was more than an academic and a theoretician; he was a clinician who saw enormous numbers of patients and recorded his observations of their illnesses in superb detail. As you know from reading them in previous chapters, his descriptions of the symptoms of bipolar disorder are vivid and insightful, and they have never been surpassed. A former professor once told me that "anyone who thinks they've discovered something new in psychiatry simply hasn't read the German psychiatric literature." I think it's fair to say that anyone who thinks he has discovered something new about bipolar disorder—at least, about its symptoms and diagnosis—simply hasn't read Kraepelin.

Kraepelin's contributions, although tremendously significant for those interested in the classification of mental disorders, offered little practical benefit in his time to those afflicted with them. I would imagine that Dr. Kraepelin's patients were more accurately informed about their illness than most patients of that time and had more reliable prognostic information, but there was really nothing he could do to help them with their symptoms. There was still no treatment for *any* psychiatric condition that offered much hope of alleviating the symptoms or altering the course of the disease. Although the English translation of the chapter on "manic-depressive insanity" in the eighth edition of Kraepelin's textbook is more than two hundred pages long, the "Treatment" section is less than five pages long—and most of that consists of warnings about the suicidal behaviors of depressed patients and cautions against discharging them too soon from the hospital. In the absence of treatments for manic-depressive illness, patients spent months, even years, in hospitals and asylums.

As the study of mental disorders entered the twentieth century, hopes for more effective treatment of psychiatric disorders rose when scientific discoveries shed some light on the causes of several mental illnesses. In 1906 the German microbiologist August Wassermann discovered a method to detect in human spinal fluid antibodies to the microorganism that causes syphilis. This may not sound like a discovery that had anything to do with psychiatry, unless you know that syphilitic infection of the central nervous system was at this time one of the most common causes of severe psychiatric symptoms, and that nearly half of the patients in mental institutions suffered from "general paresis of the insane," as syphilis with psychiatric manifestations was known. With the development of the Wassermann test, it became possible to diagnose the illness with a very high degree of reliability. For the first time, a cause of a form of "madness" had been discovered. That same year another German microbiologist, Paul Ehrlich, developed the first effective treatment for syphilis, using arsenic compounds. Although the treatment was crude and dangerous, it was effective enough in the early stages of the disease to reduce the incidence of the illness by 50 percent in several European countries.

We hardly think of syphilis as a mental illness today, but patients with syphilitic infection of the brain can suffer hallucinations, delusions, and mood changes not very different from those seen in bipolar disorder and schizophrenia. An early-twentieth-century psychiatric text describes the mania-like excitement that was sometimes seen in persons with central nervous system syphilis: "The intensity of the excitement is extreme; there is absolute sleeplessness [and] incessant restlessness. The grandiose delusions are the controlling feature of the paretic's thought. The patient . . . comes before us tremulous with emotion, his eye bright, as the overpowering visions of wealth and grandeur float before his mind."[7] The discovery of reliable and effective diagnostic techniques for general paresis of the insane—unfortunately, arsenicals had little effect on the advanced central nervous system disease—was seen by many as an enormous advance in the understanding of psychiatric disorders. Clinicians charged with the care of psychiatric patients had great hopes that the causes of other psychiatric disorders would soon be found.

As more and more powerful microscopes were invented and special tissue stains were developed for brain tissues, various microscopic structures of the brain—the many different types of neurons and the microscopic architecture of the different parts of the brain—became visible for the first time. Anatomical and chemical abnormalities were found to characterize several other diseases with prominent mental symptoms. In 1906 the Swiss neuropathologist Alois Alzheimer, who was a student of Kraepelin, discovered abnormal microscopic plaques and tangles of cellular debris in the brains of persons who had died from the progressive brain disease that was eventually named for him. Individuals with *cretinism,* a particularly severe form of mental retardation, were found to have abnormally low levels of thyroid hormones. In 1915 *pellagra,* another mysterious disease characterized by skin lesions and gradual mental deterioration, was discovered to be caused by a deficiency of vitamin B.

But blood tests and brain studies revealed nothing about manic-depressive illness. Try as they might, pathologists and anatomists could find nothing different or abnormal in the brain structures of individuals with bipolar disorder, using the tools that were available to them.

New ways of thinking seemed necessary to understand the mental illnesses for which no physical cause could be found, and shortly after the beginning of the twentieth century, new theories were advanced, most notably by Sigmund Freud, that seemed to have considerable power to explain the basis of these still-mysterious illnesses. These theories, boiled down to their essence, held that mental symptoms were reactions to life events in vulnerable individuals—not disease states caused by disruptions in biological functioning. The new theories of mental illness instructed psychiatrists to use "talking cures" to treat their patients.

By carefully exploring patients' biographies in minute detail, physicians attempted to understand what conflicts and life events their patients were reacting to with symptoms of depression or mania. It was the expectation that the proper combination of understanding, reinterpretation, and encouragement could alleviate patients' symptoms. Freud, more than any other early psychiatrist, developed elaborate theories about normal and abnormal childhood psychological development that he felt could explain why some people developed extreme psychological symptoms in response to difficult life situations and events while others did not. Manic-depressive illness and schizophrenia came to be called *functional illnesses* because it was believed that patients with depression or mania or symptoms of schizophrenia had *normal* brain and nervous system functioning. Although Freud and his disciples did not totally discount biological agents as having some role in the causation of these problems, they did not see their patients as suffering from *diseases.* A "functional illness" was believed to be an illness of the mind, not of the brain. These concepts dominated American psychiatry until well into the 1960s.

During these decades most psychiatrists believed that abnormal mental phenomena were caused by traumatic childhood events, poor parenting, repressed sexual feelings, and interpersonal conflicts. They lost interest in the classification and categorization of psychiatric illnesses; the very idea of trying to make a diagnosis in a psychiatric patient seemed a waste of time because the form as well as the cause of a psychiatric problem seemed to be as individual as the biography of the patient in whom it occurred. Then in 1949 an unknown Australian psychiatrist published an article in the *Medical Journal of Australia* called "Lithium Salts in the Treatment of Psychotic Excitement."

Dr. Cade and Lithium

By the 1930s and 1940s, most physicians interested in the treatment of mental disorders had joined psychoanalytic institutes to learn the theory and practice of psychiatry according to the teachings of Freud and his followers. They trained and practiced mostly in the big cities, mostly treating patients with mild depression or anxiety, patients who had the time, motivation, and money to attend therapy sessions four or five days a week, to explore their past and reinterpret their present to become healthier, happier, and better "adjusted." The theories of Freud revolutionized the understanding of many aspects of human behavior, and they continue to form the basis for the practice of psychotherapy. But there were many patients who benefited little from these new ideas. They were the patients Dr. Kraepelin had cared for: the victims of schizophrenia and manic-depressive illness.

For these patients, housed for months or years in (mostly public) hospitals and asylums, the therapeutic armamentarium had not changed much in two hundred years: bed rest for the depressed; physical restraint for the agitated; baths, tranquilization with morphine and bromides, and the use of

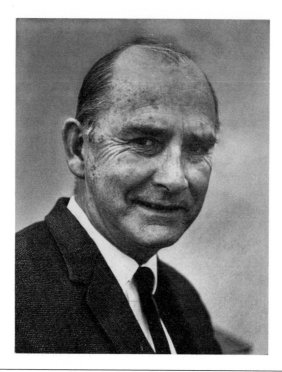

Figure 4-1 John F. J. Cade.
Source: State Library of Victoria.

numerous other substances thought to have beneficial effects, among them quinine and even cod-liver oil. None of these interventions had any but the most insignificant effects on serious mental illness.

John F. J. Cade, M.D., senior medical officer in the Mental Hygiene Department of Victoria, Australia, was convinced that manic-depressive illness was a biological disorder, not a psychological one (figure 4-1). Working in his laboratory to determine whether some toxin might be present in the urine of patients with manic-depressive illness, Cade became especially interested in urea and uric acid, by-products of protein metabolism found in urine. He was testing the toxicity of these compounds by injecting small amounts of them into guinea pigs.

One of the technical problems with this work was that uric acid is rather insoluble in water, making it difficult to prepare injectable solutions at high concentrations. Looking for a soluble urate salt to use instead of uric acid, Cade consulted prior research and discovered that uric acid was easiest to dissolve in water when it was combined with a lithium ion as lithium urate. He injected small amounts of lithium urate into the guinea pigs and noticed that uric acid seemed to be much less toxic in this form. This suggested to

Cade that the lithium component of the compound might have some sort of protective effect against urate toxicity. To determine what the effect of the lithium ion might be, he injected lithium carbonate—the carbonate ion is harmless and is found in substances such as baking soda—and discovered that "after a latent period of about two hours the animals, although fully conscious, became extremely lethargic and unresponsive to stimuli for one to two hours before once again becoming normally active."[8]

Cade admits in his original paper that "it may seem a long distance from lethargy in guinea pigs to excitement in psychotics," but asylum doctors of the time were desperate for new treatment possibilities, so Cade decided to administer lithium preparations to several patients who were chronically agitated. The effect on patients with mania was dramatic:

Case I—W.B., a male aged fifty-one years, who had been in a state of chronic manic excitement for five years, restless, dirty, destructive, mischievous and interfering, had long been regarded as the most troublesome patient in the ward. His response was highly gratifying. From the start of treatment on March 29, 1948, with lithium citrate he steadily settled down and in three weeks was enjoying the unaccustomed surroundings of the convalescent ward. As he had been ill so long and confined to a "chronic ward," he found normal surroundings and liberty of movement strange at first. He remained perfectly well and left the hospital on indefinite leave with instructions to take a dose of lithium carbonate, five grains, twice a day. He was soon back working at his old job. However, he became more lackadaisical about his medicine and finally ceased taking it. His relatives reported that he had not taken any for at least six weeks prior to his readmission on January 30, 1949 and was becoming steadily more irritable and erratic. On readmission to the hospital he was at once started on lithium carbonate, ten grains three times a day, and in a fortnight had again settled down to normal. He is now (February 28, 1949) ready to return to home and work.

Case VIII—W.M., a man of fifty years, was suffering from an attack of recurrent mania, the first of which he had had at the age of twenty. The present attack had lasted two months and showed no signs of abating. He was garrulous, euphoric, restless and unkempt when he started taking lithium. Two days later he was reported to be quieter. By the ninth day he was definitely settling down and the following day commenced work in the garden. By the end of two weeks he was practically normal—quiet, tidy, rational, with insight into his previous condition. This was in marked contrast to his condition a fortnight before when he had to be locked in a single room at night . . . and was too restless to eat in the dining room owing to his unsettling effect on the other patients.[9]

Dr. Cade had treated ten manic patients with lithium, and all ten had shown the same dramatic improvement. He had also given lithium to six patients with "dementia praecox" (schizophrenia) and three patients with "chronic depressive psychoses," but with less effect. The agitated patients with schizophrenia became less agitated but had "no fundamental improvement"; the depressed patients had "no improvement."

It is often emphasized in textbooks and articles on the history of lithium treatment that Cade's discovery of lithium's efficacy in bipolar disorder was pure accident—an observation that misses an important point. Cade, like many hospital psychiatrists, but unlike perhaps many other psychiatrists of his time, was pursuing a biological intervention for what he believed was a biological disorder. His case descriptions reveal that even though he had little specific therapy to offer them, he had taken a complete history of his patients' course of illness, carefully examined them, and, following in the footsteps of Emil Kraepelin, made a *diagnosis* based on his examination and history-taking. Cade's approach to these severely ill patients—his assumption that they suffered from diseases rather than from emotional reactions—provided the theoretical underpinning that made his discovery possible. A psychiatrist who believed in "reactions" and "functional illness" would have been unlikely to divide patients into the diagnostic categories of mania, schizophrenia, and depressive psychosis and report on the differential efficacy of a pharmaceutical in each group. Such a psychiatrist would have been even less likely to look for toxins in the urine of patients with mania.[10]

One would think that the news of Cade's discovery would have spread like wildfire. It did not. In fact, several decades elapsed before lithium was approved for the treatment of bipolar disorder by the U.S. Food and Drug Administration. Why this incredible delay?

Part of the reason was the state of world psychiatry following the end of World War II. German psychiatry, which had produced superb clinicians like Kraepelin and Freud and many other pioneers in the science of mental disorders, was in ruins, literally and figuratively. The German psychiatric establishment had been mesmerized by the Nazi movement, and prominent German psychiatrists had enthusiastically participated in the expulsion of Jewish colleagues from the profession and even in the murder of the patients they had been charged to care for. Thousands of mentally retarded and mentally ill individuals were gassed in the years leading up to the war and during the war. When Cade wrote of his work with lithium, Germany was no longer providing leaders in psychiatric medicine; rather, German psychiatry was in dire need of rehabilitation.[11]

In the United States and England, psychoanalytic theories had replaced the traditional medical practices of evaluation, diagnosis, and treatment with the prescription of the "talking cure" for all emotional problems. Accurate psychiatric diagnosis simply didn't exist; any patient with severe symptoms was usually called "schizophrenic" and admitted to a state psychiatric hospital for little more than custodial care. Ronald Fieve, the American psychiatrist who championed the use of lithium in the United States in the 1970s and who was instrumental in getting American psychiatrists to prescribe it for their patients, observed that during the late 1940s and the 1950s in New York, he "rarely met with the diagnosis of manic-depression. . . . It had virtually disappeared. Most cases of excitable, talkative, and elated behavior were being diagnosed as schizophrenia."[12]

But a Danish psychiatrist, Morgans Schou, realized that Cade's discovery represented a real breakthrough. He noted in a 1954 paper, "It is rather astonishing that [Cade's] observation has failed to arouse greater general interest among psychiatrists."[13] Schou and his colleagues did the careful clinical trials that eventually resulted in the development of recommended dosages and preparations of lithium for the treatment of symptoms of bipolar disorder. Perhaps more than any other clinical researcher, Schou established the efficacy of lithium treatment for mania. Even more important was his discovery that lithium could prevent the recurrence of symptoms in patients with bipolar disorder.

In 1957 another breakthrough occurred in the treatment of mood disorders when Roland Kuhn, a Swiss psychiatrist, described how a compound originally developed as an antihistamine had remarkable effects on depressed patients. He reported his results in a Swiss medical journal, and his paper was reprinted the next year in English as "The Treatment of Depressive States with G 22355 (Imipramine Hydrochloride)." But Kuhn also noticed that in some patients imipramine simply replaced one mood problem with another: "In marked manic-depressive psychosis, i.e., if the depressions are easily and frequently replaced by manic-like phases or actual manic states, the reaction is less favorable. . . . The tendency arises for the depression to switch over into a manic phase."[14]

In one of their first papers on the use of lithium in manic patients, Schou and his colleagues had pointed out that "the beneficial effect of lithium in cases of mania appears to offer new possibilities for a study of the *pathophysiology* [i.e., the disease mechanism] of the manic-depressive psychoses."[15] The discovery of the therapeutic effects of imipramine on depressed patients and the observation that it could precipitate mania in patients with "manic-depressive psychosis" were two more clues that bipolar disorder might be more than a psychological "reaction."

The fact that a chemical (lithium) made the symptoms of mania go away indicated that mania had at least some biochemical basis. The discovery of the different effects of imipramine on depressed persons with and without a history of mania reinforced the disease model for bipolar disorder. Persons with a history of mania became manic if they took imipramine; persons who did not have a history of mania (usually) did not. Imipramine was not simply a "manio-genic" drug, a drug that produced euphoria in everyone who took it. The fact that only bipolar individuals became manic from it suggested that their illness had a different biochemical basis from other cases of depression. The modern age of psychiatry had begun, as had the search for more and better pharmaceutical treatments and for the physical basis of these disorders.

PART II

TREATMENT

Several years ago I heard a classical guitarist being interviewed on the radio. He said he was often asked by strangers, usually people who didn't know much about classical music, whether he played the *electric* or the *acoustic* guitar. "I hate that term, *acoustic guitar.* I'd rather just say I played the guitar," he said. "But after the electric guitar was invented, I suppose somebody had to come up with a term for a non-electric guitar."

There is a term for psychiatric problems that many nonpsychiatrists use that I dislike, and that's *chemical imbalance.* It's a term that we started hearing used in the 1970s to describe psychiatric problems that were not psychological reactions or "functional" problems (as I described them in chapter 4) but rather were illnesses caused by some malfunction of brain physiology. To paraphrase the guitarist, I suppose somebody had to invent a term for psychiatric illnesses as opposed to purely psychological conditions, but *chemical imbalance* implies several things about psychiatric illnesses that are very misleading.

First is the idea that all disturbances of mental life fall into two mutually exclusive categories: "chemical" and "nonchemical" (or perhaps "chemical" and "psychological" might work better). As we shall see in this next group of chapters, such a division is not possible, because the "chemical" and "psychological" aspects of mental life interact and overlap. Second, to say that a psychiatric problem like bipolar disorder is simply an "imbalance" of brain chemicals is a monumental oversimplification of what really lies at the root of these problems. The fantastically complex human brain is not simply a cantaloupe-sized organ bathed in a soup of "chemicals" that can be adjusted by the addition of medications to achieve a "balance" (as a chef adds a little more salt or another pinch of cayenne to make a favorite recipe come out right).

In chapter 5 I'll do my best to explain what causes bipolar disorder and also touch on how we think the medications used to treat the illness work. The details here are a bit complicated, but the basics are not difficult to grasp. This chapter might require a slower, more careful reading pace for those unfamiliar with terms like *neurotransmitters,* but the effort will pay off later, allowing you to understand the use of medications in bipolar disorder much better.

Then in subsequent chapters we'll talk about treatment more specifically, beginning with a review of the pharmaceuticals used in the treatment of the disorder. We'll also cover electroconvulsive therapy and other newer brain-stimulation techniques and, last but certainly not least, the important role of counseling and psychotherapy in the treatment of the illness. We'll end part II with a brief overview of the treatment approaches and some principles of treatment that I think are important to remember.

CHAPTER 5

The Plastic Brain

I'M ABOUT TO DISCUSS SOME RATHER COMPLICATED SCIENCE. NOW, if that sentence sends shivers up your spine, you can skip this chapter. You'll still be able to understand the chapters that follow. Although no one really knows for sure exactly what causes bipolar disorder, we have some theories, based on research, that make sense. If you are interested in those theories, read on. If you're not, you can skip ahead to the medication chapters.

Some years ago, the psychiatrist and neuroscientist Nancy Andreasen wrote a book, *The Broken Brain*,[1] about the new discoveries in biological psychiatry. The title makes the point that psychiatric illnesses such as bipolar disorder and schizophrenia are caused by biological malfunctions of the brain, not by repressed memories or traumatic childhoods. Although we still don't know exactly what those malfunctions are, we are getting very close to understanding some of the biological mechanisms that might be involved. In this overview of brain functioning, I want to tell you about what scientists think might be "broken" in bipolar disorder.

Many people imagine that the human brain is a kind of wonderful computer. Although this is a vast oversimplification of the true capabilities of the brain, it's a good place to start in trying to understand how this fantastic organ of the mind works.

Like the computer that I'm using to write these words, a human brain receives input, processes the information it receives, and then delivers output. Like a computer, it stores information and often uses this stored information to help process further input. The human brain receives its input

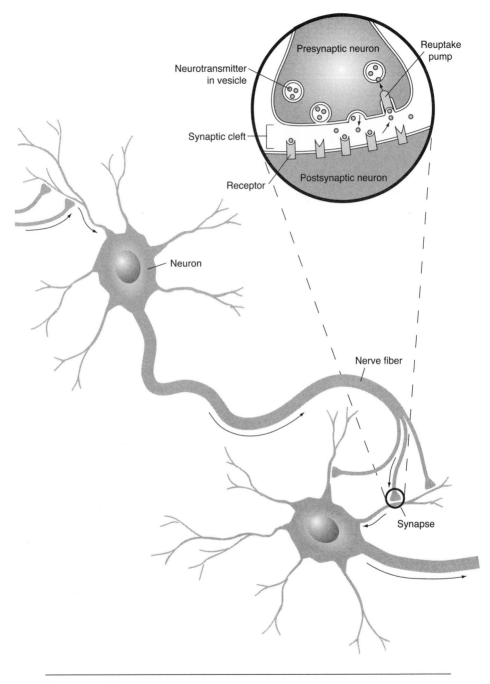

FIGURE 5-1 Synapse.

from the sense organs—the eyes, ears, taste buds, touch receptors, and so forth—and delivers output in terms of behavior.

You may know that a computer computes by means of many thousands of microscopic switches embedded in its processing chip. The pattern of "on" and "off" in the switches is what stores information; the control of the flow of signals through these switches is the processing. The human brain contains about 11 billion nerve cells, or *neurons*—but as powerful as a computer with 11 billion switches might be, our brain is many orders of magnitude more impressive than that. This is because the neuron is not just a switch that is either "on" or "off," but rather is an impressive microprocessor in its own right. Each neuron receives input from many other neurons, processes this information, and sends output to many others. The brain, then, is not like a computer with billions of switches; it is more like the Internet: a network of billions of computers, all capable of being individually programmed. Each neuron in the brain may receive input and then transmit signals to up to fifty thousand other neurons. The number of all the possible connections in the human brain is incomprehensibly large, a hyperastronomical number on the order of the number of molecules in the universe.

I'm going to jump the gun a little and tell you that there is a lot of evidence that bipolar disorder (and perhaps all mood disorders, as well as anxiety disorders) is caused by some defect in the mechanisms by which the individual neurons are programmed. Neurons have the ability to be "reprogrammed" in response to various situations (stress is one); this capability is called *neuroplasticity* (remember that the original meaning of *plastic* refers to a material that can be shaped and reshaped, like modeling clay). But before we get to that, we need to talk about neurotransmitters.

Although the human nervous system uses electrical signals to do much of its work, it uses chemical signals as well; molecules called *neurotransmitters* are the means by which nerve cells communicate with each other. Neurons send these chemical signals to each other at the *synapse*, an area where two neurons nearly touch. The first neuron releases neurotransmitters, which flow across this narrow space to link up with targets called *receptors* on the next neuron (figure 5-1). When enough of the receptors are occupied by neurotransmitter molecules, which fit into the receptors like keys fit into locks, the recipient nerve cell is activated and fires off its own signal. There needs to be some mechanism for this signaling system to be turned off and reset, of course. After neurotransmitter molecules link up with receptors across the synapse, they must somehow be removed in preparation for the next batch. This happens in a variety of ways in different cells, but one of the most important mechanisms is by reuptake into the neuron that released them. A *reuptake pump* on this neuron removes neurotransmitter molecules from the synapse and transports them back into the interior of the cell, where they can be repackaged for rerelease.

Neurons are continually communicating with each other. Neurotransmitter molecules passing from one neuron to another across synapses maintain a steady tone of chemical signal, with the signal getting stronger, or pulsing up, at times and the neuron detecting and reacting to these pulses. Thus, as I noted earlier, neurons are not just switches that can only be set to "on" or "off" but rather are tiny information-processing units that are constantly communicating with other neurons to which they are functionally linked.

Soon after Roland Kuhn discovered that G 22355 was an effective antidepressant (see chapter 4), neuroscientists started to investigate the effect of this pharmaceutical on brain chemistry. They discovered that imipramine is a powerful inhibitor of one type of reuptake pump, blocking the reuptake of a group of neurotransmitters called *neurogenic amines* (or *neuroamines*). Remember that neurons turn off their chemical signals ("turn down" is probably more accurate) by scooping up neurotransmitter molecules from the synapse and repackaging them. Just as partly closing the drain in a bathtub while the water is running will cause the tub to begin to fill, if you block the reuptake of neurotransmitter molecules into cells, the net effect will be an increase of neurotransmitters in the synapse. Neuroscientists found that nearly all the medications that are effective antidepressants cause a blockade of neurotransmitter reuptake in brain cells. This observation led to the "amine hypothesis" of the mood disorders. This theory basically stated that depression was caused by an abnormally low level of the neurotransmitter *norepinephrine* and that mania was caused by too high a level. (This may be where the unfortunate term *chemical imbalance* had its origins.)

Further work soon indicated, however, that too little norepinephrine was too simplistic an explanation. As more antidepressant medications were discovered, researchers found that some very effective ones seemed to have little effect on norepinephrine. Fluoxetine (Prozac) is one of a family of pharmaceuticals that are powerful inhibitors of the reuptake of a different neurotransmitter, *serotonin;* they have very little direct effect on norepinephrine. Other antidepressants seem to affect yet other neurotransmitters.

Another argument against a simplistic theory involving too much or too little norepinephrine comes from an observation about the time course of these chemical changes in the brain. Antidepressant-induced changes in neurotransmitter levels at the synapse occur almost immediately after the drug is taken—in a matter of hours. But, as is well known, it takes several weeks for these agents to start alleviating the symptoms of depression. If the problem were simply too little neurotransmitter in the synapses of certain brain circuits, why would it take several weeks after the drug raised neurotransmitter levels at the synapse for the symptoms of depression to improve? We now believe that antidepressant treatment, by artificially changing levels of neurotransmitters in the brain, triggers some reaction in neurons that enhances neuroplasticity, a reaction that takes weeks to occur.

It has been shown in animal studies that after several weeks of exposure to an antidepressant drug, there is an increase in the process by which stem cells in the brain develop into mature neurons. These new neurons must then integrate themselves into brain circuits. The reason antidepressant medications take several weeks to work is that it simply takes time for these cellular processes to play out. This effect is the most dramatic in an area of the brain called the *hippocampus,* a brain center known to be important in the regulation of emotions.

Antidepressants change neurotransmitter levels in the brain, but that is just a first step, the trigger for more complicated changes that involve the growth of new neurons and also the sprouting of new connections between nerve cells.

Because of the unique therapeutic effects of lithium in bipolar disorder, there has naturally been a lot of effort to figure out where this medication is active in the brain and what its effect is on brain chemistry. Lithium doesn't seem to affect neurotransmitter levels in the synapse and doesn't interact with neurotransmitter receptors or affect the reuptake pumps. In fact, it has none of the types of direct effects on cells that the antidepressants have. Only in the past few years has the probable site of lithium action been found, and it's not at the synapse at all. Lithium (and perhaps the newer mood stabilizers as well) seems to work at a different cellular level: *inside* the neuron. Several small molecules inside the neuron, with odd names like BDNF (for brain-derived neurotrophic factor) and CREB (for cAMP response element binding protein), are thought to be very important for maintaining neuroplasticity. Lithium has been found to have dramatic effects on the levels of these molecules in neurons.

There is also increasing interest in another neurotransmitter, *glutamate,* which doesn't seem to be affected by antidepressants at all, although it is affected by lamotrigine (Lamictal) and other mood stabilizers; glutamate seems to be very important in neuroplasticity.

One way to think about neuroplasticity is that it underlies the brain's responsiveness to the environment and its ability to react to change and stress. Neuroplasticity is also thought to be involved in memory and learning. If you consider the symptoms of bipolar disorder, which include thinking and concentration problems in addition to mood changes, and consider how episodes of the illness can be triggered by stresses of various types, this idea that neuroplasticity is disrupted in bipolar disorder begins to make sense. Neuroplasticity may be a necessary part of maintaining mood within a normal range, somehow "tuning" the responsiveness of our mood state to experiences and environment, allowing us to react to and then recover from stresses.

There is strong evidence that chronic stress impairs neuroplasticity. This last finding is extremely interesting because it may explain why stress triggers mood episodes in persons with mood disorders. (Much more on stress and bipolar disorder is to come in chapter 18.)

Taken together, these findings on the importance of cell plasticity and growth explain why medications that help with symptoms of bipolar disorder, especially bipolar depression, take several weeks to do so.[2]

It may be a while before we understand how all the molecular and cellular pieces of this complicated story fit together, but the work to unravel the basic cause (or causes) of bipolar disorder is proceeding very rapidly. And when we understand exactly what is "broken" in bipolar disorder, the job of fixing it will become much easier.

CHAPTER 6

Mood-Stabilizing Medications

MOOD STABILIZERS ARE MEDICATIONS THAT HAVE BOTH ANTIMANIC and antidepressant effects. Perhaps an even more important effect of this class of medications is their ability to decrease the frequency and severity of episodes of the illness. Thus, the vast majority of patients with bipolar disorder are treated with one or another of these medications, and sometimes with several.

Lithium

We've already learned about John Cade's discovery in the 1940s of the therapeutic effects of lithium in bipolar disorder. But lithium has an even older history as a pharmaceutical, and it is just as interesting as the story of Dr. Cade and his guinea pigs. In the second century AD, the Greek physician Seranus Ephisios recommended that physicians who treated patients suffering from mania should prescribe "natural waters, such as [from] alkaline springs."[1] We now know that the water from many alkaline springs is rich in lithium. Roman physicians recommended that their patients "take the waters" at various springs for various physical and mental ailments. Down through the centuries, centers for healing grew up around natural springs all over Europe, from the little town in eastern Belgium called Spa to Bath in England, Wiesbaden in Germany, and dozens of other towns in Italy and Greece. As the science of analytic chemistry developed, curious chemists and physicians evaluated these various springs and found that the waters of many were rich in lithium.

In the middle of the nineteenth century, lithium compounds were tried as treatments for gout and kidney stones. Gout is a painful arthritic condition caused by abnormally high levels of uric acid in the body; the uric acid is deposited in the form of urate crystals in the joints and other tissues. Kidney stones are also usually made up of urate compounds. It was hoped that lithium would somehow dissolve the urate crystals in the joints of gout patients and also dissolve urate kidney stones. (Remember that Dr. Cade picked lithium urate to work with because it is the most soluble of the urate compounds.) Unfortunately, lithium did not turn out to be helpful for these problems, and the approach was abandoned. But this work led to the formulation of pharmaceutical preparations of lithium compounds and to information on the range of safe doses for lithium preparations in humans.

In the late 1940s, lithium came to medical attention again when lithium chloride was introduced as a salt substitute for patients with medical problems such as heart disease and high blood pressure that required them to be on a low-sodium diet. But when heart patients were given saltshakers full of lithium salts to sprinkle on their food, the results were catastrophic for some. Because lithium is toxic in surprisingly low concentrations, substituting lithium chloride for sodium chloride turned out to be a disaster. There were many reports of severe lithium poisoning and even several deaths among these patients. The use of lithium as a salt substitute ended. This episode had the effect of giving lithium a very bad reputation among physicians, and it may have been another reason for the delay in accepting Cade's discovery of lithium as a treatment for bipolar disorder.

In the 1950s, the Danish psychiatrist Morgans Schou began what turned out to be his life work: the development and refinement of the therapeutic use of lithium for the treatment of bipolar disorder. Schou very quickly became convinced of the effectiveness of lithium in treating acute mania, and he was one of the first clinical researchers to become convinced of another therapeutic effect of the drug: its ability to prevent further episodes of illness (lithium's preventive or *prophylactic* effect). Schou had a harder time convincing his colleagues around the world that lithium could prevent recurrences of bipolar disorder, that patients should take it even after their acute symptoms had subsided. In 1967 Schou and his colleague Paul Christian Baalstrup reported on eighty-eight patients who had taken lithium for several years and who had a dramatic reduction in the frequency and duration of their mood episodes (figure 6-1 shows a sample of their results). Several patients who had been sick for several weeks out of every year experienced a complete remission of their illness that lasted more than five years; their illness had essentially ceased.[2]

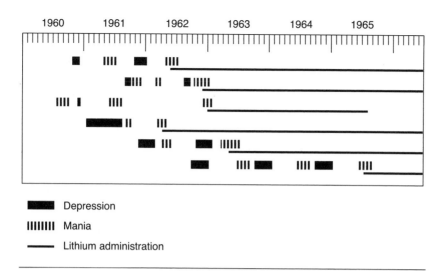

1960 1961 1962 1963 1964 1965

■■■■ Depression

|||||||| Mania

—— Lithium administration

FIGURE 6-1 This graph illustrates data from six patients in Baalstrup and Schou's early study on the prophylactic effects of lithium on bipolar symptoms. Each horizontal line represents the symptom course of one patient. In all these patients, when lithium was started, episodes of mania and depression stopped completely.

Source: Data from Paul Baalstrup and Morgans Schou, "Lithium as a Prophylactic Agent: Its Effect against Recurrent Depressions and Manic-Depressive Psychosis," *Archives of General Psychiatry* 16, no. 2 (1967): 162–72.

As they treated more and more patients with the medication, it became so apparent to Schou and his colleagues that lithium favorably altered the course of bipolar illness that they had ethical qualms about doing a more rigorous placebo-controlled study—one in which bipolar patients would be divided into two groups, some to receive lithium and the others a placebo. In a rather cranky 1968 article titled "Prophylactic Lithium: Another Therapeutic Myth?" several British psychiatrists scolded the Danes for reporting their results without a placebo group.[3] So Baalstrup and Schou did a lithium discontinuation study in which they took patients who had been stable on lithium for at least a year, divided them into two roughly equal groups, and in one group substituted a placebo for the lithium.

This was a *double-blind study,* the most powerful type of clinical trial possible—and now a required test for new medications. In this type of study, patients who are similar as to age, diagnosis, severity of illness, and so forth and who agree to be in the study are divided into two groups. One group gets the medication that is being tested, and the other group (the *control* group) gets a placebo (or in some studies the control group receives a standard medication for the disorder being studied). The patients do not know whether they are taking the new medication or the placebo, and neither do the clinicians who examine them for improvement; hence the term *double-blind*. It is only after the trial is over that the group membership of the patients is revealed and the results of the two groups compared. Improvement is measured objectively by using checklists of symptoms and various rating severity scales that have been verified as being reliable and valid.

The results of the Baalstrup and Schou study were dramatic: of the thirty-nine patients whose lithium was replaced with the placebo, twenty-one relapsed within five months; of the forty-five other patients, those whose lithium was not replaced, *none* had a relapse. In 1970 Baalstrup and Schou published their results in the same British journal in which their critics' paper had appeared, establishing once and for all that lithium's prophylactic effect on bipolar disorder was no myth.[4]

THERAPEUTIC PROFILE

It has now been shown in many more studies that lithium is not only effective in the treatment of mania and depression; it also reduces the severity, duration, and frequency of manic and depressive episodes of bipolar patients.

Lithium is a naturally occurring element found in mineral springs, seawater, and certain ores. Like its close cousin sodium, it is never found in its pure form in nature but only combined with other ions as a salt of one type or another. It is mined on an industrial scale for use in the manufacture of ceramics and batteries. Therapeutic lithium preparations usually contain lithium carbonate (the carbonate ion combined with lithium; when the carbonate ion is combined with the closely related sodium, it forms sodium carbonate, which is common baking soda).

Because it is an element, lithium is not chemically transformed (metabolized) within the body, and because lithium atoms are so similar to sodium atoms, the body handles lithium in much the same way it handles sodium. Lithium is rapidly absorbed through the gastrointestinal tract, enters the bloodstream, and is eliminated from the body by being filtered out by the kidneys. (Table 6-1 summarizes the therapeutic profile.)

Descriptions of the effects of a pharmaceutical in the body always include one vital statistic: the medication's *half-life*. This is a measure of how quickly the body gets rid of the pharmaceutical. Specifically, it is the time required for half the amount of the drug to be eliminated or metabolized by the body. Put another way, it is the time it takes for the body to reduce the level of the medication by half. The half-life of lithium in adults is between fourteen and thirty hours.[5] Another useful number that can be derived from the half-life statistic for any medication is the time it takes for the level of medication to build up to a constant level in the body, or in other words the

TABLE 6-1 Therapeutic profile of lithium

Medication class:	Mood stabilizer
Brand names:	Eskalith, Eskalith CR, Lithobid, Lithonate, Lithotabs
Half-life:	14–30 hours
Metabolism:	None
Elimination:	Kidneys
Other considerations:	Blood levels extremely important

time it takes for the amount being taken in to equal the amount being eliminated: the *equilibrium point.* By a series of mathematical steps that we don't need to detail here, it can be shown that the equilibrium point is always the same for all medications: five half-lives. This means that since the half-life of lithium is roughly one day, it will take roughly five days for a patient who starts on lithium to reach a steady level of lithium in the bloodstream. It also means that if the lithium dose is changed, it will take about five days for the blood level to stabilize at the new level.

Because of the toxicity and even deaths that were reported when heart patients sprinkled it freely on their food as a salt substitute, there was a significant delay in the acceptance of lithium as a therapeutic agent. Lithium is a powerful pharmaceutical, one that must be treated with respect. It has a very low *therapeutic index,* meaning that the difference between the therapeutic dose and a toxic dose is small.[6] Fortunately, lithium can be measured in the bloodstream accurately and cheaply, and the dosage can be adjusted according to the results.

It is important to pay attention to lithium blood levels not only to prevent toxicity but also because it has been clearly demonstrated in clinical studies that lithium needs to be present in the bloodstream at a certain level to be effective in most patients. (We speak of a "therapeutic level" in discussing the effective range of lithium in the bloodstream for treatment, not a "normal level." Lithium is a trace element in the body, normally present in undetectable concentrations. Bipolar disorder is not a lithium deficiency!) Just what that level should be has been a matter of debate, and the definition has shifted over the years. But an important study from Massachusetts General Hospital found that a level of between 0.8 and 1.0 meq/L (this stands for milliequivalents per liter and is a chemical measure of concentration) was most effective.[7] In this double-blind study, bipolar patients were divided into two groups, a "standard-dose" group, whose lithium levels were kept between 0.8 and 1.0 meq/L, and a "low-dose" group, whose levels were maintained between 0.4 and 0.6 meq/L. The researchers found that the relapse rate in the "low-dose" group was more than double that in the "standard-dose" group (table 6-2).

TABLE 6-2 Comparison of higher and lower lithium levels in relapse rates of bipolar disorder

Treatment group	Any relapse	Depressed	Manic/ mixed	Hypomanic	Withdrew from study
Standard range (0.8–1.0 meq/L)	6 (12%)	3 (6%)	3 (6%)	0	24 (51%)
Low range (0.4–0.6 meq/L)	21 (44%)	1 (2%)	17 (36%)	3 (6%)	11 (23%)

Source: Data from Alan Gelenberg, John Kane, Martin Keller, Phillip Lavori, Jerrold Rosenbaum, Karyl Cole, and Janet Lavelle, "Comparison of Standard and Low Levels of Lithium for Maintenance Treatment of Bipolar Disorder," *New England Journal of Medicine* 321, no. 22 (1989): 1489–93.

There's more to these data than may initially meet the eye, however. Many more patients from the "standard-dose" group than from the "low-dose" group dropped out of the study because of side effects. The take-home message seems to be that levels closer to 1.0 meq/L are more protective—but that many people have trouble taking that high a dose because of side effects. Many psychiatrists compromise and try to maintain their patients at levels between the "standard" and the "low" range. Dr. Schou, whom many consider to be the father of lithium therapy, recommended levels of 0.5 to 0.8 meq/L.[8] However, it's very clear that some people have good control of their symptoms on even lower levels—elderly patients, for example. Lithium levels thus need to be individualized to the patient, and Dr. Schou also points out that "changes in lithium levels as small as 0.1 to 0.2 [meq/L], upward or downward, may substantially improve patients' quality of life during maintenance treatment."[9]

The lithium level in the bloodstream rises after every dose, peaks in about two hours, then begins to fall again. If a patient takes his lithium two or three times a day, there will be several peaks and valleys. Because the level is rising and falling throughout the day, it is important that the blood for a lithium-level test be drawn at a time when it can be correctly interpreted. The convention that has been adopted is to use a twelve-hour level, making it convenient to draw blood in the mornings. For most patients this means getting to the lab twelve hours after their bedtime dose—for example, by 11:00 a.m. if the bedtime dose was taken at 11:00 p.m. the night before—with their usual morning dose in their pocket or purse.

Lithium is uniquely effective for some patients with bipolar disorder, for whom it is truly a miracle drug. In many of these patients, other medications simply don't control their symptoms as well. At the consultation clinic at Johns Hopkins, we regularly see patients who have been told they can no longer take lithium because of medical issues (usually because they have developed kidney disease, a complication of high blood pressure and diabetes as well as other medical disorders). Many of these patients have taken lithium for decades with complete control of their illness. Some have been so stable that they haven't seen a psychiatrist in years, getting their lithium treatment and monitoring from their family doctor instead. These patients come to us desperate to start taking lithium again because other medications they've tried since stopping lithium simply haven't kept them well. Fortunately, most of them can resume lithium treatment despite their kidney disease (there have even been case reports of patients with such severe kidney failure that they require dialysis being safely treated with lithium).[10] Their desperation and the great lengths these patients go to in order to get back on lithium are explained by its unique effectiveness for them. Usually they are patients with classic bipolar I disorder, characterized by severe manias requiring hospitalization, often with psychotic features. Another illness characteristic is that their between-episode recovery is usually quite complete, that is, they do not have smoldering residual mood symptoms for long periods when they are not acutely ill. This group of patients, for whom lithium is fantastically effective and for whom nothing else works quite so well, has prompted a number of research projects searching for genetic markers for lithium's therapeutic effect. The hope is that this research will eventually lead to a test that will help physicians select medications for individual patients with mood disorders. In this case, physicians want a test that will predict whether a particular patient is or is not likely to benefit from taking lithium.

SIDE EFFECTS

Individuals vary widely in their sensitivity to the side effects of lithium (and all other medications, for that matter). Some patients will have no side effects; others will have several. Fortunately, almost all the side effects of lithium can be eliminated or managed (table 6-3).

Many of lithium's side effects are *dose-related,* meaning that the higher the dose, the more severe the side effect. One side-effect management strategy, then, is to lower the lithium dose. The advantages of higher levels are clear, as noted above, but most physicians will try to maintain patients at the lowest dose that controls their symptoms.

Because of its similarity to sodium, lithium has some of the same effects that an increased sodium (salt) intake would have: increased thirst, increased urination, and water retention. These side effects are often temporary and subside as the body adjusts to the medication. Many patients notice this slight and temporary increase in urination and thirst when they

TABLE 6-3 Treatable side effects of lithium

Side effect	Remedy
Nausea, diarrhea	Take immediately after meals
	Switch preparations
Weight gain	Diet and exercise
Thirst, frequent urination	Diuretics helpful, but must be prescribed by an M.D. (see text)
Tremor	Beta-blocker medications
Flareup of preexisting dermatologic conditions	Dermatologic preparations
Hypothyroidism	Thyroid medications

start taking lithium. For some patients, however, it's after taking lithium for many years that they notice they need to urinate much more often and find that they are frequently thirsty. This occurs because lithium can affect the functioning of the kidneys over time. Remember that the kidneys' job is to remove waste products from the bloodstream; they filter nearly twenty gallons of blood every hour to do this, and they recycle nearly all of this fluid back into the bloodstream. When taken for many years, lithium can impair this recycling function, so that large amounts of urine are produced. The term for this problem is *diabetes insipidus* (which has nothing to do with diabetes mellitus, the common "sugar diabetes"). This problem develops very slowly, is easy to diagnose with a few laboratory tests, and is treatable with amiloride, a drug that changes how the kidney reabsorbs water and other agents. When caught early on, this problem is usually completely reversible, so it's very important that patients taking lithium let their doctor know if they find themselves awaking more often to urinate during the night.

When lithium was first being prescribed, concern arose based on case reports that lithium disrupted the kidneys' filtering system, causing the kind of damage that can result in the need for dialysis. This has now been shown to be extremely rare, occurring almost entirely in persons who are already at risk for kidney damage from other causes, such as poorly controlled high blood pressure or diabetes. Fortunately this problem is also very slow to develop.[11]

Because of these potential problems, blood tests that measure kidney functioning are routinely ordered for patients taking lithium, in addition to blood tests to monitor their lithium blood levels.

Lithium is irritating to the gastrointestinal tract and can cause nausea or diarrhea. Taking it on a full stomach can ease these problems considerably. A fine shaking in the hands (tremor) can occur at higher dosage levels.

These problems can sometimes be alleviated with slow-release preparations of lithium, which reduce the peak blood level that occurs after each dose. Medications used to treat tremors, called *beta blockers,* are frequently prescribed and can be very helpful. Weight gain can be an annoying side effect and unfortunately has an equally annoying remedy: diet and exercise.

Between 5 and 35 percent of patients treated with lithium develop depressed thyroid gland functioning (hypothyroidism).[12] When hypothyroidism develops, it seems to be able to cause an increase in mood cycling in addition to the symptoms of too little thyroid hormone (low energy, dry skin, sensitivity to heat, and puffiness around the eyes are some of the early signs). If a person's lithium seems to "stop working"—that is, if the person suddenly seems to have an acceleration in her illness—hypothyroidism should be suspected. When it does occur, hypothyroidism can be treated by thyroid-replacement medications. A test of thyroid functioning is the third in the battery of blood tests routinely ordered for lithium patients.

Lithium can cause flareups of preexisting skin conditions but only rarely causes new dermatological problems. Patients with psoriasis, acne, and other such problems may need closer follow-up from their dermatologist.

Another side effect that troubles a significant number of patients taking lithium is a noticeable dulling of mental functioning and coordination. Patients complain that their ability to memorize and learn is affected and that they have a difficult-to-explain sense of mental sluggishness. For years these complaints were downplayed by clinicians, many of whom tossed them off as coming from patients who simply weren't used to feeling "normal," who missed the mental alacrity of hypomania. This view seemed to be supported by research using psychological tests on bipolar patients taking lithium, research that has been inconclusive. But when nonpatient volunteers were given lithium and similarly tested, there was a small but definite drop-off in their performance, proving that lithium-induced mental sluggishness is a very real problem for some patients.[13] This is a dose-related side effect and is another reason to strive for the lowest possible maintenance dose of lithium that still controls mood symptoms adequately.

Lithium has been associated with birth defects, especially certain heart defects. At one time, it was recommended that women never get pregnant while taking lithium, but more recent research has shown that while lithium increases the risk of serious heart problems in the fetus, the risk is still very low. What to do about taking lithium during pregnancy is a complicated decision that should be discussed well beforehand with your psychiatrist and your obstetrician. (See chapter 14 for a more complete discussion of medications and pregnancy.) Lithium is secreted in breast milk, so patients taking lithium should not breast-feed.

Lamotrigine (Lamictal)

Several years ago, I was riding in a cab with a colleague of mine as we returned to our hotels after spending the day at an international conference on bipolar disorder in Pittsburgh. We were talking about the seminars we had attended that day, discussing how we might better classify bipolar disorders, whether lithium is safe during pregnancy, and other bipolar topics of that day's sessions. During a pause in our conversation, the cab driver looked back at us in his rearview mirror and asked, "Do either of you guys prescribe Lamictal?" We were both a bit surprised by the question, since lamotrigine had not yet been approved by the Food and Drug Administration (FDA) to treat bipolar disorder, but we replied that yes, we had prescribed the new drug for several of our patients at Johns Hopkins. The cabbie paused for a short moment and then said, "That's good. . . . Ya know, Lamictal saved my life."

Lamotrigine (brand name Lamictal) is something of a child prodigy among medications used to treat bipolar disorder. Unlike other medications, which became common treatments for bipolar disorder only after many years of investigation and testing, lamotrigine proved its value in treating bipolar disorder very quickly. As a result it went from an uncommonly used drug prescribed mostly at research medical centers to a mainstay of the treatment of bipolar disorder in only a few years. Like several other medications we will discuss, lamotrigine was introduced as a medication to treat seizure disorders. The first studies on lamotrigine appeared in the 1980s, describing it as a useful "add-on" therapy for epilepsy patients who were already taking other antiseizure medications. During the early investigations of this use, researchers noted that patients who took lamotrigine for seizure control reported an improvement in their mood and sense of well-being—even if it hadn't helped much with their seizures. These observations led to clinical trials in patients with mood disorders, which quickly revealed that lamotrigine is an effective medication for many such patients.

Lamotrigine has several effects on the brain that might explain its efficacy in bipolar disorder. It inhibits the release of the neurotransmitter glutamate, an amino acid that causes stimulation of various neural circuits. Glutamate is also the signal that the nervous system uses to trigger a kind of cellular suicide called *apoptosis* that inactivates and removes malfunctioning neurons. There is evidence that abnormally high levels of glutamate are present in several brain areas of persons with bipolar disorder, suggesting that lamotrigine's effectiveness is due to a dialing back of glutamate activity in the brain to more normal levels.[14]

The most exciting aspect of lamotrigine's profile is its effectiveness in bipolar depression. One of the first reports on its use in the treatment of bipolar disorder told of a patient who had suffered from rapid-cycling bipolar I disorder since he was fourteen years old.[15] In the year before starting lamotrigine, he had been either depressed or manic continuously, with no period of normal mood. When the research team first saw him, he had been severely depressed and had not responded to lithium, to other mood stabilizers, or even to antidepressants. After beginning to take lamotrigine, his depressive symptoms gradually improved, and eleven months later he'd had no recurrence of either depressive or manic symptoms. Case reports and studies of lamotrigine as a medication added to other agents started to accumulate and continued to look promising.

In 2003 two large studies were published that compared the efficacy of lamotrigine with lithium (and also with a placebo) in keeping patients with bipolar disorder from having another mood episode; each study lasted eighteen months. In one study, the patients were recovering from a manic or mixed episode as they entered the study; in the other, patients were recovering from a depression.[16] In the section on lithium, I mentioned that the best way to tell whether a medication is truly effective is to do a double-blind, placebo-controlled study. Both of these studies comparing lamotrigine with lithium and a placebo were carried out in just this way; they also were large studies that included hundreds of patients, and they lasted for a year and a half—much longer than most medication trials. So when both studies reported that lamotrigine was just as effective as lithium in keeping patients well, this new medication suddenly came into the spotlight and became one of the foundations of the treatment of bipolar disorder.

The exciting finding from these studies was that lamotrigine is especially effective against depression in bipolar disorder—extremely good news. This was such an important finding because, as you will see later, the depression of bipolar disorder is much more difficult to treat than manic or mixed states (see "Treating Bipolar Depression" in chapter 7). You may remember from chapter 2 that individuals with bipolar II disorder have more problems with depression than with mania and that these depressions can be especially long, debilitating, and difficult to treat. Lamotrigine can often fill an important therapeutic need for these patients, because for them lithium is often less effective.

Lamotrigine has a half-life of about twenty-four hours, and its metabolism is affected by taking carbamazepine and valproate (table 6-4). Blood-level tests are not routinely ordered for lamotrigine because of its low toxic-

TABLE 6-4 Therapeutic profile of lamotrigine

Medication class:	Mood stabilizer (anticonvulsant)
Brand name:	Lamictal
Half-life:	15–24 hours
Metabolism:	Affected by carbamazepine, valproate
Elimination:	Liver
Other considerations:	Rarely causes severe skin rashes, but otherwise has good side-effect profile

ity and because therapeutic effects have not been correlated with particular amounts in the blood.

SIDE EFFECTS

In contrast to the other mood stabilizers, lamotrigine causes only minimal side effects. Patients taking it may have some initial nausea or gastrointestinal upset and the sort of side effects that many medications affecting the brain can cause: sleepiness, light-headedness or dizziness, and headaches. At higher doses, some patients complain of concentration problems similar to those often reported by patients taking lithium. In my experience, lowering the dose usually takes care of this problem.

A very rare but very serious problem that has been associated with lamotrigine is a dangerous type of allergic skin rash called *toxic epidermal necrosis* (TED). TED is the most extreme form of a group of allergic skin reactions that are lumped together under the term erythema multiforme. These problems were reported right after lamotrigine was introduced as a treatment for epilepsy in the early 1990s. When research was done to see which patients were at highest risk for these serious reactions, it was discovered that children and patients who started the drug at high doses were more likely than others to develop a serious rash. Subsequently, the drug's manufacturer recommended against prescribing lamotrigine to children except under special circumstances and also changed the dosing recommendations for starting the drug in adults. Now patients start lamotrigine at a very low dose and gradually increase it over a period of weeks. Although this means that it may take five weeks or more to get to the usual therapeutic dose of 200 to 400 mg/day, the risk of serious skin reactions to lamotrigine has virtually been eliminated. Since these dosing recommendations were put into effect, the number of patients developing serious rashes has dropped to the number in the general population. In the pivotal clinical trials where lamotrigine was prescribed to several thousand patients for the treatment of bipolar disorder, none of the patients developed a serious rash.[17]

Nevertheless, many individuals develop minor skin reactions to med-

TABLE 6-5 The Stanford protocol for patients starting lamotrigine

Do not start lamotrigine within 2 weeks of any rash, viral infection, vaccination
During first 3 months of treatment, avoid new
    Medicines, foods
    Soaps, cosmetics, conditioners, deodorants
    Detergents, fabric softeners
During first 3 months of treatment, avoid
    Poison ivy/oak, sunburn

ications and lots of other things as well, so it's important when a person starts taking lamotrigine to take precautions against developing a rash from another source. If a rash develops in a patient taking lamotrigine, it presents something of a therapeutic dilemma: Is the patient's rash erythema multiforme or a minor skin reaction? If the rash is a serious one, is lamotrigine the culprit? The patient might be told to stop the drug unnecessarily, perhaps missing out on a medication that might be very effective. For this reason, patients starting on lamotrigine should consider the protocol developed at Stanford University to prevent skin rashes from other sources (table 6-5). I had one patient who had been told by her previous psychiatrist to stop lamotrigine, which up to that point had seemed very helpful for her bipolar depression, because she had developed what in retrospect was probably a reaction to poison ivy. She was able to restart lamotrigine and move up to a therapeutic dose with no problems. I tell my patients as I hand them the prescription, "No gardening, no hiking, no new restaurants or shampoos or clothes detergents; stay out of the sun and take care of your skin!"

A corollary to the start-low protocol for lamotrigine is that a person who stops taking it for a period of time should not resume taking it at the same dose. Experts recommend that patients who are off lamotrigine for one week or more should restart the drug at the low beginning dose.

Valproate (Depakote, Depakene, Epival)

The development of valproate (brand names include Depakote and Depakene) for the treatment of bipolar disorder is another convoluted study in serendipity. Valproic acid is a carbon compound similar to others that are found in animal fats and vegetable oils: it is a fatty acid. It was first synthesized in 1882 and was used for many years as an organic solvent for a variety of purposes. (Remember that a solvent is a liquid that other substances easily dissolve into.) Many decades ago pharmacists used it as a solvent for bismuth salts, which were used to treat stomach and skin disorders.

In the early 1960s, scientists looking for treatments for epilepsy were working with a group of new pharmaceutical compounds that appeared promising but were difficult to dissolve. (Is this beginning to sound familiar?) They discovered that valproic acid was an effective solvent for the compounds they were testing, and they started using it to dissolve their test drugs for animal experimentation. As they tested various new pharmaceuticals, the results they obtained seemed to be confusing—until someone realized that it didn't matter *which* of the new pharmaceuticals was used. As long as *any* of them was dissolved in valproic acid, the drug was found to be effective in stopping epileptic seizure activity. It soon became obvious that it was the valproic acid that was stopping the seizures, not what was dissolved in it. By 1978 valproate had been approved by the Food and Drug Administration for use in treating epilepsy.[18]

In the 1960s there were some reports that valproate might be helpful in treating mood disorders, and throughout the late 1960s and early 1970s, a French psychiatrist named Lambert published a series of papers about using it to treat bipolar disorders. After the discovery that another anti-epilepsy medication, carbamazepine, was effective in treating mania (see the next section of this chapter), interest in the possibilities of valproate as a mood stabilizer grew. In the mid-1980s, there were several studies by American psychiatrists of the use of valproate in treating bipolar disorder, and ten years later valproate had become firmly established as an effective antimanic medication and a mood stabilizer.

Valproate's therapeutic action in bipolar disorder—or in epilepsy, for that matter—is still unknown. It is known to improve neuronal transmission in the brain that is mediated by the neurotransmitter gamma aminobutyric acid (GABA). GABA seems to have an inhibitory or modulating effect on many brain circuits, and valproate's effect may be to enhance this modulator in some way.

THERAPEUTIC PROFILE

The half-life of valproate is between six and sixteen hours in adults (table 6-6). Thus, it reaches equilibrium in the body more quickly than lithium, in two to three days. Valproate seems to have some advantages over lithium in the treatment of acute manic episodes. First, it appears to work more quickly. Whereas lithium may take up to three weeks to have its full effect, valproate has been shown to start working within five days. Second, valproate also seems to be more effective than lithium for certain subgroups of manic patients: patients with rapid cycling (four or more mood episodes per year) and patients with mixed mania (a mixture of manic hyperactivity and pressured thinking with depressed or unpleasant mood).[19] Third, valproate is much less toxic than lithium.

Controlled studies of the use of valproate to treat acute depression and

TABLE 6-6 Therapeutic profile of valproate

Medication class:	Mood stabilizer (anticonvulsant)
Brand names:	Depakene, Depakote, Epival
Half-life:	6–16 hours
Metabolism:	Affected by other antiepilepsy drugs
Elimination:	Liver
Other considerations:	Blood-level tests helpful; blood tests for liver inflammation are needed

to prevent recurrences of bipolar disorder have been less impressive.[20] In fact, if one sticks to the more rigorous controlled studies, it can be said that valproate should be used only to treat acute mania and that the lack of strong evidence for its benefit in depression or for maintenance treatment argues against any other use in bipolar disorder.[21] Nevertheless, any psychiatrist with experience in treating mood-disorder patients will tell you that some patients need and benefit from valproate and that for them it is extremely and sometimes uniquely effective. It may be that these patients have an unusual variant of bipolar disorder and that the benefit of valproate for these patients gets lost in large studies, where they are vastly outnumbered by patients who do not respond to valproate.

Like lithium, valproate can be measured in the bloodstream; blood levels above 45 mcg/ml (micrograms per milliliter) have been shown to be necessary for the therapeutic effect to occur, and side effects become more problematic at levels greater than 125 mcg/ml.[22] Several studies show that valproate is helpful in cyclothymia, bipolar II, and "soft" bipolar disorders and that lower doses and lower blood levels are required than in the treatment of bipolar I.[23] As with lithium, blood for a test of valproate levels should be drawn twelve hours after the last dose of medication.

SIDE EFFECTS

Side effects that are common as a patient starts taking valproate include stomach upset and some sleepiness. These problems usually go away quickly. Increased appetite and weight gain are perhaps the most serious side effects. Mild tremor occurs as well and can be treated with beta-blocker medication. A few patients report hair loss, usually temporary, which resolves even more quickly with the use of shampoos and vitamin preparations containing the minerals zinc and selenium.[24]

Several cases of severe liver problems have been reported in patients taking valproate, but these have occurred almost exclusively in children taking the drug for control of epilepsy, most of whom had other medical problems and were taking several different medications. A 1989 review article states that no fatalities from liver problems caused by valproate had ever been reported in patients over the age of ten who were taking only valproate. Just to be on the safe side, however, patients taking valproate for the first time are given a blood test that can detect liver inflammation and the test is repeated at appropriate intervals while they are taking it. Since valproate can also, in rare cases, cause a drop in blood counts, a complete blood count is usually done as well. These are very rare problems, and even when they do occur, they develop slowly and usually during the first six months of therapy. Thus, they can be detected with routine blood tests. Nevertheless, patients on valproate should be on the lookout for signs of liver or blood-count problems, which include unusual bleeding and bruising, jaundice (yellowing of the eyes and skin), fever, and water retention.

Valproate has been associated with birth defects, and women of child-bearing age should practice birth control while taking valproate if there is any possibility of becoming pregnant.

Carbamazepine (Tegretol, Equetro, Epitol)

After the introduction of carbamazepine for the control of epilepsy in the 1960s, several reports appeared indicating that epilepsy patients taking carbamazepine who also had mood problems not only had good control of their seizures but had improvement in their psychiatric symptoms as well. It was a small step to test carbamazepine in patients with mood problems who did not have epilepsy. Much of the early work on the use of carbamazepine in bipolar disorder was done by Japanese clinicians looking for an alternative to lithium, which was not approved for use in Japan until years after it was available in the United States. In 1980 a study appeared in the *American Journal of Psychiatry* titled "Carbamazepine in Manic-Depressive Illness: A New Treatment," and the race was on to refine the use of this medication in bipolar disorder and to define the group or groups of patients whom it helped the most.[25]

THERAPEUTIC PROFILE

Although carbamazepine has been used to treat bipolar disorder for several decades, less research has been done on its efficacy in this illness than for other medications. This gap is slowly being filled, however, and newer studies have appeared, prompted by the development of a sustained-release preparation of carbamazepine.

Every once in a while a patient of mine requests that I prescribe the "best" mood stabilizer or antidepressant medication there is. I usually respond by saying that if there were a "best" medication in a particular class of medications, it would be the only pharmaceutical manufactured and prescribed. What would be the point of using anything else? The reason there are so many drugs of a particular type is that some work better or have fewer side effects in particular patients. Many newer medications don't seem to be more effective than available ones when studied in large groups of patients, but they are clearly better for certain patients who can't take or don't respond to an older agent.

Carbamazepine is one such medication: it doesn't seem to have any big advantage in most studies of groups of patients, but it works *very* well—in fact, works when other medications do not—for some patients. In one well-designed double-blind study, manic patients who took carbamazepine actually seemed to do worse than patients taking lithium.[26] But most psychiatrists have had a patient like "Ms. B.," whose case history was reported in a paper from the National Institute of Mental Health (NIMH) in 1983:

> Ms. B., a 53-year-old woman, had a history of treatment resistant, rapid cycling manic-depressive illness that required continuous state hospitalization from 1956 to her admission to NIMH in 1978. She had been non-responsive to [antipsychotic medications, tricyclic antidepressants] and lithium. . . . After institution of carbamazepine, both mood phases improved dramatically and she was able to be discharged. . . . During a subsequent hospitalization her severe mania again did not respond to [antipsychotic medications] and she was not able to leave the hospital until she was treated with carbamazepine.[27]

In this study the authors noted that "additional improvement appeared to occur when [antipsychotic medications] were used in conjunction with carbamazepine or when lithium and carbamazepine were used in combination."[28] This had become carbamazepine's niche: a second-line mood-stabilizing agent for patients who do not respond to other agents; it was often used in combination with other agents. However, at least one placebo-controlled study using carbamazepine alone to treat patients hospitalized with mania supported the idea that this medication may be underused and can be helpful for many patients.[29]

Like the other mood-stabilizing medications, carbamazepine can be measured in the bloodstream, and blood-level tests can be used to adjust the dose. Unfortunately, not much work has been done on carbamazepine blood levels in bipolar patients, so the therapeutic range used for the treatment of epilepsy is usually the target that psychiatrists aim for in their patients.

Carbamazepine is metabolized in the liver (table 6-7), and like some other drugs, it causes the liver to increase the level of the enzymes that metabolize it. This means that the longer a person takes carbamazepine, the more quickly the liver gets rid of it. So after a few weeks, the blood levels may go down and the dose may need to be increased. This increase in liver

TABLE 6-7 Therapeutic profile of carbamazepine

Medication class:	Mood stabilizer (anticonvulsant)
Brand names:	Tegretol, Equetro, Epitol
Half-life:	18–15 hours (shortens over time)
Metabolism:	Complex; affects and is affected by other drugs
Elimination:	Liver
Other considerations:	Blood-level tests helpful; blood tests for liver inflammation and blood abnormalities needed

enzymes can also affect other medications that the patient might be taking, including certain tranquilizers, certain antidepressants, other epilepsy medications, and some hormones. The change in hormonal levels is very important for women using birth control, since some oral contraceptives that use very low hormone levels lose their effectiveness if taken with carbamazepine. It is very important that all physicians involved in a person's care know when the person has started taking carbamazepine so that dosage adjustments for other medications can be made.

SIDE EFFECTS

Carbamazepine can cause the same sort of general side effects as many other medications that affect the brain: sleepiness, lightheadedness, and some initial nausea. These problems tend to be short-lived and dose-related.

As with valproate, there have been rare cases of liver problems associated with carbamazepine, so blood tests for liver inflammation are routinely done. There have been even rarer reports of dangerous changes in blood counts, so blood cell counts are also done, especially in the first several weeks of therapy. Cases of a dangerous skin reaction called Stevens-Johnson syndrome have been attributed to carbamazepine; this is another of the severe variants of erythema multiforme that I mentioned in the discussion of lamotrigine. All these problems are quite rare, but patients should be on the watch for the development of a rash, jaundice, water retention, bleeding or bruising, or signs of infection.

Oxcarbazepine (Trileptal)

As its name suggests, oxcarbazepine (brand name Trileptal) is very similar to carbamazepine. It is another medication used to treat epilepsy, and it seems to work similarly to carbamazepine but has several advantages over it. Oxcarbazepine is not associated with the blood-count problems that can be caused by carbamazepine or with the changes in liver enzymes that affect the metabolism of other drugs. This makes it significantly easier to take, with less need for monitoring blood tests and changes in dosage. It also appears less likely to cause Stevens-Johnson syndrome. Much of the early work on oxcarbazepine in bipolar disorder was done in Europe, and studies by German investigators in the mid-1980s suggested it was as beneficial as carbamazepine in treating mania. More recently, American clinicians have also published favorable reports on its safety and efficacy, especially as an "add-on" to other mood stabilizers, and the effectiveness of oxcarbazepine for breakthrough manic symptoms has been especially well established.[30]

Many clinicians have been reluctant to prescribe oxcarbazepine's parent compound, carbamazepine, because of the possibility of severe adverse reactions. Given the much less significant problems associated with oxcarbazepine, we will probably see it prescribed more often and studied more closely.

Other Mood Stabilizers

Several other agents show promise for the treatment of bipolar disorder. For the most part, the promise of these medications is based on clinical trials in which the medication is added to the regimen of patients already taking an established mood stabilizer such as lithium, but sometimes a few case reports of a therapeutic effect are enough to attract the attention of psychiatrists.

Pramipexole (Mirapex) is a medication that is usually used to treat Parkinson's disease and restless-leg syndrome; it activates dopamine circuits in the brain. Several studies have shown pramipexole to be an effective add-on treatment for bipolar depression not responding to mood stabilizers alone.[31] As with other treatments that are especially helpful for bipolar depression, there is a risk of developing hypomanic or manic symptoms from taking pramipexole.

Because this medication has already been approved to treat other disorders, physicians may prescribe it to patients with bipolar disorder, a practice known as "off-label" prescribing. One of the roles of the FDA is to approve how manufacturers market pharmaceuticals to physicians. Companies may only advertise drugs to physicians for the treatment of specific symptoms or a particular diagnosis, and even then only after the agency has been presented with mountains of data supporting the drug's effectiveness for that condition. The details of that data are used to prepare the "label" of the drug, actually a pamphlet-sized document called the "package insert." But since the FDA does not regulate the practice of medicine, physicians may prescribe any available drug for other conditions if, based on their review of available research and their judgment and experience, the drug is appropriate to treat the patient. When they use it to treat a condition not listed in the FDA "label," this practice is called "off-label prescribing."

If taking a medication for an off-label disorder seems risky, it may reassure you to learn that most new mood stabilizers, including valproate and lamotrigine, were widely prescribed "off-label" for years before they received FDA labeling for bipolar disorder.

There is evidence that N-acetyl cysteine (NAC), an amino acid available in vitamin stores as a nutritional supplement, may be useful as a mood stabilizer.[32] A small handful of studies examining NAC as an add-on medication to other mood stabilizers have shown very promising results, especially in bipolar depression. This discovery is especially exciting because the mechanism of action of NAC is very different from that of any other mood stabilizer. NAC is a metabolic precursor to glutathione, a powerful antioxidant that occurs in brain tissue, suggesting that NAC, like other mood stabilizers, may work through neuroprotective mechanisms.

Another promising agent is riluzole (Rilutek), a medication approved for the treatment of amyotrophic lateral sclerosis (ALS, sometimes known as Lou Gehrig's disease, after the famous baseball player of the 1930s who suffered from it). Riluzole has a protective effect on neurons, and this is why it helps slow the progression of ALS, a disease characterized by progressive deterioration of the nerve cells that control muscles. (Lithium has long been known to have a similar protective effect.) Riluzole works through the same chemical pathways that lamotrigine does. Some of the most promising studies on the use of riluzole in bipolar disorder have been those showing that it is helpful in bipolar depression.[33]

Tiagabine (Gabitril) and zonisamide (Zonegran) are other anti-epilepsy drugs that have attracted the interest of clinical researchers on bipolar disorder. Ongoing work may result in these drugs also being introduced as mood-stabilizing medications.

On the Horizon: Promising New Approaches

In the past decade, science has made almost unbelievable progress in understanding the intricate workings of the human brain. This new understanding means that, for the very first time, pharmaceuticals are being developed based on how they interact with specific biological systems in the brain. Thanks to work in the fields of genetics and neuroscience, molecular pathways have been identified that seem to be involved in the development of the symptoms of mood disorders. Many new pharmaceutical agents now being tested have been selected because they are known to have certain molecular effects. In some cases, clinical trials are being carried out on older medications that have been used for decades to treat other medical problems. No one suspected that these pharmaceuticals might help persons with bipolar disorder, but they are substances that are known to work through some particular biochemical process that we now know can go awry in mood-disorder patients.

A good example of this "old becomes new" approach is the interest in allopurinol, a drug introduced in the 1960s to treat gout. Several small clinical trials have demonstrated that it helps some people with bipolar depression.[34] An even older agent is scopolamine, a drug originally extracted from a family of poisonous plants in the nightshade family (jimsonweed is one) that was first used at the beginning of the twentieth century as an obstetrical anesthetic and is now used to treat motion sickness. A 2006 study at the National Institute of Mental Health demonstrated "rapid, robust antidepressant responses" in patients with bipolar depression who were given scopolamine intravenously.[35] In both of these cases, clinical scientists went looking for an agent that was known to affect a particular biological pathway in neurons after studies by neuroscientists implicated that pathway in the development of bipolar disorder. They were fortunate to find just the medications they were looking for, though perhaps not where they expected to find them: among older treatments for, of all things, gout and motion sickness.

Entirely new pharmaceuticals are being developed as well, drugs that, for now at least, bear only code names assigned to them by the pharmaceutical companies working on them, names like AZD6765 and EVT 101.[36]

Maybe the days of accidentally stumbling upon effective treatments for bipolar disorder, as happened in the case of lithium and valproate, are coming to an end. Older drugs are being redeployed and entirely new drugs are being developed based on knowledge and understanding of the biochemistry of bipolar disorder. After decades of nearly aimless searching in the dark for new treatments, bright lights are indeed on the horizon.

CHAPTER 7

Antidepressant Medications

THE ROLE OF ANTIDEPRESSANT MEDICATIONS IN TREATING THE depression of bipolar disorder has been debated for several decades now. This is because these medications can push a bipolar patient from depression into a manic state. (The development of manic symptoms in patients being treated for tuberculosis with a medication called iproniazid is what led to the development of the class of antidepressants called *monoamine oxidase inhibitors*.) In some patients, antidepressants seem to increase the cycling of their illness.

Yet, despite the risks associated with antidepressants for persons with bipolar illness, some patients with bipolar disorder appear to benefit from them and can take them safely. Unfortunately, we don't yet have any way of identifying who those patients are, so caution is the byword when it comes to prescribing these drugs.

Tricyclic Antidepressants

Although tricyclics are now less frequently used as antidepressants, our discussion starts with this group because these were the first antidepressant medications developed and because they still provide the standard by which all promising new pharmaceuticals for the treatment of depression are judged.

These drugs are called *tricyclics* because of the three rings in their chemical structure. Although some tricyclics have an effect on serotonin systems in the brain, their primary effect in the brain seems to be inhibiting reuptake of the neurotransmitter norepinephrine by neurons. Remember that the reuptake of neurotransmitters into the neuron after they have been released into the synaptic cleft, and have done their work signaling the next cell, is the means by which the synapse is "reset." Norepinephrine is usually quickly removed from the synapse and pumped back into the cell that released it in order to turn off and reset the system. By blocking the removal of norepinephrine, tricyclics seem to prolong or intensify norepinephrine's message to the next cell in some way.

This effect of tricyclics on norepinephrine in neurons was one of the first chemical effects of a medication active in the brain to be measured in the laboratory. The observation that tricyclics *increased* the amount of norepinephrine in the synapse, along with the discovery that certain other medications used to treat high blood pressure *reduced* norepinephrine—and were observed to cause depression in some patients—led to the early amine hypothesis of the mood disorders: the theory that depression was caused by too little norepinephrine and mania, presumably, by too much. However, further research indicated that tricyclics increased amines in the synapse within *hours* of taking them but took *weeks* to begin to help with depressive symptoms, and this led to a search for an alternative explanation. That search is still going on. Table 7-1 lists the common tricyclics.

The principal reason that tricyclic antidepressants are now less frequently prescribed is their many side effects. As with all medications, some patients can take tricyclics easily and without unpleasant side effects, but many patients have to put up with a few days or even weeks of troublesome side effects to get the benefits. Fortunately, all the side effects are dose-related, and most are temporary.

You may remember that Roland Kuhn found imipramine, the first tri-

TABLE 7-1 Tricyclic antidepressants

Pharmaceutical name	Brand name
Amitriptyline	Elavil
Amoxapine	Asendin
Clomipramine	Anafranil
Desipramine	Norpramin
Doxepin	Sinequan
Imipramine	Tofranil
Maprotiline	Ludiomil
Nortriptyline	Pamelor
Protriptyline	Vivactil

cyclic, among a group of compounds that had some antihistamine effects. It's not surprising, then, that these medications affect some people the way antihistamines do, causing mild sleepiness and sometimes what some of my patients have called a "weird" or "spacey" feeling for the first day or two after starting them. Tricyclics block another neurotransmitter called *acetylcholine*, which is used in the part of the nervous system that regulates many "automatic" functions of the body such as digestion. These *anticholinergic* side effects include a slowing down of the gastrointestinal tract, causing constipation and dry mouth. The focusing of the lens of the eye and emptying of the urinary bladder are also controlled by this system, and tricyclics can cause blurry vision and urination difficulties also, although usually only at high doses. Patients with a history of glaucoma or urinary-tract problems should be monitored closely by their physician while taking these medications. Tricyclics also cause weight gain in many patients.

Tricyclics are toxic in larger amounts and overdoses are very dangerous. Although the lethal overdose is up to twenty times the normal dose for an adult, children are more sensitive to the toxic effects of these medications; just a handful of tablets can be fatal in a small child. For this reason, tricyclic medications must be scrupulously safeguarded in households with children.

Selective Serotonin Reuptake Inhibitors

It will come as no surprise that a new pharmaceutical that had none of the tricyclic side effects listed above and was not toxic in overdose caused something of a sensation when it was introduced in 1988. That pharmaceutical was fluoxetine (Prozac). For a time it seemed that everyone you talked to was either taking Prozac or reading about it. A Prozac capsule showed up on the covers of *Newsweek* and *New York* magazines, and the drug was featured in innumerable other magazine and newspaper articles.

Unlike the tricyclics, this class of antidepressants has little direct effect on norepinephrine in the brain but instead blocks the reuptake of another neurotransmitter, serotonin, into neurons. The very potent and specific serotonin-reuptake-blocking effects of these agents give this class its name: *selective serotonin reuptake inhibitors,* or *SSRIs* (table 7-2).

The side-effect profile of the SSRIs is very benign. Some patients experience nausea for the first couple of days after starting one of the SSRIs, and a very few have diarrhea or vomiting. Headaches are not uncommon. These problems can often be alleviated by restarting the medication at a lower dose, and they tend to pass quickly. SSRIs can be somewhat stimulating in some people, and while this is just what is needed by some depressed patients, others feel unpleasantly nervous or "wired" when taking these medications. The converse can also be seen, and sleepiness is sometimes a side effect. Many

TABLE 7-2 Selective serotonin reuptake inhibitors

Pharmaceutical name	Brand name(s)
Citalopram	Celexa (Cipramil)
Escitalopram	Lexapro (Cipralex)
Fluoxetine	Prozac, Sarafem (Erocap, Fluohexal, Lovan, Zactin, and others)
Fluvoxamine	Luvox
Paroxetine	Paxil, Paxil CR* (Aropax, Seroxat, and others)
Sertraline	Zoloft (Altruline, Aremis, Gladem, Besitran, Lustral, Sealdin, and others)

Note: Names in parentheses are brands marketed outside the United States.
*Slow-release preparation.

patients report that SSRIs seem to curb their appetite a bit and notice some weight loss, especially soon after they begin taking an SSRI. Weight gain can also be a problem, however. All of these side effects are usually noticed by patients pretty much immediately, if they are going to occur; none of them sneak up after a person has been on an SSRI for weeks or months.

One problem that might not be noticeable to patients until they've been taking an SSRI for weeks or months is a change in sexual functioning, specifically a noticeable decrease in sexual interest (loss of libido) or a difficulty in reaching or inability to reach orgasm. This is a significant problem affecting about one-third of patients. A variety of strategies are available for dealing with these problems when they occur, so they should be reported to the physician. Weekend "vacations" from the medication have been reported to be helpful, as well as the addition of other medications that seem to block these effects, but sometimes a switch to an antidepressant in another class is the only solution.

When I asked one of my male patients whether he was having any sexual dysfunction from his new antidepressant, he replied that he thought fluoxetine had *improved* his sex life, increasing his sexual stamina and causing him to have more intense orgasms—a reminder that a list of potential medication side effects should never be a reason not to try a particular medication. Pleasant surprises sometimes do occur. Also, a medication effect that causes problems for some patients can actually be helpful for others; for example, SSRIs have been reported to be helpful in treating premature ejaculation.[1]

New Antidepressants

Since the early 1990s, many other new antidepressants have come onto the market that aren't tricyclics and aren't SSRIs. Since most of these phar-

TABLE 7-3 Other antidepressants

Pharmaceutical name	Brand name(s)
Bupropion	Wellbutrin, Wellbutrin XL,* Wellbutrin SR*
Desvenlafaxine	Pristiq
Duloxetine	Cymbalta (Davedax, Xeristar, Yentreve, and others)
Mirtazapine	Remeron (Remergil, Zispin, and others)
Nefazodone	Serzone† (Dutonin)†
Trazodone	Desyrel (Azona, Molipaxin, Sideril, Thombran, and others)
Venlafaxine	Effexor, Effexor XR* (Efexor, Efexor XR,* and others)
Vilazodone	Viibryd

Note: Names in parentheses are brands marketed outside the United States.
*Slow-release preparation.
†Brands withdrawn by manufacturer because of reports of liver failure.

maceuticals don't share many common features, there is no good class name for them, although you'll sometimes see many of them listed as "atypical" or "second-generation" antidepressants (table 7-3). They have a variety of effects on norepinephrine, serotonin, and other neurotransmitters. Some have more than one effect on these systems, and so they are thought to provide different ways of manipulating the chemical systems in the brain that are concerned with mood. Venlafaxine and duloxetine, for example, inhibit the reuptake of both norepinephrine and serotonin and are referred to as dual reuptake inhibitors or SNRIs, for *serotonin and norepinephrine reuptake inhibitors.* Bupropion is most active on a different neurotransmitter altogether, dopamine. The side-effect profiles of these medications vary widely. Some have a profile more like that of tricyclics, others more like that of SSRIs.

Monoamine Oxidase Inhibitors

In the early 1950s, a new drug that had been developed for the treatment of tuberculosis was observed to cause mood elevation in some patients who took it for their lung disease. After more years of investigations, mostly in England, several papers appeared that confirmed the therapeutic effects of iproniazid in patients suffering from depression. Shortly afterward it was discovered that iproniazid causes inactivation of an enzyme in the body that metabolizes amine compounds in the nervous system. This enzyme, called *monoamine oxidase,* is responsible for gobbling up molecules of norepinephrine, serotonin, and several other neurotransmitters. Inactivating monoamine oxidase has the effect of increasing the amounts of these neurotransmitters in the nervous system, and this effect—in some as yet poorly understood way—may be how these medications alleviate the symptoms of depression. This class of pharmaceuticals is called *monoamine oxidase inhibitors*, or *MAOIs* (table 7-4).

There are two forms of monoamine oxidase in the body, MAO-A and MAO-B. Until recently, all of the pharmaceuticals used to treat depression were active in blocking MAO-A. In addition to its activity in the nervous system, MAO-A is also present in the lining of the intestine. Some naturally occurring substances in foods are close enough chemically to norepinephrine to need deactivation before they are absorbed into the bloodstream, and intestinal MAO-A serves this purpose. The importance of this becomes clear when I tell you that another name for norepinephrine is *adrenaline*—a name that is probably more familiar to you. Tyramine, an amino acid that has adrenaline-like effects on blood pressure and heart rate, is present in high enough concentrations in some foods to cause dangerous cardiovascular problems in individuals taking MAOIs. Numerous pharmaceuticals, including the ingredients of many over-the-counter remedies, also have adrenaline-like effects. People taking MAOIs therefore need to observe certain dietary restrictions and, even more importantly, must *scrupulously* read the labels of any over-the-counter medication they are considering—or better yet, consult their pharmacist before taking any pharmaceutical they buy over the counter.

MAOIs also interact with other medications that are prescribed or commonly used in emergency rooms for various problems. People taking MAOIs must be sure to inform all physicians who treat them that they are on this type of medication. And they should consider wearing an alerting bracelet so that, should they be brought into an emergency room unconscious or otherwise unable to communicate, the bracelet can communicate to ER personnel that they are taking an MAOI.

Recently a pharmaceutical has been developed that blocks primarily MAO-B, the other form of MAO in the body. MAO-B is present almost entirely in the brain and is not involved in blocking tyramine absorption in the intestine. The big advantage of an MAO-B inhibitor over an MAO-A inhibitor, then, is that persons taking it wouldn't have to be on a special diet. This

TABLE 7-4 Monoamine oxidase inhibitors (MAOIs)

Pharmaceutical name	Brand name(s)
Phenelzine	Nardil
Tranylcypromine	Parnate
Selegiline	Eldepryl, Emsam transdermal system*

*The selegiline patch.

drug, called *selegiline,* has been used for the treatment of Parkinson's disease for several years. There were early attempts to use it as an antidepressant, but it was discovered that the required doses were so high when taken in pill form that selegiline affected *both* forms of MAO (A and B)—that is, the specificity for MAO-B is lost. This meant that patients taking it would still need to watch their diet for sources of tyramine—no advantage there! Then someone came up with the idea of making a selegiline *patch,* so that the drug is absorbed through the skin rather than taken orally. The patch turns out to have two important advantages. First, because the selegiline is more directly absorbed into the bloodstream, it can be given at a lower dose and maintain its specificity for MAO-B. Second, since it doesn't travel through the intestine, it doesn't affect the MAO-A located there nearly as much as the older MAOIs did. Thus, the selegiline patch is an easier way of taking an MAOI, with fewer side effects and less worry about tyramine-rich foods.

MAOIs can have other side effects, too. They can be stimulating and cause insomnia. For this reason, taking the oral preparations at bedtime should be avoided. Dizzy spells, especially when one suddenly gets up from lying down, can occur. MAOIs block a blood-pressure reflex that usually maintains blood pressure when we stand up, and the sudden drop in blood pressure on standing (called *orthostatic hypotension*) causes lightheadedness. Weight gain and sexual dysfunction are other side effects.

Because of these issues, MAOIs are most often prescribed to patients who have failed to benefit from other antidepressants. This said, they are sometimes uniquely effective, indeed are "miracle drugs," for some patients who have been helped by no other antidepressants. I think every psychiatrist I've ever spoken with has had the experience of effectively treating a particular patient with an MAOI after no other antidepressant had helped.

Treating Bipolar Depression

The observation that antidepressants can cause manic symptoms in persons with bipolar disorder has been confirmed again and again. Perhaps more worrisome is the observation that antidepressants may cause an acceleration of the illness in some patients. Some persons with bipolar disorder experience increased cycling of their mood episodes and even switch to a period of rapid cycling.

In the late 1990s, the National Institute of Mental Health sponsored a large, multicenter study of the treatment of bipolar disorder called the Systematic Treatment Enhancement Program for Bipolar Disorder (STEP-BD). This study enrolled more than 4,000 people with bipolar disorder, followed them over several years while they were receiving treatment, and evaluated the success or failure of various interventions. One of the surprising findings of the study was in a subgroup of 350 patients who developed depression during the course of the study. About half of these patients were then prescribed an antidepressant in addition to their mood stabilizer, while the others stayed on the mood stabilizer alone. At the end of about six months, antidepressant medications appeared to have offered no benefit whatsoever—nor did the patients who took an antidepressant have any more problems with manic symptoms than the patients who took only a mood stabilizer.[2] Now, this seems to fly in the face of decades of research and clinical experience demonstrating what I said at the beginning of this chapter—that some bipolar patients need, benefit from, and can safely take antidepressants. But it makes the point strongly that those patients are the exception, not the rule, and that most bipolar patients should probably avoid taking antidepressant medications.

Studies on the issue of increasing mania and rapid cycling indicate that some patients are at more risk than others for a worsening of their situation with antidepressant treatment. Unfortunately, it is not possible to say with certainty who is and who is not at risk. Bipolar I patients seem to be at greater risk than bipolar II patients; women are at greater risk than men; and patients who already have a history of more rapid cycling—either more full-blown episodes or a tendency toward cyclothymia (continuous low-amplitude cycling) between full-blown episodes—are at greater risk. Moreover, some antidepressant medications seem to be riskier than others. A few studies indicate that bupropion, paroxetine, and MAOIs may be safer than other antidepressants—that is, less likely to precipitate mania (and, by implication, perhaps less likely to increase cycling).

Another finding from the STEP-BD study was that after some patients with bipolar disorder take an antidepressant and seem to recover from a severe depression, they may notice more of the feelings of tense uneasiness that psychiatrists call "dysphoria," along with a smoldering irritability and sleep disturbances. The researchers referred to this set of symptoms as "ACID," short for *antidepressant-associated chronic irritable dysphoria,* and they found that these patients were quite impaired by these symptoms.[3] The researchers had already suspected that antidepressants were the cause of this problem, and so when they looked for patients with the triad of chronic irritability, dysphoria, and sleep disturbances among STEP-BD patients, they noted who had or had not taken an antidepressant along with a mood stabilizer. The results were unequivocal. They found that the patients with these symptoms who had taken an antidepressant outnumbered patients taking only a mood stabilizer by ten to one.

So what do we conclude from all this? I think a reasonable approach is to recommend a cautious and closely observed trial of one of the safer antidepressants for patients who still have serious depression despite optimization of mood-stabilizer treatment, but only if they have never had a previous problem with an antidepressant. At the first sign of irritability, dysphoria, or sleep disturbance, strong consideration should be given to stopping the antidepressant. I think it's also fair to conclude that trying one antidepressant after another in bipolar patients should be avoided; the research literature really does support the idea that most bipolar patients will *not* benefit from an antidepressant.

Perhaps more than any other treatment issues, the questions surrounding the use of antidepressants in bipolar disorder emphasize the need for individualization of treatment for every patient. There are no hard-and-fast rules for when, why, or how to use an antidepressant for bipolar patients. Patient and physician need to communicate clearly and honestly about every aspect of symptoms and treatment to achieve the best treatment outcome.

CHAPTER 8

Antipsychotic Medications

A DIFFICULTY THAT IMMEDIATELY ARISES IN DISCUSSING THE antipsychotic medications is their unfortunate name. *Psychotic* is an imprecise term at best, and these medications have many more uses than simply treating psychotic symptoms.

A psychosis can be thought of as a mental state or disorder in which the affected person's ability to comprehend his or her environment and react to it appropriately is severely impaired. The layman's definition of *psychotic* might be "out of touch with reality." The person who is hearing voices (having hallucinations) or who has bizarre idiosyncratic beliefs (delusions) is psychotic. The word also connotes a severe disorganization of thinking and behavior, usually with restlessness and agitation. The manic syndrome is a good example of a state of psychosis, and we have already talked about "psychotic features" in depression.

In the 1930s a group of pharmaceutical compounds called *phenothiazines* were synthesized in Europe and were found to have antihistamine and sedative properties. One in particular, chlorpromazine, was found to be very useful in surgical anesthesia because it deepened anesthetic sedation more safely than other available agents. In the early 1950s, two French psychiatrists carried out several clinical trials using chlorpromazine to treat highly agitated patients suffering from schizophrenia and mania. They had hoped the drug would provide sedation for these very sick patients, which it did—but these astute clinicians noticed that the medication did much more.

In addition to its quieting and sleep-promoting effects, chlorpromazine made the hallucinations and bizarre delusional beliefs of many patients with schizophrenia practically disappear. It also decreased the severity of the disorganization of thinking and agitated behavior seen in patients with acute mania. Chlorpromazine, in other words, had a *specific* effect on the cluster of symptoms usually referred to as "psychotic" symptoms, and thus the name for this group came about: *antipsychotic medications*. Occasionally they are still referred to as *neuroleptic medications* (or *neuroleptics*), from *neuroleptique*, the French word (coined from Greek roots) that means roughly "affecting the nervous system." The term *major tranquilizers* was frequently used for these medications at one time (with the term *minor tranquilizers* used for sleep and anxiety medications), but these agents are much more than just "tranquilizers," and this term has, fortunately, fallen out of favor.

In the 1980s a new antipsychotic medication was developed that had much more effect on the neurotransmitter serotonin than the other antipsychotics did. In the years since, many more of these drugs have been developed. This group of medications has been a very important development in psychiatry, for reasons I'll discuss below. Now antipsychotic medications are usually divided into two groups, the original group of medications being called the *typical antipsychotics*. The newer group, which have more effect on the serotonin system than their predecessors, are called the *atypical antipsychotics*. In this chapter we'll take a look at each group in turn.

Typical Antipsychotic Medications

As we saw in part I of this book, episodes of bipolar disorder—both depression and mania—can sometimes include extremely frightening mental symptoms and dangerously disturbed behaviors. And, as we saw in chapters 6 and 7, mood stabilizers and antidepressants sometimes take weeks to begin working. What can be done to slow down the racing thoughts, the pressured, bursting overactivity of the manic patient, before lithium starts working? This is where the typical antipsychotic medications have been useful (table 8-1). Because their calming effects begin almost immediately, these medications are especially useful in acute mania and are frequently part of the treatment for the severely ill manic patient. In cases of depression where the patient is highly restless and agitated, they can have similar beneficial effects.

The main chemical effect of all antipsychotics is to block dopamine receptors in the brain. Neural circuits that use dopamine as their neurotransmitter may be dysfunctional in some way in people with schizophrenia, and this situation may cause the bizarre hallucinations and disorders of thinking typical of that illness. Antipsychotic medications may work by affecting

Table 8-1 Typical antipsychotic medications

Pharmaceutical name	Brand name
Chlorpromazine	Thorazine
Fluphenazine	Prolixin
Haloperidol	Haldol
Loxapine	Loxitane
Molindone	Moban
Perphenazine	Trilafon
Thioridazine	Mellaril
Thiothixene	Navane
Trifluoperazine	Stelazine

Note: Side effects include sedation, anticholinergic effects, and extrapyramidal effects (see text).

these systems in some as yet unknown way. Whether the medications alleviate the psychotic symptoms that sometimes complicate bipolar disorder in a similar fashion is unknown.

SIDE EFFECTS

The typical antipsychotic medications were once called "major tranquilizers" because they are, well, tranquilizers—in a major way. Some are more sedating than others, but all can be pretty powerful sedatives, especially in higher doses. They can cause some of the same anticholinergic side effects as tricyclic antidepressants: dry mouth, constipation, and blurred vision. People seem to accommodate to these side effects after a period that ranges from days to weeks.

The main problem with most of these medications is their effect on muscle tone and movement, side effects that are caused by the dopamine blockade that they cause. In textbook discussions of these medications, you will see these problems referred to as *extrapyramidal symptoms,* or simply *EPS.* Dopamine is the main neurotransmitter used in a complex circuit of brain areas called the *extrapyramidal system,* which coordinates movement. (The term *extrapyramidal* contrasts this system with another system, called the *pyramidal system* because its main fibers are carried in triangular bundles into the spinal cord [the "spinal pyramids" or "pyramidal tract"].) The pyramidal system controls the quick, accurate execution of fine muscle movement, and the extrapyramidal system makes sure that the rest of the body moves as needed for the smooth and graceful execution of these movements. Antipsychotic medications, by blocking the dopamine receptors in these centers, can cause a variety of side effects that affect movement.

One of these is *pseudo-parkinsonism.* You may know that persons suffering from Parkinson's disease have a slowed and shuffling walk, seem to lose facial expression because of stiffness of their facial muscles, and also have trembling of their hands. Pseudo-parkinsonism consists of these same symptoms.

Another extrapyramidal side effect is the *acute dystonic reaction.* This is a sudden muscular spasm, more common in young males than in other patients, that usually involves the tongue and facial and neck muscles. People taking antipsychotic medications can also develop a very uncomfortable restlessness called *akathisia.* This is felt mostly in the legs, so that the individual feels the need to walk or pace.

Fortunately, all these side effects are treatable, either by lowering the dose of medication or by adding one of several medications that are also used to treat Parkinson's disease. Although uncomfortable, these side effects are not dangerous and usually respond quickly to treatment once they are encountered and identified.

Most of the typical antipsychotic medications can, over a period of years, cause a side effect called *tardive dyskinesia,* or *TD* for short. This consists of repetitive involuntary movements, usually of the facial muscles—usually chewing, blinking, or lip-pursing movements. There is no good treatment for TD other than lowering the dose of the medication; and occasionally it will need to be discontinued. We used to worry a lot about TD because some patients who developed it seemed to continue to have these movements even after the medication was stopped. But two factors are calming these worries: the discovery that most TD symptoms *do* eventually go away with time and, more importantly, the development of the atypical antipsychotic medications, which do not seem to cause TD very often.

I want to emphasize that extrapyramidal symptoms are usually easily treated and are not dangerous. But the symptoms of bipolar disorder that the antipsychotic medications are usually used to treat *are* extremely dangerous. These medications are powerful agents, and they need to be used carefully and for the shortest period of time possible, but for the present, at least, they are nearly irreplaceable in treating the most dangerous and most terrible symptoms of severe mania and psychotic depression.

Atypical Antipsychotic Medications

As is probably apparent from the foregoing paragraphs, there is room for improvement in the antipsychotic medications. Not only are the extrapyramidal symptoms uncomfortable, but it is usually necessary to add another medication to control them—and the more different medications a

TABLE 8-2 Atypical antipsychotic medications

Pharmaceutical name	Brand name(s)
Aripiprazole	Abilify
Asenapine	Saphris
Clozapine	Clozaril
Iloperidone	Fanapt
Lurasidone	Latuda
Olanzapine	Zyprexa, Zyprexa Zydis
Paliperidone	Invega
Quetiapine	Seroquel
Risperidone	Risperdal
Ziprasidone	Geodon

person takes, the more likely he is to have problems with side effects and drug interactions. So it created quite a stir when a new group of antipsychotic medications was introduced, antipsychotics that don't seem to cause EPS. Even more good news was that these medications seemed to work better than their predecessors. One article in the *American Journal of Psychiatry* called the first of these new agents "arguably the most significant development in antipsychotic drug therapy since the advent of chlorpromazine."[1]

These atypical antipsychotic medications (table 8-2) are designated *atypical* because, although they block dopamine receptors, just as their predecessors do (though not as potently), they differ from the typical antipsychotics in that they are also active at serotonin receptors. Their double action seems to have two effects: extrapyramidal symptoms do not appear nearly as often, and these medications seem to have significant mood-stabilizing effects.

The first atypical antipsychotic, *clozapine,* was synthesized in the laboratory in the 1960s but was not marketed in the United States until 1990. One of the reasons it took so long for clozapine to get onto the market is that, in about 1 percent of patients who take it, it causes a very dangerous drop in the number of white blood cells (called *agranulocytosis*).[2] This problem might have meant the end for clozapine as a new medication, except that it was found to be highly effective in treating patients with schizophrenia who had derived little benefit from traditional antipsychotic medications. Dramatic case studies of patients with chronic treatment-resistant schizophrenia who basically "awakened" from years of unrelenting psychotic symptoms after they started clozapine sustained the interest of clinicians and pharmaceutical researchers. When it was discovered that the risk of agranulocytosis could be substantially reduced if the patient had her white blood cell count monitored monthly, clozapine treatment became available to larger groups of patients, and before long, treatment-resistant mood-disorder patients were treated with it as well.

There are now many studies of the use of clozapine for people with treatment-resistant bipolar and schizoaffective disorder. A year after clozapine came onto the market, a letter to the editor of the *Journal of Clinical Psychopharmacology* reported that clozapine had been effective in treating two rapid-cycling bipolar patients "who were resistant to all conventional treatment."[3] One patient was a forty-eight-year-old woman who had been very ill for more than thirty years, had started rapid cycling about five years previously, and had been almost constantly cycling between delusional depressions and dysphoric mania for a whole year before starting on clozapine. The authors stated that after the woman had been taking clozapine alone for three months, "her mood swings completely stopped." The case report indicates that there were episodes of breakthrough manic and depressive symptoms, but the patient had done remarkably better on clozapine. (This case illustrates why some patients, at least, are willing to pay the price of the needed blood tests.)

Another study looked at the use of clozapine in twenty-five acutely manic patients "for whom lithium, anticonvulsants and [traditional] neuroleptics had been ineffective, had produced intolerable side effects, or both."[4] Almost three-quarters of the patients had "marked improvement" in their manic symptoms. The answer to the question posed in a 1995 article title, "Is Clozapine a Mood Stabilizer?" seems to be an emphatic yes.[5]

In the years since the introduction of clozapine, many other atypical antipsychotic medications that do *not* cause blood count problems have come along, and their introduction has substantially expanded the number of treatment options for bipolar disorder. More and more evidence is emerging that the atypical antipsychotic medications are helpful in all phases of bipolar disorder—mania *and* depression—as well as for ongoing treatment to prevent relapse (sometimes known as maintenance treatment). The really good news is that these medications have very significant antidepressant effects in many patients (another reason why calling them "antipsychotic" medications is inaccurate). In 2002, just after the first atypicals introduced after clozapine appeared, the *Journal of Clinical Psychopharmacology* published a letter to the editor titled, "Are the Atypical Antipsychotic Drugs Antidepressants?"[6] Once again the answer is a definite yes, and in subsequent years, this fact has been borne out in study after study.

Practicing psychiatrists (including this one) will tell you that some of the atypicals seem to be more antimanic and others more antidepressant in their effect. Unfortunately, research that might bear this out by comparing the effects of different atypicals for mania and for bipolar depression has not been done.

I should also mention that several of the newer atypicals are not labeled by the Food and Drug Administration for use in bipolar disorder, meaning that prescribing them to bipolar patients is technically "off-label." (Remember that physicians may prescribe any available drug for a condition if, based on their review of available research and their judgment and experience, the drug is appropriate to treat the patient. When this is for a condition not listed in the FDA "label" the practice is called "off-label prescribing.")

SIDE EFFECTS

Of the atypical antipsychotics, only clozapine causes the blood-count problem that requires frequent blood counts. None of the atypical antipsychotics cause EPS except at high doses. High doses can also trigger the other side effects that the traditional antipsychotic medications cause: anticholinergic side effects and sedation.

The most significant side-effect problem with the atypical antipsychotic medications has been their tendency to make some individuals gain weight and develop such obesity-related problems as high cholesterol and even diabetes (table 8-3). Not all individuals develop these problems, but attention to diet and weight issues is very important for persons taking these medications, especially for patients who take them over a long term. The primary mechanism for the weight gain associated with the atypical antipsychotics seems to be stimulation of the appetite center of the brain, although it has also been suggested that these medications affect several hormones that control how the body handles calories and stores fat.[7] Some of the atypical antipsychotics are more likely to cause weight gain than others; in fact, several seem relatively weight neutral—that is, they seem to have little or no effect on weight.

TABLE 8-3 Weight gain risks of atypical antipsychotics

Higher risk	Clozapine
↑	Olanzapine
	Quetiapine
	Risperidone
	Ziprasidone*
Lower risk	Aripiprazole*

Source: Data from T. Baptista, N. M. Kin, S. Beaulieu, and E. A. de Baptista, "Obesity and Related Metabolic Abnormalities during Drug Administration: Mechanisms, Management, and Research Perspectives," *Pharmacopsychiatry* 35, no. 6 (2002): 205–19.
*Negligible effect on weight.

The weight-neutral agents would seem to be preferable for already obese patients and for patients with diabetes or a family history of diabetes. Blood tests for diabetes and high cholesterol should be done at the beginning of treatment and regularly thereafter in patients taking antipsychotics for maintenance treatment. All patients taking atypical antipsychotics should take steps to control possible weight gain by paying attention to their diet and getting regular exercise.

CHAPTER 9

More Medications, Hormones, and Dietary Supplements

THERE ARE MANY OTHER PHARMACEUTICAL AGENTS THAT HAVE proved helpful in the treatment of bipolar disorder. Some are *symptomatic treatments,* meaning that they treat symptoms rather than the underlying disorder and therefore are usually used for only a short time. Others are medications that affect functioning in another body system that is important for normal mood regulation.

Sleeplessness and anxiety are very common problems for persons with bipolar disorder. As we will see in chapter 16, sleep deprivation is often very destabilizing for such persons. Anxiety raises the levels of stress hormones like cortisol in the body, and therefore keeping this uncomfortable symptom in check is an important part of staying well.

Medications for Anxiety and Sleep Disturbances
BENZODIAZEPINE MEDICATIONS

The benzodiazepine medications represented a major advance in the treatment of psychiatric symptoms when they were first developed, and they continue to be widely prescribed (table 9-1). They often have a place in the treatment of bipolar disorder because they are highly effective for the treatment of anxiety and insomnia and, in higher doses, are safe and effective sedatives. If this sounds too good to be true and you're wondering if there's a hidden drawback, there is. These medications can be abused; it's possible to become psychologically dependent on them and even physically addicted to

TABLE 9-1 Benzodiazepine medications

Pharmaceutical name	Brand name
Alprazolam	Xanax
Chlordiazepoxide	Librium
Clonazepam	Klonopin
Clorazepate	Tranxene
Diazepam	Valium
Lorazepam	Ativan

Note: These medications are best thought of as temporary agents and are frequently prescribed for occasional "as-needed" use.

them. (Withdrawal symptoms in persons taking high doses of these medications can include very serious problems such as seizures.) Moreover, their sedating effects decrease over time, and after several weeks of use, their effectiveness as tranquilizers decreases. For these reasons benzodiazepines are best thought of as temporary measures.

Benzodiazepines really have two main uses in treating bipolar disorder: they are used to treat patients who are very sick and to treat patients who are doing very well. This seems to be a contradiction, doesn't it? The explanation is in the doses used and how the medications are combined with other medications. In acutely manic patients, the short-acting benzodiazepine lorazepam (Ativan) can be an effective short-term tranquilizer, especially in combination with a typical antipsychotic medication like haloperidol (Haldol). This combination is very familiar to psychiatrists working in emergency settings, because it works quickly and effectively in calming even the most agitated patients. A very ill manic patient, perhaps delusional and agitated, who hasn't slept for days can be asleep less than an hour after receiving this combination, especially by injection. The longer-acting benzodiazepine clonazepam (Klonopin) has also been used and extensively studied in the treatment of acute manic symptoms and appears to be another effective adjunct medication.

These medications are not mood stabilizers and are not effective in treating hallucinations or delusions, but as sedatives they are unsurpassed. Remember that before effective psychiatric medications became available, patients with severe mania died of the physical stress of the manic state. By simply slowing manic patients down for a few hours or days until antipsychotic medications and mood-stabilizing medications start working, benzodiazepines can be literally lifesaving.

At the other end of the spectrum of illness severity, patients who are not having severe mood symptoms can safely take these medications for anxiety symptoms and insomnia. During periods of unavoidable psychological stress, such as after the death of a loved one, benzodiazepine medications can help with the insomnia and lessen the psychological tension that may bring on mood symptoms in bipolar patients. It's important to emphasize here that these medications should *not* be used as substitutes for making changes to chronically stressful situations. A person who finds that he feels the need to take a sedative to deal with everyday situations is well on his way to psychological dependence on tranquilizers, medication abuse, and addiction. We'll discuss this in more depth in chapter 15.

There's another way these medications are used, and that is in treating patients who have anxiety disorders. Anxiety disorders (such as recurrent panic attacks) are effectively treated with benzodiazepines. The connections between the mood disorders and anxiety disorders are poorly understood, but there are certainly some people who need treatment for both. The treatment of panic disorder and other severe anxiety disorders sometimes involves taking benzodiazepine medications on a longer-term basis, but prolonged use of benzodiazepines is the exception rather than the rule in treating bipolar disorders, and any use requires close monitoring.

NOVEL ANXIETY MEDICATIONS

Two medications developed as treatment for epilepsy have proved to be very helpful in patients with anxiety problems. Both are active in a neuro-receptor system that is known to be involved with anxiety, the GABA pathway (for gamma aminobutyric acid), and their names reflect this: *gaba*pentin (Neurontin) and pre*gaba*lin (Lyrica). These medications have several advantages for treating the anxiety that can be associated with bipolar disorder. The first is that there is little or no risk of developing a psychological dependence on them. Gabapentin is not a "controlled substance" in FDA parlance, and although pregabalin is, it has been assigned the lowest possible risk rating, schedule V (other schedule V drugs include cough preparations with very small amounts of codeine). Also, gabapentin and pregabalin can be taken over the longer term without losing effectiveness. For these reasons, they can be very helpful for persons with prolonged anxiety problems that have no clear precipitant, a pattern that is often called "generalized anxiety."[1]

Thyroid Hormones

In several sections of this book we're going to talk about the interrelationships of mood and hormones. The pulsing daily rhythms of melatonin from the pineal gland that may be involved with the seasonal mood changes of seasonal affective disorder (SAD), the mood fluctuations that can follow changing levels of female reproductive hormones (important in understanding postpartum mood symptoms and premenstrual syndromes), the stress hormones secreted by the adrenal gland—all these hormonal changes seem to be important in the regulation of mood. But perhaps the most important hormones in this respect are the thyroid hormones.

The thyroid gland plays a major role in the body's energy regulation. Too little thyroid gland activity leads to sluggishness and weight gain, and too much leads to metabolic overdrive—rapid pulse, nervous energy, and anxiety. While the precise role of thyroid hormones in the regulation of mood remains unclear, it's very clear that normal thyroid functioning is essential for effective treatment of mood disorders. Put another way, if a patient's mood symptoms don't respond to the usual treatments, or if a treatment that has been effective seems to lose its effectiveness, a thyroid problem, especially abnormally low thyroid functioning (hypothyroidism), should be suspected.

Several studies have shown that hypothyroidism is surprisingly common in patients with rapid-cycling bipolar disorder.[2] One group of scientists tested for thyroid abnormalities in stored blood samples from almost four thousand patients who had been hospitalized for psychiatric problems over a period of four years. They found a high association between thyroid abnormalities and a diagnosis of rapid-cycling bipolar disorder.[3]

But it is also clear that some patients with bipolar disorder whose thyroid hormone levels prove to be in the "normal range" when blood tests are done can nevertheless benefit from treatment with thyroid medications. Studies have demonstrated that many patients with bipolar depression symptoms that are not responding to treatment have thyroid function that is "normal" by the usual criteria, but blood tests show them to be in what might be called the "low normal" or even "barely normal" range.[4] It may be that depressed individuals need a higher level of thyroid hormones than those who are not depressed. Perhaps the extra thyroid hormone somehow makes these patients more responsive to other treatments. Patients who have a partial response to lithium or other mood stabilizers may have better control of their mood symptoms when a small dose of thyroid replacement hormone is added, even if their thyroid hormone levels are normal. As a paper on treating rapid-cycling bipolar disorder put it, "Normal thyroid [blood test results] should not discourage the clinician from pursuing thyroid supplementation" in bipolar patients.[5]

Notice that I haven't used the term *thyroid medication* in this discussion. That is because it has been possible for many years to synthetically produce the very same molecules that the thyroid gland itself naturally produces. (Hence the brand name, Synthroid, of the most commonly prescribed brand of levothyroxine.)[6] What dose of hormone to prescribe is determined by measuring hormone levels in the blood, something that should be done several times a year for anyone who takes a thyroid hormone replacement.

Herbal Preparations and Nutritional Supplements

There are some nutrients that we must include in our diet to remain healthy. These are compounds that our body cannot manufacture but are nevertheless necessary for normal cellular functioning. The most familiar of these are, of course, the *vitamins,* compounds manufactured by some plants and animals but not by humans. Their name, from the Latin word *vita* meaning "life," indicates just how important to health they are. Unless we eat foods that contain the vitamins we need, serious illness results. Scurvy, beriberi, and pellagra are three illnesses—now, thankfully, unfamiliar—that result from deficiencies of vitamin C, vitamin B1, and niacin, respectively. All these illnesses have significant central nervous system symptoms, especially B1 deficiency, which causes severe central nervous system degeneration.

There are other naturally occurring substances that our bodies are not very good at producing but that are important for health. These are substances that modern diets, as opposed to ancient human diets, tend not to include in the amounts that some believe are necessary for optimal health. A good example of these substances is the *essential fatty acids,* a collection of complex fat molecules that are found in some vegetables and other plant sources (such as flaxseed) and in large amounts in some fish. Nutritionists have long touted the health benefits of diets rich in seafood, and the lower incidence of breast cancer and heart disease in the Japanese population has been attributed to a diet rich in seafood.

Botanicals are plant-derived naturally occurring substances that have pharmaceutical effects in the body; that is, although they have no nutritional value, they interact with some biological system in the body so as to treat a symptom or an illness. A good example of this group is *digitalis,* derived from the foxglove plant (*Digitalis purpura*), which happens to be a very effective treatment for heart failure. It is thought that the foxglove produces this chemical in its tissues as chemical protection against animals and insects. Digitalis is fatal in high doses, but tiny amounts have beneficial effects. Similar plant "toxins" form the basis of many modern pharmaceuticals, for example, pain medications from the opium poppy and the antimalaria drug quinine from the bark of the cinchona tree.

Finally, there are substances that are normally present in the body and have some biological function that, taken in larger amounts, may enhance that function. An example is *melatonin,* a hormone, secreted by the pineal gland in a daily rhythm, that is important in sleep regulation. It also happens to be synthesized by a variety of plants; it is found in the seeds of sunflowers and corianders. Although it can be argued that melatonin is a true pharmaceutical, the FDA tends to be reluctant to regulate such naturally occurring substances. They are considered "nutritional supplements" and are regulated as foods, even if, as with melatonin, the manufacturing process takes place in a pharmaceutical manufacturing facility and doesn't involve food or plants or anything one would think of as "natural."

Omega-3 Fatty Acids and Fish Oil

Some evidence suggests that essential fatty acids, especially a subgroup called *omega-3 fatty acids,* may be useful in the treatment of mood disorders, especially bipolar disorder. The particular compounds thought to have the most health benefits have tongue-twisting names typical of complex organic compounds: eicosapentaenoic acid (EPA) and docosahexaenoic acid (DHA).

Numerous studies have indicated that omega-3 fatty acids, taken as fish-oil capsules, are beneficial for individuals with mood disorders. A review article that analyzed five studies in persons with bipolar depression concluded that there is "strong evidence that bipolar depression may be improved by the adjunctive use of omega-3."[7] Studies of omega-3 in mania have not shown any benefit.

Omega-3 fatty acids are incorporated into cell membranes in association with molecules that are known to be involved in cell signaling. They seem to be active at some of the same points in cellular signaling mechanisms where lithium and valproate are thought to work. Since valproate is, after all, a *synthetic* fatty acid, the idea that natural fatty acids might have benefits in mood disorders shouldn't seem strange at all. Other circumstantial evidence has been cited to support the importance of omega-3 fatty acids for good mental health. Archaeological and epidemiological studies suggest that modern humans consume much less food that is rich in fatty acids than ancient peoples did and that we may be deficient in these important compounds compared with our ancestors. This fact, combined with evidence that the prevalence of depression is increasing and the age of onset of mood disorders is decreasing, has been cited as further evidence of a link between these important compounds and mental health. Omega-3 fatty acid therapy is an adjunctive treatment, added to other agents such as lithium; it should *not* be substituted for proven treatments. However, given the apparent low risk of these compounds, supplementation of standard treatments for mood disorders with omega-3 preparations under the supervision of one's physician is an option some patients will want to explore.

N-Acetyl Cysteine

The health benefits of foods that are high in *antioxidants* are well-known. Sales of green tea, which is high in naturally occurring antioxidants, have soared in recent years, and green tea has been studied as an adjunctive treatment for everything from diabetes to cancer.

So just what are antioxidants? Although oxygen is a vital ingredient for biological functioning, it is very reactive chemically, combining with just about anything in a reaction called oxygenation, often with untoward results. When oxygen rapidly combines with the organic compounds in gasoline, we call it "fire." When oxygen combines with various molecules in the body, a much less dramatic but still damaging process called *oxidative damage* can occur. Plants and animals all have substances, the antioxidants, that essentially prowl about scooping up these damaging oxygen-containing molecules when they occur. You can think of oxidative stress as a kind of biological overheating, requiring antioxidants to step in and cool things down.

In humans, the main antioxidant in the brain is a substance called *glutathione,* which the body manufactures by combining several ingredients, including N-acetyl cysteine (NAC). High levels of oxidative stress deplete glutathione in the brain, but since glutathione is not well absorbed from the gut, the best way to increase levels is to take in the more easily absorbed NAC. Intravenous NAC is routinely used to halt the oxidative damage to the liver caused by overdoses of acetaminophen (Tylenol) as well as in other situations when the antioxidants of the body are overwhelmed.

A placebo-controlled study of adjunctive NAC (that is, as an add-on to standard medications such as lithium) in bipolar depression found a significant benefit, and a follow-up study in which all the subjects took NAC for another two months showed continued benefit.[8] Like omega-3, NAC is clearly an adjunctive medication, the benefits of which should be considered promising rather than firmly established. Nevertheless, it is an option some may wish to explore—again, with the guidance of their physician.

St. John's Wort

Hypericum perforatum, commonly known as St. John's wort, is one of about three hundred species of shrubby perennial plants (of genus *Hypericum*) with bright yellow flowers; the plants grow in most of the temperate regions of the world. Teas and other extracts of St. John's wort have been recommended by herbalists for centuries to treat everything from insomnia to the painful viral skin infection called shingles. In the late 1980s hypericum (*H. perforatum*) was investigated as a possible treatment for HIV infection when it was found to have activity against retroviruses, but its activity unfortunately did not translate into clinical usefulness against HIV infection.

A 1996 article in the *British Medical Journal* that systematically reviewed twenty-three different studies involving a total of 1,757 patients concluded that "extracts of hypericum are more effective than placebo for the treatment of mild to moderately severe depressive disorders."[9] More recent studies have been less encouraging. When St. John's wort was compared with a placebo in two hundred patients who had been rigorously evaluated and diagnosed with major depression, the herbal preparation was no better than the placebo in treating depression. This study concluded that "the results do not support significant antidepressant or anti-anxiety effects for St. John's wort when compared to placebo in a clinical sample of depressed patients" and that "persons with major depression should not be treated with St. John's wort, given the morbidity and mortality risks of untreated or ineffectively treated major depression."[10] In a follow-up study, the same researchers reported that when the individuals who had not responded to St. John's wort were given standard antidepressants, most of them improved, suggesting that the herbal preparation had failed not because these were "treatment-resistant" patients but simply because St. John's wort wasn't effective against their depression.[11]

Questions about the effectiveness of St. John's wort are one thing, but reports of it making things worse are unfortunately not hard to find:

A 53-year-old man without prior psychiatric treatment presented to our clinic with depression. His history was significant for hypomania cycling into depression every June and December for 20 years, consistent with a diagnosis of bipolar II disorder. . . . Of note, his 18-year-old son is treated for bipolar I disorder with lithium. He had no medical history and had never been prescribed psychotropics, although in May 1998, he bought a bottle of St. John's wort with the hope that it could improve his mood.

Shortly after taking St. John's wort 900 mg/day, he noticed a surge in self-esteem. His thoughts raced, he was more talkative, his sleep decreased, his sex drive increased, he spent money excessively, and he drove faster than usual. Two months later, his behavior changed dramatically. He missed work because he just "didn't care," he angrily lashed out at his wife, he shoplifted from the supermarket, and he surfed the Internet for romantic intrigue. He communicated with many women by e-mail, later met these women, and engaged in unprotected sexual relationships with as many as four women in 1 week. He regarded these affairs as a "hobby," lacking any appreciation for their impact on his marriage. He had visual illusions and believed that people at work were trying to undermine him. Although he had experienced mood elevations in the past, he explained that this episode was particularly long and severe and admits that he was doing things which "didn't make sense."

Subsequently, he reduced his SJW to 300 mg/day, and his depression recurred. His treatment team discontinued the SJW and initiated lithium [and] he reports steady improvement in mood.[12]

I think it's fair to say that St. John's wort isn't good enough as an antidepressant to help persons with bipolar disorder, but that it's enough of an antidepressant to cause problems for them, and so is best left alone, except perhaps in the garden.

CHAPTER 10

Brain-Stimulation Treatments

IF YOU'RE UNFAMILIAR WITH THE TERM *BRAIN-STIMULATION treatments,* you're not alone. It's a relatively new term for a variety of treatment techniques, one of which has been around for many decades. These techniques involve using tiny electrical impulses to stimulate areas of the brain. The oldest of these is electroconvulsive therapy, in which a very small electrical current is applied directly to the scalp while the patient is under general anesthesia. Some newer techniques use even smaller electrical impulses and require no anesthesia. The details of how these treatments work is still far from certain. However, it is fairly clear that they all work by affecting the levels of electrical activity in certain areas of the brain, areas that are underactive or overactive during episodes of abnormal mood. They bring activity levels into a more normal balance, in much the same way that very small electrical impulses are used to reregulate heart rhythms in individuals who have a cardiac pacemaker.

Electroconvulsive Therapy

Although the effectiveness of electroconvulsive therapy (ECT) in mood disorders was not a completely accidental discovery, its original theoretical basis has been shown to have no validity, so the development of modern ECT, like so many other treatments in psychiatry, was a kind of happy accident. In the early 1930s the Hungarian physician Joseph Ladislas von Meduna proposed that there was a mutual antagonism between epilepsy and schizophrenia: patients who suffered from epilepsy did not suffer from schizophrenia and vice versa. Modern research has shown that this is not the case, but von Meduna was convinced of the truth of this assertion on the basis of his microscopic post-mortem examination of the brains of persons with the two conditions. He conducted animal experiments attempting to find a way to produce seizure activity artificially. In 1935 he published a paper reporting a dramatic improvement in symptoms after artificially inducing seizures in several patients who suffered from what he thought to be schizophrenia (in retrospect, it's probable that at least some of them had severe mood disorders with psychotic symptoms). Von Meduna used injections to produce seizures, but several years later two Italian psychiatrists reported that seizures could be produced by briefly passing a low-voltage electrical current through the skull by means of electrodes applied to the scalp. Ugo Cerletti and Lucio Bini first developed their technique in animals and then tried it on several patients with "schizophrenia," and they also reported remarkable success.

Although patients with some forms of true schizophrenia do indeed often show improvement in some of their symptoms after these treatments, it quickly became apparent that it was the severely depressed patients who showed improvement—improvement that was little short of miraculous. Decades previously, Emil Kraepelin had described patients in a catatonic state from depression: "The patients lie in bed taking no interest in anything. They betray no pronounced emotion; they are mute, inaccessible; they pass their [bowel movements] under them; they stare straight in front of them with [a] vacant expression of countenance like a mask and with wide open eyes."[1] In the 1940s, after receiving "electroshock" treatments, such patients had complete recovery from their symptoms within a matter of days. The most recent major breakthrough in the treatment of psychiatric problems— the discovery of the Wassermann test for syphilis in 1906—now seemed almost insignificant compared with this astonishing new therapeutic technique. Naturally, interest in ECT spread quickly around the globe.

But ECT's success was also nearly its downfall. Like many other seemingly miraculous treatments, it was overprescribed at first and probably was administered to many hundreds of persons it had little chance of helping. It's important to remember, however, that those were desperate times in psychiatry. With the discovery of antipsychotic medications nearly a decade off and the discovery of antidepressants nearly two decades in the future, "little chance" of helping was better than no chance at all. Since, as we shall see, ECT is a highly effective treatment for mania, some institutions were inclined to use it for any highly agitated patients and sometimes on merely uncooperative ones (a misuse that was dramatized—with a few inaccuracies unfortunately thrown in—in the film *One Flew over the Cuckoo's Nest*). Another negative factor was that in the first decade or so after its development, ECT could have some very serious complications. An epileptic seizure is a violent event: all the muscles of the body contract simultaneously for a few moments, sometimes with such force that broken bones result. Breathing stops as well, and heart-rhythm irregularities can occur.

The nearly indiscriminate overprescription of a therapy with serious potential side effects led to a backlash. By the late 1960s and 1970s, although modern anesthetic techniques were making ECT safer, and more careful research was being done to determine which psychiatric disorders the treatment helped with and which it did not, the damage to ECT's reputation had already been done. (*Cuckoo's Nest*, awarded the Oscar for best movie in 1975, depicted ECT as it would have been administered circa 1945 and certainly didn't help.) State hospitals drew up regulations sharply curtailing its use, and legislation was in effect briefly in California banning the procedure completely.

Fortunately, the pendulum has swung back to center. ECT is now safer than most surgical procedures, side effects are minimal, and guidelines for when it should be used have been clarified. A 1980 survey of 166 ECT patients reported that about half of them thought a trip to the dentist was more unpleasant than an electroconvulsive treatment.[2]

MODERN ECT

Improvements in ECT have been due both to changes in the way the electrical stimulus is used and, perhaps even more, to modern anesthesia. Many psychiatric hospitals have treatment suites for ECT; in general hospitals, ECT is often administered in the recovery room of the hospital's surgical suite (the area where patients waking up from surgery are taken for observation). The ECT treatment lasts only about sixty seconds; most of the "treatment" time is the ten minutes or so it takes to administer general anesthesia before the actual treatment and another ten minutes for the patient to awaken from it.

The crucial anesthetic advance for ECT was the introduction in the 1950s of agents called *muscle relaxants,* or more properly *neuromuscular blocking agents,* which temporarily paralyze the patient by blocking nerve fiber signals to the muscles. These medications prevent the violent muscle contractions during seizures that characterized early ECT use.

After an intravenous medication is given to put the patient to sleep, the neuromuscular blocking agent is given so that the patient's muscles are almost completely relaxed. Electrode disks similar to those used for cardiac defibrillation are applied to the scalp. Modern ECT equipment designed for the purpose delivers a precisely timed and measured electrical stimulus. In *bilateral* treatments, an electrode is applied over each temple. In *unilateral* treatments, wherein the object is to stimulate only half of the brain, one electrode is placed in the middle of the forehead or the crown of the head and the other at the temple. (Unilateral treatment causes less post-ECT confusion and memory problems and is now used almost exclusively, although patients for whom unilateral treatments are ineffective often switch to receiving bilateral treatments.)

The electrical stimulus is applied for two to eight seconds, triggering seizure activity in the brain. The "seizure" in modern ECT is pretty much an electrical event only, with few or no jerking movements such as those that usually characterize seizures, and thus what ECT causes is usually called a modified seizure. The ECT equipment also records an electroencephalogram (a measurement of the electrical activity of the brain), allowing the physician to monitor the seizure activity, which usually lasts less than a minute. There might be some muscle contractions observed during this time, but the muscle relaxant keeps the patient nearly motionless. Usually a quickening of the heart rate and an increase of blood pressure occur, which also signal that the "seizure" has occurred. The anesthetist uses a face-mask breathing device to deliver oxygen until the patient wakes up five or ten minutes later, and the treatment is over. As with other short procedures done under general anesthesia, the first words the patient usually says upon awakening in the recovery area are, "When will I have my treatment?" That is, patients have no memory of the procedure.

About the only patients who absolutely must not receive ECT are the few individuals with medical conditions so severe that even ten to fifteen minutes of general anesthesia is too dangerous—people with severe cardiac or lung diseases, for example. ECT is safe in elderly persons and during pregnancy.

Patients awakening from anesthesia after ECT are a bit groggy, of course, and many are also slightly fuzzy-headed and feel "spacey" for another hour or so. This effect is probably related to the treatments themselves, not just the anesthesia, and it resembles the mild postseizure confusion that patients with true epilepsy often experience. Occasionally a more prolonged period of confusion called *delirium* is seen, especially after bilateral treatments and especially toward the end of a course of treatments. Sedatives can treat this problem, but when it occurs, consideration should be given to stopping the treatments or giving them less often.

The most troublesome possible side effects of ECT relate to its effect on memory: about two-thirds of patients report that ECT affects their memory, at least temporarily. The most common memory problem is with *visuo-spatial* memory, the type needed to get places and find things. In a famous article in the *British Journal of Psychiatry,* a practicing psychiatrist who received a course of ECT to treat depression wrote of his experiences and noted that after his course of treatments, he could no longer remember how to get where he needed to go using the London Underground (the subway).[3] He suddenly found that he had forgotten where the different lines went and needed to consult route maps even for routine trips that he had taken for years. After a time, everything became familiar again, and he was knowledgeable enough about what was going on to find the whole thing amusing rather than worrisome (or at least that's what he wrote in the article). If patients are not prepared to expect this possible side effect, they can be quite alarmed when they return home and find their house oddly unfamiliar or find that they can't put their hands on their favorite frying pan or remember where in the world those darn hedge-clippers are. The experience of the English psychiatrist is a reminder that being forewarned and prepared for these potential problems is important so that if and when they occur, they are not so frightening.

Another type of memory loss sometimes seen with ECT affects the memory of events occurring during the several weeks when the patient was receiving ECT. Since treatments are typically given three times a week and a patient usually needs six to twelve treatments for complete recovery, a course of ECT will last two to four weeks. Patients not infrequently lose the memory of some events that occurred during those weeks. Patients sometimes also suffer *retrograde amnesia* as well: memory loss for a period of time before they actually started ECT. This is thought to occur because ECT somehow disrupts the process by which shorter-term memories become incorporated into longer-term memory. (If you've ever lost an hour's worth of computer work because you failed to save your work before something untoward "froze" your computer, you get the idea of what retrograde amnesia is. The short-term memories that are still in the brain's memory "buffer" are lost because of the ECT.) Patients who have successfully completed a course of ECT may say they don't remember checking in to the hospital, or they might not recollect a home visit or a trip they took with their family during the treatments. This problem seems to be worst just after a patient receives ECT. In a study of forty-three patients who were interviewed about their memory a few weeks after completing ECT, some reported difficulty remembering events for a period up to two years before their ECT. But when these patients were tested again seven *months* after their treatment, the more distant memories had been almost completely recovered.[4]

As you might suspect, these kinds of memory problems are almost impossible to pick up on tests, and so despite many years of memory research on ECT patients, it has been difficult to quantify precisely the effect of ECT on long-term memories. Another factor that confuses the issue is the effect that severe depression has on memory. Several studies indicate that complaints of memory problems after ECT correlate better with the severity of the patient's depression than with how they do on memory tests.[5]

ECT FOR BIPOLAR DISORDER

Electroconvulsive therapy can be thought of as a symptomatic treatment for both phases of bipolar disorder: although it can quickly interrupt an episode of depression or mania, it does not have a long-term effect as a mood stabilizer (a *symptomatic* treatment treats *symptoms* but not the underlying disease). Medication treatment will still be necessary to sustain the benefit of ECT and to keep the patient's mood state stable after the treatments are finished.

Typically, when the decision is made to give a course of ECT, medications are stopped or their doses reduced. (Sedative medications often shorten and otherwise interfere with the ECT "seizure," and so do the anticonvulsant mood stabilizers—they are anticonvulsants, after all. Lithium seems to make patients more prone to episodes of confusion after their treatments.)

ECT is generally considered to be the most effective antidepressant treatment available. Naturally, it should be a treatment consideration whenever a bipolar patient continues to be severely depressed despite antidepressant medication treatment. It is also *rapidly* effective. Often, patients are dramatically improved after just three or four treatments—that is, after five to seven days. Severely suicidal patients or those who have stopped eating and drinking and are in danger of malnutrition and dehydration—any patients for whom profound depression has become an imminently life-threatening illness—are candidates for ECT. Pregnancy is also considered to be an indication for use of ECT to treat bipolar depression because of the risk most mood-stabilizing medications pose to the fetus.[6] Because depression can be highly resistant to antidepressant medications and also risky in some elderly patients, ECT is frequently recommended as a first-line treatment for severe depression in older people as well. Depressed bipolar patients who receive ECT can become slightly hypomanic. When this occurs, obviously it's time to stop the treatments. Unlike the antidepressants, ECT does not seem to increase the cycling of the illness.[7]

ECT is also a highly effective treatment for mania. A 1994 review of fifty years' experience of the use of ECT for treating mania found that it provided complete symptom remission or marked improvement in 80 percent of the manic patients studied. Many of the patients in these studies had failed to respond to many other available treatments—making this success rate all the more impressive.[8] ECT seems to work more quickly in mania than in depression. One study found that patients recovered after an average of six treatments, about half the usual requirement for the treatment of depression.[9] Severely manic patients whose highly agitated state becomes physically dangerous are obvious candidates for ECT, as are pregnant manic patients.

ECT is a valuable therapeutic tool for any bipolar patient who is very sick and seems to be getting sicker despite aggressive treatment with medication. It is perhaps the most effective treatment there is for severe depression and severe mania, and it often works more quickly than medications.[10] If you're beginning to wonder why ECT isn't used more often in bipolar disorder, you're in very good company. It is certainly much more complicated to go through general anesthesia two or three times a week for two to four weeks than it is to take medication, but ECT may well still be underutilized, especially for patients sick enough to need hospitalization. We also know that bipolar depression can be less responsive to medication treatment, and there is the risk of antidepressants accelerating the cycling of bipolar illness. These facts make the use of ECT for severe bipolar depression even more compelling.

Transcranial Magnetic Stimulation

Transcranial magnetic stimulation (TMS) is a new therapeutic technique similar to ECT that is effective in treating mood disorders. The great advantage of TMS over ECT is that TMS is much simpler to administer: no seizure activity is induced by the treatment, and therefore no anesthesia is necessary.

This novel technique takes advantage of a principle of electromagnetism called *induction* to deliver an electrical stimulus to the brain without applying electrical energy to the scalp (as in ECT). During TMS treatments, a magnetic coil is held against the scalp, and the magnetic field that develops in the coil causes electrical current to flow through nearby neurons within the skull. No electricity passes through the skull, as in ECT; rather, the magnetic field "induces" a tiny electrical current in the underlying brain tissue. Since the electrical current that is generated in the brain tissue by TMS is very small, no seizure occurs; thus, no anesthesia is needed. Pulses of magnetic energy are delivered over a period of about twenty to forty minutes while the patient simply sits in a chair, awake and alert throughout the whole procedure. Other than some soreness from muscle stimulation, there appear to be no side effects of any kind.[11]

TMS has been used for years to do brain mapping. The mapping of motor areas of the brain involves stimulating an area and then measuring electrical activity in the muscles controlled by that area. Stimulating a sensory area of the brain can cause a person to feel tingling in the part of the body that sends sensory nerves to that area. Sophisticated TMS techniques are also being used to study language functions and the organization of complex movements as well.

It is possible to give a placebo TMS treatment, facilitating valid research on the efficacy of TMS in depression. (A true placebo-controlled study of ECT would require giving two groups of patients anesthesia but giving the electrical stimulus only to patients in one of the groups. Risking anesthesia to receive a fake ECT treatment is something few people would volunteer for, and ethically it is a rather dubious idea.) When the TMS coil is applied to the scalp at a slightly different angle from that normally used to give treatments, it does not cause electrical current to flow through the brain tissue and thus does not have the usual TMS effect. However, because stimulation of the muscles still occurs, the slight muscle soreness associated with the treatment occurs as well, and so research subjects have no way of knowing whether they are getting a sham treatment or the real thing. This makes the all-important double-blind placebo-controlled studies fairly easy to do.

As we shall see in chapter 18, various studies indicate that the left prefrontal lobes of the brain are less active than normal in depression. This finding has led researchers to try TMS treatments on depressed patients by stimulating the left prefrontal lobes. One of the first studies on TMS in the treatment of depression appeared in the *American Journal of Psychiatry* in 1997.[12] In this study from the National Institute of Mental Health, twelve patients received TMS stimulations over a period of twenty minutes every weekday for two weeks. Either before or after the two weeks of therapy, the patients were given two weeks of "sham" treatments (the placebo), during which the TMS coil was held at an angle that would not cause brain tissue stimulation. The patients were tested for depressive symptoms by trained investigators, using a standardized questionnaire. Neither the patients nor the investigators giving the mood questionnaire knew whether the patients were receiving real or sham TMS (making the study *double* blind). There was a statistically significant mood improvement in these patients after the real TMS treatments, but not after the sham treatments. Several patients continued TMS after the completion of the study and experienced further clinical improvement in their depressive symptoms. In several studies, depressed patients with drug-resistant depression have shown improvement after TMS.[13]

TMS is in its infancy. The strength of the magnetic stimulation that is most beneficial, the exact placement of the coil, the number of magnetic impulses delivered per treatment session, the total number of treatments, and the duration of therapy are all under investigation at various centers around the world. Will TMS, like ECT, be effective in bipolar depression as well as in unipolar depression? How about in mania? These and many other questions remain to be answered. It is clear, however, that TMS is a very promising development in the treatment of mood disorders and may open up a whole new array of treatment options.

Vagal Nerve Stimulation

Vagal nerve stimulation (VNS) is another new approach for treating depression that has now been approved by the FDA.

The vagal nerve (or *vagus*) is a long nerve that emerges from the base of the brain and travels down the neck and into the chest and abdomen. It regulates some vital bodily functions such as digestion and heart rate. Its connections in the brain occur through important centers thought to be involved with emotional regulation and specifically with mood regulation. VNS is done by means of a pacemaker-like device that must be surgically implanted; it is connected to the vagus nerve and constantly delivers tiny electrical signals. The connection is made where the nerve travels through the neck, making it a simple surgical procedure that is usually done on an outpatient basis.

Animal studies done as early as the 1930s demonstrated that electrical stimulation of the vagal nerve produced changes in the electrical activity of the brain, and studies in the 1980s demonstrated that VNS could control epileptic seizures in dogs.

In the 1990s VNS became available for the treatment of intractable epilepsy in humans, first in Europe and then in the United States. By the end of 2000, about six thousand patients worldwide had received VNS, almost all of them for the treatment of epilepsy. As with anti-epileptic medications that later turned out to be effective mood stabilizers, VNS was noted to have beneficial effects on mood in several patients who had received it to treat their seizures. Some had substantial antidepressant effects from VNS, even though the treatment didn't improve their seizure control.

In one of the first studies of the VNS treatment of depression, thirty adults received VNS for severe treatment-resistant depression; nine of the patients had a diagnosis of bipolar I or bipolar II disorder. Some of these patients had taken dozens of different medications and undergone ECT, with little benefit. About half of the patients benefited from VNS.[14] In a follow-up study, most of the patients who had shown a response were continuing to do well, and several were found to have experienced continued improvement when they were evaluated after one year of VNS treatment.[15]

Emerging Technologies

Several other methods of delivering small electrical stimuli to areas of the brain are being investigated as possible treatments for mood disorders.

One of these is *deep brain stimulation* (DBS), a technique that has been used since the mid-1990s to treat Parkinson's disease, tremor, chronic pain, and other neurological conditions. Like vagal nerve stimulation, DBS uses electrodes powered by a pacemaker-like device in the chest wall. Unlike VNS, however, the electrodes are implanted directly into deep brain centers. A very invasive neurosurgical procedure is required, and so DBS has been investigated in only a small number of patients with the most treatment-resistant mood disorders, including some with bipolar disorder, but the results have been very promising.

Another investigational treatment is *transcranial direct current stimulation* (tDCS), in which a small electrical current is delivered over a period of time by means of electrodes applied to the surface of the scalp. This technique resembles electroconvulsive therapy in that an electrical current is passed directly through the skull, but the current is much smaller. Whereas the current delivered by an ECT device is usually 800 mA, tDCS devices deliver only 2 mA. As with transcranial magnetic stimulation, the patient can remain awake, simply sitting in a chair, during the treatments, and no anesthesia is required. These treatments, like TMS, last about twenty minutes and are repeated daily for several weeks. A big advantage of tDCS over TMS is that the equipment is much simpler and hence less expensive. Several sham-controlled clinical trials of tDCS have been published, and the results have been very encouraging.

CHAPTER 11

Counseling and Psychotherapy

ALTHOUGH MEDICAL TREATMENTS SUCH AS PHARMACEUTICALS are the foundation of the treatment of bipolar disorder, counseling and psychotherapy are important, perhaps indispensable, additional therapeutic interventions. Some people still picture psychotherapy as something that happens in a richly paneled, dimly lit office where a bearded psychiatrist sits taking notes in a high-backed leather chair behind a patient lying on a couch who is trying to remember what she dreamed about last night. Or perhaps they think of talk-radio therapists, dispensing sound-bite-sized advice to the lovelorn and lonely between car commercials on the AM dial. All of this is psychotherapy of a sort, but the practice of psychotherapy is a serious and well-studied clinical intervention for individuals in psychological distress that requires years of training and experience to master. Many types of counseling and therapy are enormously helpful in bipolar disorder. By reading this book to this point, you've already received several hours of a kind of therapy. You've allowed an objective but sympathetic individual with knowledge and experience about mental illness and psychological processes (that's me) to present facts about bipolar disorder to increase your understanding of the illness. This understanding has, I hope, helped you make sense of your thoughts and feelings about this problem as it affects you. It has also, perhaps, helped prepare you to make decisions based on knowledge rather than on emotions such as fear of or anger about the illness. This is, in large measure, what therapy is all about: not interpreting dreams, not simply doling out advice, and certainly not supplying all the answers, but providing good information, objective feedback, and solid encouragement in a supportive, confidential setting.

Brain and Mind

In chapter 4 I described how manic-depressive illness came to be called a "functional" psychiatric illness in the early twentieth century. After the discovery of the biological causes of mental illnesses, such as general paresis (central nervous system syphilis) and cretinism (mental retardation caused by thyroid deficiency), psychiatric illnesses came to be divided into two categories: *organic* and *functional*. Organic psychiatric illnesses were "real" illnesses, caused by germs or abnormal hormone levels or something else that could be seen under a microscope or measured in a blood test. In functional illnesses, on the other hand, it was assumed that there wasn't anything wrong with the person's brain functioning in a physical sense. Patients with manic-depressive illness or schizophrenia were thought to be having some kind of abnormal reaction to life events.

The question then became, Why do some people have these very abnormal reactions while others with very similar backgrounds and experiences do not? It was at this point that the attempt to understand and treat these illnesses turned away from medicine and toward psychology. Sigmund Freud spent his lifetime treating and trying to understand patients who were unhappy in their relationships, disappointed in themselves for the choices they had made, perhaps confused and anxious about decisions they were facing. Freud and his followers developed a large and sophisticated system for understanding human behavior based on understanding childhood development. Their treatments in essence consisted of helping patients understand themselves better, let go of grudges, resentments, and fears rooted in their past, and learn better, more mature strategies to cope with life's challenges. This approach has come to be called *dynamic* psychology or psychiatry and is based on the belief that mental life is best understood as a dynamic interplay between emotions and intellect, present circumstances and unconscious memories of past experiences, and many other psychological factors.

Although this approach was extremely successful in helping people with a wide variety of problems and symptoms, practitioners of dynamic psychotherapy soon discovered that it didn't make much of an impact on the symptoms of illnesses like schizophrenia or bipolar disorder. Psychological theories arose to explain their symptoms, but these patients were simply considered too intrinsically disturbed or too psychologically stunted or their families too dysfunctional for them to benefit from therapy. This was a dark time for patients with mental illnesses and their families, who in effect were blamed for causing these terrible illnesses in the first place.

Then a revolution occurred: lithium, chlorpromazine, and other effective medications for "functional" illnesses came along. In the 1970s, persons with bipolar disorder and schizophrenia left therapists behind and made tracks for a new kind of doctor: the *biological* psychiatrist, a "pharmacotherapist," someone who would treat them like real people dealing with a "real" illness. For a time there was a kind of schism in American psychiatry between those who believed that dynamic psychology best explained mental illnesses and those who believed that biology was the key that would unlock the mysteries of psychiatric disorders.

When I was interviewing for psychiatric training programs in the mid-1970s, this biological psychiatry–dynamic psychiatry split was at its most pronounced. Many university medical center departments of psychiatry proudly identified themselves to me as either "biological" or "psychodynamic" in their approach. Usually each camp denigrated the other: psychodynamic psychiatry was "touchy-feely" soft science based more on nineteenth-century literary theory than on medicine; biological psychiatrists were "pill-pushers" who didn't even talk to their patients and had no appreciation for the human experience. But a few departments of psychiatry—Johns Hopkins's was one—were teaching their residents that mental experiences were neither a series of chemical reactions nor simply a collection of dynamically interrelated thoughts and feelings, but both. We learned at Hopkins that people with bipolar disorder are still people, still subject to disappointments and loss, to relationship problems and blows to their self-esteem. To regard their moods as just the expression of so many chemicals to be fine-tuned with more chemicals was to do them a great disservice. (Maybe that's how I came to dislike that phrase "chemical imbalance.") Fortunately, this schism has now healed for the most part, and even the most ardent biological psychiatrists realize that psychodynamic understanding of the patient is *always* important. Perhaps the most important development has been the conclusion, now supported by decades of research, that the most effective treatment for persons with mood disorders (and, indeed, most other psychiatric illness) combines *both* approaches, which are now understood to be complementary rather than competing therapeutic approaches.

The variety of available psychological treatments has broadened tremendously in the past twenty-five years or so. Sophisticated techniques have been developed that work for particular kinds of problems. Some involve individual sessions with a therapist, others a group setting. Some are focused on a particular problem, such as marital or family difficulties or addiction, others on a particular symptom, such as depression or panic attacks. Some are designed to last only a few sessions; others are more open-ended. Some are not "therapy" in the traditional sense at all: support groups, made up of individuals who offer guidance and support to each other, don't even include a "therapist." Moreover, a lot of research has been done to determine which psychological treatments work best for which problems. The prescription of a particular kind of counseling or therapy for a particular kind of problem is often backed up by as much research as is the prescription of a particular medication.

What Can Therapy Do?

No one today would even think of recommending counseling or therapy as the only treatment for bipolar disorder; to do so would constitute malpractice. But because we have highly effective medications for this illness, some doctors, and perhaps many more patients, want to turn away from counseling and therapy altogether and approach the illness as a purely "chemical" problem that has a purely "chemical" solution. This is a mistake, for several reasons.

First of all, the diagnosis of bipolar disorder is almost always a traumatic event, not only for patients but for their family members as well. In addition to the emotional turmoil that is the symptom of the illness itself, there is an emotional reeling that results from coming face to face with fears about how this diagnosis will affect one's life. Vaguely familiar terms like *manic-depression* and all-too-familiar terms like *mental illness* conjure up all sorts of confused and confusing ideas and feelings. "Why has this happened to me?" (or perhaps "This *can't* be happening to me!") and "My life will never be the same" and "Whose fault is this?" are only some of the thoughts and questions that start spinning through the minds of people affected by this diagnosis. Remember that I described therapy as "providing good information, objective feedback, and solid encouragement in a supportive, confidential setting." It becomes obvious, doesn't it, that this kind of psychological treatment is going to be necessary and very helpful? Some research suggests that the first year after a diagnosis of bipolar disorder is a crucial time for persons with the disorder and that the education, support, and encouragement that psychotherapy provides are very important in making treatment successful in the long term.[1]

Another traumatic event that persons with bipolar disorder face all too frequently is relapse. The management of bipolar disorder is still far from perfect, and despite everyone's best efforts, relapse can and does occur. Many patients feel that they're "back to square one"; they blame themselves or their medication or their doctor; they become angry, disappointed, discouraged, and confused about what to do next. Again, counseling helps the person put things back into perspective, get over the setback, and move on. I shall discuss individual therapy in more detail later in this chapter.

Group Psychotherapy

Psychotherapy can be very effective in a group setting. The worry I often hear expressed by patients for whom group therapy is recommended is that they don't want to "sit around listening to other people's problems" week after week. But no group therapist worth his salt is going to let the group deteriorate into a "pity party"; instead, he will guide the group members onto the track of learning from, and helping solve, one another's problems—not just ventilating about them. An excellent way to become a better problem solver is to see how other people are solving, or failing to solve, their own problems. By observing and being asked to objectively react to another person's problems, group members learn how to think more objectively, and less emotionally, about their own.

In traditional group psychotherapy, the groups are usually made up of persons with a variety of problems. In the treatment of bipolar disorder, however, *homogeneous* groups (composed exclusively of persons with bipolar disorder) have been studied more and have been shown to be effective. Several studies show that bipolar-disorder patients in group therapy have fewer relapses and improved productivity at work or school.[2] The research suggests that the shared aspect of the problems seems to be very important to the therapeutic experience. Persons with bipolar disorder who are in groups with other bipolar-disorder patients report that the practical advice they receive about living with the disorder is very helpful. Their understanding of the disorder, of how it affects their relationships and self-attitudes, is enhanced, and the guidance they receive from group members is perceived as very valuable.[3] This aspect of group therapy—sharing and learning from one another—is the basis of another type of "therapy," one that doesn't require a therapist: peer support groups. We shall discuss this helping format in chapter 20.

Another psychotherapeutic group approach developed for persons with bipolar disorder is the *psycho-educational group*, which can be thought of as combining more traditional group therapy with a didactic, instructional approach. This kind of group often includes reading materials and discussion questions about bipolar disorder and information about symptoms, about the warning signs of relapse, and about how to better communicate with family members, employers, and co-workers regarding the illness, among other topics. A presentation of facts about the illness or techniques for dealing with it becomes a taking-off point for a discussion of the individual's experiences and using new knowledge to feel better and function more effectively. A study of patients who were "minimally symptomatic" compared how effective attending a psycho-educational group was, compared to receiving individual cognitive behavioral therapy. The researchers found that each treatment improved the patients' functional level and residual symptoms—and the group treatment was much less expensive. For this and other reasons, this approach is gaining favor. Dr. David Miklowitz, who has spent more than a decade investigating the effectiveness of psycho-educational treatment, has even developed a program called "Facilitated Integrated Mood Management" that can be completed in only five sessions.[4] Numerous studies have shown psycho-education to be a valuable adjunct to other treatment approaches to bipolar disorder.

Individual Therapy for Depression

As we saw in earlier chapters, available pharmaceutical treatments for the depressed phase of bipolar disorder are less than perfect by a long shot. The mood stabilizers are not completely effective as antidepressants for some patients, and antidepressant medications carry the risk of precipitating mania or accelerating the frequency of cycles. But psychotherapy has a proven track record in helping with depression and, as far as we can tell, has no risk of precipitating mania or of accelerating the course of bipolar disorder.

"Now wait a minute," I can hear you say, "I've been reading through this entire book that the moods of bipolar disorder are caused by abnormal brain chemistry, and now you want me to believe that psychotherapy can treat the depressive phase of bipolar disorder?" Well, perhaps "psychotherapy can treat the depressive phase of bipolar disorder" overstates the case a bit, but there is some research showing—by implication, at least—that it may be very helpful.

In the 1960s Dr. Aaron Beck and his colleagues developed a theory of depression and psychotherapeutic treatment for it called *cognitive-behavioral therapy,* or CBT for short.[5] This type of psychotherapy has been researched more thoroughly than most others and has a proven track record in helping with symptoms of depression; in some studies—though not in others—it has been found to work as well as antidepressant medication for some patients, or even better.[6]

The theory of cognitive therapy maintains that people who are chronically or frequently depressed have developed a distorted view of themselves and of the world and have adopted certain patterns of thinking and reacting to challenges that perpetuate their problems. This emphasis on thinking, or *cognition,* lends the theory and the therapy its name. As we saw in chapter 1, depressed persons tend (1) to think negatively about themselves, (2) to interpret their experiences in a negative way, and (3) to have a pessimistic view of the future. Cognitive theory calls this the "cognitive triad."[7] The theory further proposes that all this negative thinking causes a person to develop a repertoire of mental habits called "schemas"[8] or "negative automatic thoughts" that spring into action and reinforce the negative thinking.

John is a thirty-two-year-old computer specialist whose idea for a new project has just been turned down by his company. He comes to his therapy session and brings along a lengthy handwritten critique of the project that the senior vice-president of his division left behind after coming by John's cubicle to tell him that the project had been turned down.

"You see, I should have known better than to take on that big a project. The senior vice-president, no less, comes by with the bad news. 'Better luck next time,' she said. Now I'm never going to move up in this company."

"Why do you say that?" I asked.

"If someone that high up thinks I'm incompetent, I'm done for. That's the last time I bother trying something I'm not cut out for."

"Did she say she thought you were incompetent?"

"Well, no, of course not."

"I see. This vice-president doesn't tell people what she thinks."

"Oh, no, that's not true at all. She's got a reputation for coming right out with her opinions about things."

"But she treats you differently from everyone else?"

John began to get a little annoyed. "Well, I wouldn't think so, but how should I know? I'd never talked with her before."

"What do you make of that?" I asked. "The fact that she came in person to give you the news about your proposal?"

"Well, I did think it was unusual."

"Could it mean she was impressed with some aspects of your proposal and wanted to meet you?"

"Well, I suppose that's possible."

I continued reinterpreting John's negative assumptions: "And how about the handwritten critique?"

"It was really negative," John went on glumly. "She went through every point and shot them down one by one."

"When had you sent the proposal to Ms. Kaiser? How long did she have to look at it?"

"Oh, I didn't send it to Kaiser; she's over the whole division. I had sent it to Bob Rodney, my team leader. I guess he sent it up to her, but I don't know how long she spent with it."

"Well, she must have spent several hours with it if she gave you back such a carefully organized critique. Don't you think?"

"Yeah, I guess she wouldn't have taken all that time and trouble if she had thought it was worthless."

"And your team leader must have thought it had some potential if he sent the proposal to *his* boss. Have you asked him for some feedback?"

"No, I assumed he'd be down on me for it, too."

"But do you see how your negative assumption stopped you from checking in with your team leader and prevented you from getting what could have been positive feedback and encouragement from him?"

"I see what you mean. If I hadn't jumped to conclusions, I might have gotten some positive strokes."

John is down on his talents and assumes everybody else is, too. In situations that can be interpreted many different ways, both positive and negative, he tends to go for the negative rather than to seek alternative positive explanations. This in turn sometimes causes him to do things that reinforce his negative thinking, and the vicious cycle repeats itself. This might seem to be a trivial example, but it's not difficult to come up with several negative schemas that people with bipolar disorder are prone to:

Negative: "I got manic even though I was taking my lithium. It doesn't matter what I do. What's the use?"

Realistic: "Relapses occur even with medication. It might have been much worse and lasted much longer if I hadn't been on medication. Perhaps this new medication will be more effective for me."

Negative: "Everyone will be avoiding me when I go back to work. No one wants to work with a mentally ill person."

Realistic: "Some people might avoid me at work, perhaps many at first. But when they see that I'm the same old me, they'll come around. And those who don't are people I don't want as friends anyway."

Cognitive-therapy techniques more specifically focused on bipolar disorder have also been developed. Part of the treatment deals with the negative automatic thoughts that interfere with treatment by medication. For example, if a person with bipolar disorder is troubled by the negative automatic thought "Taking mood-stabilizing medication is a sign of personal weakness" every time she takes a dose of lithium, she might be more likely to skip doses or stop taking the medication altogether. Cognitive therapy works on the psychological barriers to proper treatment by replacing automatic negative thoughts with realistic ones.[9]

Cognitive therapy has been proven to be effective in the treatment of depression. Clearly it cannot replace medication treatment for bipolar disorder, but perhaps more than any other form of psychotherapy, it holds great promise for bipolar patients.

New Psychotherapies for Bipolar Disorder

For many years psychiatrists and the therapists who work with them in treating patients with bipolar disorder have had a sort of intuition that there are fewer relapses among patients who understand their illness and their treatment better, who work on learning to cope better with the stresses and difficulties that everybody faces, and whose family members are also informed and supportive. Psychiatrists have also observed that life stresses, difficult relationships at home, and even disruptions of sleep cycles seem to bring on symptoms and affect the course of the illness. Often, though, they find it hard to persuade patients—and sometimes hard to persuade themselves, perhaps—that a course of traditional psychotherapy is what's needed.

Psychiatrists have done their best to spend time with patients and their families, answering their questions about bipolar disorder and its treatments; trying to persuade patients with marital problems to get marital therapy and patients with job problems to get career counseling; and encouraging them to learn about stress management, watch their sleep habits, and steer clear of conflict and difficult situations whenever possible. But such interventions are time-consuming or expensive (or both), they are difficult to put into practice ("Steer clear of conflict? How do I do *that*, Doc?"), and until recently we have had only the impression that these are important interventions, with little hard data to back up our recommendations.

But now several research teams are developing treatment models of psychological therapy for bipolar patients that draw on these sorts of impressions. The treatment models take into account the available research about the particular kinds of stresses that cause symptoms in bipolar patients, and they incorporate the experiences of clinicians who have treated many, many bipolar patients. Those treatments emphasize issues such as patient and family education about the illness, stress management and conflict resolution, and close attention to the strains in family and marital relationships that are often caused by this illness in even the healthiest family units. These research teams are testing their ideas with well-designed clinical studies, and the results have been very encouraging. One or another or a combination of the therapies they are testing may well become standard recommendations for patients with bipolar disorder in the future.

The treatments in question differ from standard psychotherapy in several ways. Traditional psychotherapy is often unfocused and "exploratory"; the patient and the therapist work on the issues that the patient identifies (for example, "I want to learn to make better choices in my relationships"), and treatment is open-ended: the patient is in therapy as long as he finds it beneficial and has an issue to work on. These new treatments, however, are very focused. The focus varies slightly in the two current models: one focuses on family education and communication and the other on lifestyle regularization and stress management. In both kinds of treatment, the therapist often acts more like a teacher or coach than a counselor, and the goals are to develop concrete solutions to real problems and to learn about and master new problem-solving techniques. Since the patient often doesn't bring "issues" to the therapy, there is a specified time course to the treatment; the main work of the treatment is finished within a certain time period, although there is a maintenance phase that can be indefinite.

Behavioral family management for bipolar disorder emphasizes the patient's family unit. To some extent this model has grown out of research showing that patients with schizophrenia had more illness relapses if there were conflicts and stresses at home and within the family. This therapy works hard at family support. Educating the patient and her family members about the symptoms of bipolar disorder and its treatments is a priority, emphasizing that bipolar disorder is indeed an illness and that its symptoms are not under voluntary control. Family sessions are held to identify difficulties and conflicts within the family unit—whether caused by the illness or by other, perhaps preexisting, factors or situations. Conflict resolution and problem-solving techniques are presented and practiced, and healthy communication skills are developed through role playing and rehearsals.

Interpersonal and social rhythm therapy (IP/SRT) puts more emphasis on patients as individuals and on their "social rhythm." Based on the observation that sleep deprivation and other disruptions of body rhythms can bring on symptoms, this treatment emphasizes stability and stress management. It involves having patients track their mood states on a daily basis and also their daily routine with a sort of checklist of activities called the *social rhythm metric.*

In their sessions the patient and the therapist review these diaries and also the patient's "interpersonal inventory" (a list of the persons in the patient's social network) with an eye toward identifying conflicts and stresses in relationships. The therapist and the patient work on identifying emotional or physical stresses and factors in the environment that upset daily rhythms and emotional stability. The goal is to "find a healthy balance between daily rhythm stability, social activity, social stimulation and mood states."[10] Although it's still too soon to know the impact of IP/SRT on the course of bipolar disorder over time, early results of the research indicate that IP/SRT patients made more healthy lifestyle changes and showed greater stability in daily routines and rhythms than a control group of patients did.[11]

"Traditional" Individual Psychotherapy

I hope I haven't given you the impression that traditional psychotherapy isn't useful for patients with bipolar disorder. Quite the contrary. Kay Redfield Jamison has written: "At this point in my existence, I cannot imagine leading a normal life without both taking lithium and having had the benefits of psychotherapy. Lithium prevents my seductive but disastrous highs, diminishes my depressions . . . and makes psychotherapy possible. But, ineffably, psychotherapy *heals.* It makes some sense of the confusion, reins in the terrifying thoughts and feelings, returns some control and hope and possibility of learning from it all."[12]

So far in this chapter we've talked about "situational" supportive counseling focused on episodes of illness, either the first one or a relapse. The goal of this counseling is to help patients deal with the acute stresses of diagnosis, hospitalization, reintegration back into their job, or other specific issues related to an episode of illness. We've discussed the cognitive therapy of depression, a course of treatment that might be recommended for chronic or smoldering depressive symptoms that medication alone doesn't seem to quite take care of. In the preceding section we discussed some new therapies that aim to teach patients and their families how to smooth out the bumpy spots in their relationships, improve communication and conflict-resolution skills, and regularize their social rhythms. These treatments are perhaps more preventive than the others and might be thought of as providing psychological immunization against future problems as well as ways of dealing with present ones.

What, then, of traditional psychotherapy? By *traditional psychotherapy* I mean individual meetings with a therapist, usually over an extended period of time (months or years), in which the person in treatment discusses his past and present experiences and feelings with the goal of self-understanding, self-acceptance, and personal growth. (*Dynamic* or *insight-oriented psychotherapy* is the same thing.) Disappointments and accomplishments, affections and enmities, fears, inspirations, passions, and worries—all are "grist for the mill" of therapy, as psychotherapists are fond of saying. The patient and the therapist will, of course, talk about symptoms like sadness and anxiety too, but traditional therapy sees symptoms as indicators of underlying psychological conflicts rather than as the focus of treatment in and of themselves. Traditional psychotherapy emphasizes exploration of the *meaning* of symptoms, the development of self-awareness and maturity.

So when would we recommend traditional psychotherapy to a person with bipolar disorder? For what types of problems would it be helpful? Basically, for the same types of problems that people without bipolar disorder go to therapists for: dealing with psychological traumas and setbacks—past and present—that, understandably, cause feelings of sadness, anger, or anxiety, or thought patterns, self-attitudes, and interpersonal styles that disrupt a person's ability to be happy in relationships, effective at work, carefree in play, and confident in making decisions about the future. Sounds like a tall order, doesn't it? Well, of course it is. That is why psychotherapists often study and train in their profession for as many years as physicians train in theirs. That is why people are sometimes in therapy for months or even for years at a time. That is why psychotherapy is such an intense, powerful experience and the therapeutic relationship between patient and therapist a unique one.

Bipolar patients often have had more than their share of setbacks and psychological traumas—both past and present. Persons with bipolar disorder, because it is a genetic illness, often have had difficult, even traumatic childhoods. Perhaps a parent was afflicted with the illness, perhaps the parent could not or would not receive proper treatment, and the child may have suffered disruptions to family life, periods of poverty or homelessness, or even physical or emotional abuse. Psychotherapy can be enormously beneficial in helping people face and work through their difficult pasts, let go of the anger, resentment, and fear that often comes out of these experiences, and move on with their lives.

The fact that a person has bipolar disorder can make ordinary life decisions seem complex and important life decisions seem overwhelming. There is no better way of dealing with these sorts of anxieties and apprehensions than traditional psychotherapy. I remember a young woman who came to see me for a routine medication-monitoring appointment when I was working in the very busy medication clinic of a community mental-health center, a clinical setting in which patients were scheduled every twenty minutes. "I've been dating a man for several months now, and I think he might ask me to marry him," she told me. She looked worried. "I haven't told him about my illness. I don't know what to tell him. How do you think I should handle this?" I stared at her helplessly for a moment and panicked just a little when I heard the nurse slipping the chart of the next patient into the bin outside the interviewing-room door. I hope I didn't sound as rushed as I felt when I tried to convince her that the situation raised an enormous number of complex issues. Adequately dealing with the questions of how, when, where, why, and with whom she discussed her diagnosis was going to need much more than one—or a dozen—twenty-minute appointments with me.

I doubt very much that this was the first time this young woman had been confused about what to tell someone about her diagnosis. Perhaps she had muddled through other situations at work, at church, or in her neighborhood, maybe saying nothing about her diagnosis because of feelings of shame, or maybe blurting out too much about herself and then feeling vulnerable and exposed. Perhaps being diagnosed with bipolar disorder reactivated feelings she had struggled with in childhood or adolescence about being teased for being too fat or too skinny—or perhaps, more likely in a bipolar patient, for being "hyper" or "weird." I was sure that since we had discussed the fact that bipolar disorder is a genetic illness, a possible marriage proposal raised questions in her mind about having children who might be affected by the disorder. How had the diagnosis affected her identity as a potential parent, as a woman? Or perhaps none of these issues needed to be explored but instead other, completely different ones. Well, all these issues are what good old-fashioned once-a-week "How do you feel about that?" psychotherapy is all about.

Psychotherapy in Bipolar Disorder: Is It Really Necessary?

All the psychiatrists I know talk about how much time they spend trying to persuade their bipolar patients to supplement their medication treatment with some form of therapy. There are many reasons why persons with bipolar disorder are reluctant to do so. Some patients have made uneasy peace with taking medication for a psychiatric illness (or, as they might say to themselves, for a "chemical imbalance"), but they see going to psychotherapy as confirmation of the "mental" aspect of their "mental illness." But if you think about it, the treatment of even the most "medical" of medical illnesses—heart disease, say, or a ruptured lumbar disk—usually requires nonmedical interventions, and sometimes these turn out to be just as important as the pharmaceutical or even surgical interventions prescribed by the doctor. The patient with diabetes would hardly regard staying on a healthy diet and watching her weight as unnecessary adjuncts to the insulin injections she receives. The recovering coronary-bypass surgery patient wouldn't ignore the physician's recommendation for a cardiac-hardening exercise program. Would anyone have an operation for lumbar disk problems and skip the physical therapy sessions afterward? I don't think so.

We know that chronic psychological stresses make a whole variety of physical illnesses more difficult to treat: asthma, high blood pressure, irritable bowel syndrome. Psychological stresses will make mood-disorder symptoms more difficult to control as well.

The research results on the psychotherapeutic treatments of bipolar disorder aren't all in, so we can't yet specify particular therapies for a particular duration of time for particular mood syndromes. But the available research and many years of clinical experience indicate that psychotherapy and counseling have been enormously helpful to countless patients with bipolar disorder. If a particular type of therapy or counseling is available, is affordable, and has been recommended by the physician or treatment team, persons with bipolar disorder owe it to themselves to take advantage of the unique healing powers of these marvelous therapeutic techniques.

The Psychiatrist-Psychotherapist: An Extinct Species?

You have probably noticed that I have been referring to the psychiatrist and the psychotherapist as two different individuals. Unfortunately, most patients in America do not find one person serving both functions. It would, of course, be preferable for all sorts of reasons for the person prescribing medication and the person doing psychotherapy to be one and the same individual. But for a variety of complicated reasons, most people with bipolar disorder will see a psychiatrist for medication management and a nonphysician therapist—often a social worker or psychologist—for therapy. Some of the reasons for this state of affairs are the changes in medication management of bipolar disorder that have come about with the development of new medications; there are now so many different pharmaceuticals used in psychiatry that staying skilled in their use has become more and more time-consuming. Perhaps even more significantly, as more and more effective medications become available for more psychiatric problems, more and more patients want (and need) to see a psychiatrist for their treatment. There simply aren't enough psychiatrists to do both medication management and therapy, especially in busy clinics. Since medical school and psychiatric training take longer and cost more than the training required to become a psychotherapist, psychiatrists are usually more expensive than other professionals. When the administrator of a busy clinic or Health Maintenance Organization (HMO) is looking to staff the organization's mental-health program, "split" treatment—psychiatric treatment split between a psychiatrist for medication management and a nonphysician therapist for psychotherapy or counseling—means more cost-effective treatment for patients.

The superior cost-effectiveness of "split" treatment allows so many more patients to receive psychiatric treatment so much more cheaply that it's difficult to envision a return to the days when psychiatrists did therapy and prescribed medications, too. Fortunately, there are excellent training programs for clinical social workers, psychologists, and counseling professionals that are producing superb psychotherapists. And as we have seen in this chapter, psychotherapy is becoming more specialized, too. It has become nearly impossible to be an expert therapist and at the same time an expert psychopharmacologist. For all of these reasons, the medication management and the therapy of the person with bipolar disorder will usually be handled by two professionals rather than one.

CHAPTER 12

Treatment Approaches
in Bipolar Disorder

THE CAUSES OF BIPOLAR DISORDER REMAIN UNKNOWN. TREATMENT approaches have been stumbled upon more or less by accident—for example, the discovery of the therapeutic effects of lithium—and although they have been refined by decades of experience, they are still largely what physicians call *empirical.* This means that the treatment is based on accumulated clinical experience rather than on a true understanding of the mechanism of the disease or symptom in question.[1]

Therapeutic Results as a Guide to Treatment

Although we have a tremendous amount of experience in the use of pharmaceuticals to treat bipolar disorder and have data on their effectiveness in large groups of patients, the treatment of individual patients with the illness is often guided by treatment results rather than by the kinds of hard data physicians use to treat other illnesses. What do I mean by this? Let me explain by looking at a very different kind of illness, pneumonia.

A young man is rushed to the emergency room with a high fever, a pain in his chest, difficulty breathing, and a congested cough. The doctor orders a chest x-ray. A specimen of the young man's sputum is rushed off to the laboratory, and a tiny droplet is spread on a microscope slide, immersed in a special dye called a Gram stain, and examined under the microscope. More tiny droplets are spread over the surface of several flat dishes (petri dishes) containing mixtures of proteins and other nutrients that are known to cause various bacteria to grow. On one of the dishes are a some little paper disks that have been soaked in different antibiotics.

The lab results start coming in. The young man's chest x-ray shows that one of the lobes of his right lung is filled with fluid. The Gram stain reveals that his phlegm is loaded with bacteria aligned in pairs and linked into short chains: the pneumococcus. The diagnosis is clear: pneumococcal pneumonia. The doctor starts the young man on penicillin, an antibiotic known to be effective against most strains of pneumococcus, and within eight hours his fever is dropping. The dose of penicillin and the length of time the young man will need to take it have been determined by years of experience, calculated to the milligram and to the hour.

In a day or so the lab reports that the petri dish containing the pneumococcus's favorite food is full of colonies of bacteria that other, more sophisticated techniques now definitely confirm as pneumococcus. The best news of all is that in the dish containing the little disks of antibiotics, there is a wide, clear halo around the penicillin disk: the penicillin is inhibiting the growth of the strain of bacteria causing this particular case of pneumonia. The young man does not have a pneumonia caused by a penicillin-resistant bug. Thus, his speedy recovery is assured.

The doctor treating this young man had quite a bit of hard data on which to base her treatment decisions. The x-ray indicated that this was probably a typical bacterial lobar pneumonia rather than viral pneumonia, tuberculosis, or any of the various other conditions with similar symptoms but that look different on x-ray images. Also—and very important for prognostic purposes—the x-ray showed that only one lobe was involved. With the results of the Gram stain, the likely identity of the bacterial culprit was determined within minutes, allowing the quick choice of a drug known to be effective most of the time against this type of germ. The identity of the bacterial culprit was solidly confirmed several days later when it grew in the culture dish and could be further tested. Most important, the lab results showed exactly which drugs would work against the germ causing the problem in this particular patient.

In contrast, when a patient with manic symptoms comes into the ER, there are no tests to order—just the eyes and ears and experience of the psychiatrist. Fortunately, or perhaps unfortunately, full-blown mania often leads to an unmistakable diagnosis, and effective antimanic drugs are readily available. But what of the person who comes to the office and says, "I'm depressed," or complains of "mood swings." There are many more diagnostic possibilities. We know that antidepressant medications can sometimes make a patient with bipolar symptoms worse. How is a physician to know whether or not a person who comes in with symptoms of depression will turn out to have a bipolar illness? There are hints, of course, such as family history, but wouldn't it be fantastic if we could order a test for bipolar disorder before considering an antidepressant for a person who is having symptoms of depression? But we can't.

How about the treatment, once the acute symptoms of mania have been controlled? Emil Kraepelin described some patients who had remission of their bipolar symptoms that lasted for decades (it was apparently quite rare for this to happen, but he observed them, nevertheless). Do we prescribe a mood stabilizer for a patient who might not get sick again for ten or even twenty years? Wouldn't it be great if we could stop the medication after a period of time and have the patient come in every couple of months for some kind of scan that could pick up changes in brain functioning before symptoms became apparent? That way the patient would take medication only as it became necessary. Sometimes patients respond to one mood stabilizer but not another, or to a combination of two mood stabilizers but not to either one when used alone. How to choose? Wouldn't it be fantastic if we could take a blood sample and look for some kind of chemical reaction around little paper disks soaked with lithium or Prozac in a petri dish to help us choose effective medications for a particular patient?

At the present moment, we don't have any blood tests, scans, or other laboratory tests to make the treatment approach to bipolar disorder as informed and logical as our approach can be in many other illnesses (although this, fortunately, may change in the not-too-distant future—more on this later).

Because we do not yet understand the causes of bipolar disorder, the medical approach to the treatment of the illness can be discussed only in general terms. Patients are started on one of the medications that have proved effective in many other patients with similar symptoms, and if these patients' symptoms are not effectively treated, other interventions are tried. We can't yet pick from among similar medications knowing beforehand which one of them will work best. There is unfortunately a lot of "trial and error" and "wait and see" when it comes to prescribing medications for a specific patient. This can be tremendously frustrating for all involved—for the patient, of course, and for family members, and, yes, for the physician, too.

But the good news is that more and better medications are becoming available all the time. Twenty-five years ago there was only one mood-stabilizing medication, lithium. Ten years ago there were three. Now we have at least five and several more on the way. There are easily twice as many antidepressants on the market as there were only fifteen years ago. The newer antipsychotic medications have fewer side effects and also have mood-stabilizing properties that the older agents lacked. As of this writing, there are medications being developed that have entirely different mechanisms of action than currently available medications. Even more options are on the horizon.

Electroconvulsive therapy is one of the most effective treatments for mood disorders and one of the safest medical procedures available—and it is probably underutilized in bipolar disorder. Transcranial magnetic stimulation and other brain-stimulation treatments may come to replace ECT (and perhaps even medications) if they are able to deliver what they seem to be promising.

Don't forget counseling and psychotherapy. Research has proved how very important this unique treatment is in controlling the symptoms of mood disorders. More effective therapy programs for bipolar disorder are being refined by researchers with studies that are as rigorous as those used to evaluate any pharmaceutical.

And I haven't even talked about light therapy and sleep manipulation yet (those are coming in chapter 16). Researchers have discovered that exposure to bright light and changes in sleep patterns can help regulate mood and perhaps help medications work better and faster.

Some Principles of Treatment

Now and then, one of the medical journals publishes a "treatment algorithm" for an illness or disorder. An algorithm is a step-by-step procedure for solving a specified problem with mathematical precision. A treatment algorithm for acute mania might look something like this:

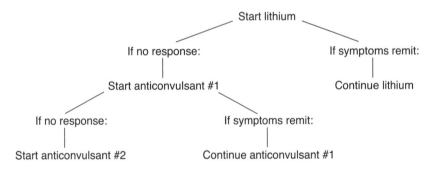

Well, you get the idea. I don't find treatment algorithms helpful in treating individual patients except in a very general way. Their "if this happens, then do that" approach never captures the myriad manifestations of the disorder and the inevitable twists and turns of the world of real treatment and real patients, not to mention the specific situations and needs of the individual. Between 1999 and 2005, a major clinical trial that included more than four thousand patients was carried out to attempt to address these complexities. Although it did include an algorithm (several of them, in fact), one of the main purposes of the study was to investigate how "real world" patients, as opposed to carefully selected patients with uncomplicated illness, would do when given treatment based on using "best practice" evidence-based approaches. This was the STEP-BD (the Systematic Treatment Enhancement Program for Bipolar Disorder) that I discussed in chapter 7.[2] The STEP-BD generated more than sixty scientific papers on every aspect of the treatment of bipolar disorder and also on the course of the illness, common complications, the prognosis, and even genetics. The STEP-BD confirmed the effectiveness of many accepted approaches to the treatment of bipolar disorder but also called into question some equally accepted approaches (the most important of these being the significant doubt that the STEP-BD cast on the effectiveness of antidepressant medications in treating bipolar patients). Much of this chapter is based on findings of the STEP-BD; I will review some of the principles of treatment that serve patients (and their physicians) well.

TINCTURE OF TIME

With so many powerful and effective medications available in psychiatry now, it's easy to become impatient when symptoms don't subside as quickly as one would wish. But in the treatment of mood disorders, a crucial principle to remember is to *take the long view.*

The medications we use to treat mood disorders usually take at least two to four weeks to even begin helping, and sometimes much longer to have their full effect. One of my mentors, to drive home just this point, is fond of telling his patients, "The *second* year on lithium is always better than the first." When treating an episode of bipolar disorder, it simply doesn't make sense to change medications quickly. Even hospitalized patients are rarely well served by adding too many medications too quickly—patients simply wind up taking more medications than they need and at higher doses than may be necessary.

When a diagnosis of bipolar II or cyclothymic disorder is being considered, the time line should stretch out even more. The mood changes in these variations of bipolar disorder can sometimes be much more subtle than those of bipolar I. It may take three to six months of taking a mood stabilizer for its beneficial effects on a subtly unstable mood to become apparent.

I saw Craig about two weeks after he had been discharged from a hospital in another city. He had been on a business trip and started to have fairly severe manic symptoms: insomnia, racing thoughts, angry irritability. He had been having good control of his symptoms on a mood stabilizer, but a series of high-stress job interviews in several different cities, jet lag, worry, and poor sleep had activated his illness, and he soon found himself hospitalized in a city several hundred miles from home.

He pulled a fistful of medication bottles out of his pocket and put them on the desk in my office. "I brought all these new medicines, but I have to admit, I've only been taking the lithium."

I picked up the bottles one by one: lithium, valproate, an antipsychotic, an anti-anxiety agent, and a sleeping pill.

"How long were you in the hospital?" I asked.

"Eight days."

"And you were discharged on *all* this?"

"That's right. I can't believe I really need all this. I was so drugged when my wife came to pick me up, I couldn't work for another week and a half. I think this is the first day I've felt safe to drive."

Craig's illness had always been very responsive to medications; it was hard for me to believe that all these medications had really been necessary. How had this happened?

When I asked Craig about his treatment in the hospital, a sadly familiar story emerged: a new medication had been added to the mix almost every other day while he was there. He was started on the antipsychotic medication as soon as he was admitted. Well, that wasn't unreasonable; I might have recommended that myself—for a while, at least. But when he didn't sleep well the next night, a sleeping pill was added. A few days later, when he mentioned that he had been worried about his finances lately, an anti-anxiety medication was added. After a week he told his doctor he was feeling less hyper but still not back to his usual self—so the valproate was added to the lithium. By the time he left the hospital, he wasn't complaining of mood problems anymore because he was too sedated to know *what* kind of mood he was in.

"Craig, you know I want you to call the clinic before you make any changes in your medication on your own," I said with a smile. "But I have to admit, in the end you did exactly what I would have recommended that you do. You certainly don't need all this."

Craig smiled back.

In Craig's case it was the doctor who forgot to take the long view, but I think it's probably even easier for patients or their family members to fall into the trap of expecting results too quickly.

"Cindy's still having mood swings, Doctor," Jim said as he sat down beside his wife in the office. "The Lamictal isn't working. Is there something else we can try?"

Jim and Cindy were a couple in their thirties. They had two small children, and Cindy usually cared for her attorney sister's little boy during the day as well as her own children.

Cindy was tense and quiet as her husband continued. "She's been on this medication for two weeks now, and things are no different. She started arguing with me about the television being too loud the other night, and when I tried to reason with her, she picked up the remote control and threw it at me. This has got to stop."

"What do you think, Cindy?" I asked. "Do you think the medication has helped any?"

"Well, I'm not sure, but I think maybe it has."

"Well, I'm sure it hasn't," said Jim. "The night before the remote incident she—"

"Jim," I said, "it's much too early to be sure about anything yet. I know Cindy's been taking the Lamictal for several weeks, but she's been at a full therapeutic dose for less than one week." I turned to Cindy. "What have you noticed that makes you think the Lamictal might be helping?"

"Well, Jim was out of town for a few days last week, and so was my sister. I had the three kids twenty-four hours a day the whole time again. You know how keyed up I got the last time that happened."

In fact it had been a similar situation that had brought Cindy into treatment in the first place. About three weeks before our first meeting, Cindy had been with the three boys, six, five, and three years old, because of coinciding business trips taken by Jim and her sister. She had needed to call Jim and get him to fly back home because she was becoming more and more irritable with the children, snapping at them, slamming doors, starting to feel out of control.

The next week she had come to see me, and as we talked about her past history, it emerged that she had experienced episodes of depression after both of her children were born, that she had had these "hyper" episodes about once a year since college, and that her mother had suffered from "mood swings" and alcoholism. A diagnosis of bipolar II or perhaps a "soft" bipolar disorder seemed likely, and we decided on a trial of a mood stabilizer.

"The kids just didn't get to me this time," Cindy continued. "First I thought they were being on their best behavior because of what had happened that last time, and maybe they were for an hour or so. But by evening I realized that they were really about as active as they usually are, and that there was something different about *me*. I wasn't as, you know, sensitive. Several times now I've noticed that I can handle things better."

"Not the other night," Jim chimed in. "I'm not noticing much difference."

"Well, maybe Jim's right," Cindy went on. "Maybe you could give me something for the times when I'm feeling really stressed? Some Valium or Xanax? I never used . . . I don't know what to call them—nerve pills? And I'm sure I wouldn't need them often."

"I don't think we should add more medication until we're sure you're getting the maximum benefit from the one you're on. And from what you're telling me, I think that's beginning to happen," I said. "The fact that you've never felt the need for tranquilizers before makes me think that the bipolar disorder explains all your symptoms and needs to be the focus of our attention. It's absolutely too early to expect the Lamictal to have had its full effect. Let's talk about this a bit more."

Cindy and Jim are very anxious for Cindy's symptoms to stop. Who can blame them? But to give up on a mood stabilizer because it hasn't completely controlled every symptom so soon is foolish. It's unlikely that another would work any faster—and it might not even work as well, in which case Cindy would be right back to square one after another couple of weeks.

DIAGNOSIS, DIAGNOSIS, DIAGNOSIS

Cindy's situation also serves to illustrate another principle of treatment: *remember the diagnosis*. If the three most important words in the real estate business are *location, location,* and *location,* then the three most important words in medicine are *diagnosis, diagnosis,* and *diagnosis*. Because we have so many effective medications, it can be tempting to consider prescribing one even though there isn't really a justification for it based on the patient's underlying diagnosis. There was a tendency at one time in psychiatry to see medications as *symptomatic treatments*. This means picking a medication and making the decision to use it based on identification of *symptoms,* not underlying *diagnoses*. Cindy wants to try another medication for "stress"—that is, for feeling tense and irritable. But the symptoms of our working diagnosis, bipolar disorder, include periods of tension and irritability. If Cindy's poor stress tolerance is a symptom of her mood disorder, and she takes an anti-anxiety medication to cover it up rather than getting more intensive treatment of the mood disorder, she'll end up taking a medication she doesn't really need for a symptom that isn't going to get much better because the underlying problem, bipolar disorder, isn't being properly treated. Insomnia is a similar symptom, very commonly a symptom of the mood disorder but all too commonly treated with sleeping medications as if it were an isolated symptom.

Every once in a while I see a patient with bipolar disorder who has read a magazine article about attention-deficit hyperactivity disorder and requests medication for ADHD. Some of the symptoms of ADHD—like impulsivity; impatience; fast, disorganized thinking; and poor concentration—are, of course, also seen in bipolar patients. These are distressing symptoms that deserve attention, but they deserve the right kind of attention. If they are an expression of the mood changes of bipolar disorder, then medication for ADHD won't help. (In fact, the medications used to treat ADHD, stimulants and antidepressants, can make things worse.)

Making a diagnosis is the process of identifying the one disease that can explain all the patient's symptoms. This is a variation of the scientific principle called Occam's razor, named after William of Occam (or Ockham), the medieval theologian-philosopher credited with coining this principle: The simplest explanation for a phenomenon is always preferable to a more complex one and is most likely to be correct. Obviously a patient may have two different disorders that require two different treatment approaches. But if all the patient's symptoms can be understood as expressions of *one* disorder, treating that one will likely alleviate all the symptoms.

I see this problem of multiple diagnoses and symptomatic treatments even more commonly in depressed patients. In depression, anxiety and insomnia can be thorny and uncomfortable expressions of the mood disorder—and physical symptoms can be as well, especially in the elderly. I have seen elderly patients taking antidepressant medications (often at an inadequate dose) who are also taking sleeping pills, tranquilizers, anti-inflammatory and pain medications for arthritis pain, stool softeners and laxatives for constipation, and sometimes some vitamins and tonics thrown in for good measure (perhaps because of complaints of "low energy"). All these problems are symptoms of depression (even the arthritis pain, because depressed patients become more distressed by painful problems like arthritis), but sometimes it's hard to see the forest for the trees. Before you know it, the patient is taking a dozen or so different medications for all the different symptoms of depression, and the disease that underlies them all, a mood disorder, has been missed. It is an amazing experience to see all these symptoms that have not been helped by perhaps a dozen medications disappear after a course of electroconvulsive therapy in an elderly patient.

THE ROLE OF ELECTROCONVULSIVE TREATMENT

This leads me to another principle: *ECT should not be a treatment of last resort for bipolar disorder.* ECT should be considered whenever symptoms are very severe, or when they are severe enough to interfere with work and family life and have gone on for an extended period of time. Some geriatric psychiatrists recommend ECT as the *first-line treatment* for serious mood-disorder symptoms in the elderly. If the patient is having symptoms day after day, has been on medical leave from work for weeks, and is still not getting relief from his medication, it's time to seriously consider ECT. When symptoms are disabling, ECT should probably be considered after the failure of the first medication, not after the failure of the second or third or fourth.

WHAT IS THE ROLE OF ANTIDEPRESSANTS IN BIPOLAR DISORDER?

Perhaps the most unexpected finding to come out of the STEP-BD was the surprising lack of evidence that antidepressant medications are helpful in treating bipolar disorder. One of the studies within the STEP-BD compared depressed patients treated with a mood stabilizer plus an antidepressant (either sertraline or bupropion) with patients treated with a mood stabilizer and a placebo. The main patient-outcome goal for this part of the study was "durable recovery" from depression, defined as maintaining a normal mood for at least eight weeks. Using this standard, antidepressants were no more effective in these bipolar patients than the placebo (the patients taking the antidepressant with their mood stabilizer did no better than those who took only a mood stabilizer). Not only that: when some secondary measures were assessed, there was the suggestion that the patients on mood stabilizer alone did somewhat *better* than the patients who took an antidepressant. For example, it appeared that depressed patients with bipolar II disorder actually did a bit better *without* the antidepressant. Furthermore, as a follow-up to the placebo-controlled study, the patients who *did* recover and who were taking the antidepressant with their mood stabilizer were divided into two groups: one group continued on both medications, and the other group stopped taking the antidepressant. Again, the group that stopped taking the antidepressant did just as well as those who did not: taking an antidepressant did not keep patients well longer and did not delay a relapse, compared with taking a mood stabilizer alone. Although it did not reach the level of statistical significance, there was also the suggestion that patients who had rapid-cycling symptoms (several episodes of mania or depression in a year) had a relapse of depression *sooner* than those who stopped taking the antidepressant: that is, continuing on an antidepressant increased the risk of getting depressed. Talk about counterintuitive!

It has been known for many years that antidepressants can trigger manic or mixed symptoms in bipolar patients. Clinicians have also long suspected that antidepressant medications increase cycling in bipolar patients, causing them to have more episodes of depression and manic or mixed symptoms.

The STEP-BD appears to reinforce both of these impressions. However, every psychiatrist cares for patients with bipolar disorder who can safely take an antidepressant and who require it to stay well.

So what should we conclude about the use of antidepressant medications in bipolar patients? I think it's fair to say that antidepressants should be used with extreme caution in patients with bipolar disorder, and that an antidepressant should be discontinued as soon as possible over the longer term of treatment. Antidepressants should be stopped immediately if the patient develops insomnia or feels overactivated or "wired" after she starts taking an antidepressant. I have had patients describe this as feeling "anxious," and while it may be a feeling that is similar to anxiety, when I see a bipolar patient taking an antidepressant who reports severe "anxiety," I have a very low threshold for stopping the antidepressant.

Sometimes there don't seem to be any immediate untoward effects from starting an antidepressant, but it may become clear over time that the patient is cycling more often. If, in the months (or even years) after a patient starts taking an antidepressant, he notices *new* mood symptoms, such as mixed symptoms or problems with "rages" for the first time, the continued use of the antidepressant should be seriously questioned.

DON'T FORGET PSYCHOTHERAPY

Finally, I can't stress enough that *every bipolar patient needs psychotherapy* at one point or another. Several weeks or months of counseling is absolutely essential after the diagnosis and initiation of treatment for bipolar disorder. Just as a person with diabetes needs to follow dietary recommendations to get the best control of her glucose levels, and a hip-fracture patient needs physical therapy for optimal functioning, persons with bipolar disorder need psychotherapy at times to have the best possible control of their mood symptoms.

Psychotherapy is one intervention for the depression of bipolar disorder that I can confidently state does *not* have any risk of triggering manic symptoms or increased cycling. Many persons with bipolar disorder go through a period of depression after they recover from a period of mania or hypomania. It can be very tempting to think about using an antidepressant to deal with this problem. For the reasons noted above, however, this is not usually a good idea. During some periods of bipolar depression, the intervention that needs to be started, or given at a higher "dose," is psychotherapy.

PART III

VARIATIONS, CAUSES, AND CONNECTIONS

In this group of chapters we'll explore several variations on the theme of bipolar disorder. We'll look first at how the course and symptoms of the illness can differ in children and adolescents and then note the differences in symptoms between men and women (with special attention to premenstrual mood symptoms, the challenge of postpartum mood disorders, and the dilemmas faced by women who have the illness during their childbearing years).

Chapter 15 deals with the complicated relationships between bipolar disorder and substance abuse. Individuals with bipolar disorder seem to be especially vulnerable to substance-abuse disorders, so much so that it's reasonable to think of chemical dependency as a complication of the illness. The symptoms of substance abuse and of bipolar disorder can become so intertwined that it is impossible to figure out which is which. We'll look for a way out of this confusion and discuss the treatment approaches that work in such cases. It's extremely important to confront chemical dependency head on, because research shows that alcoholism and drug abuse are often *fatal* complications of bipolar disorder.

In the subsequent chapters, we'll go from one extreme to the other as far as causes and connections are concerned, looking first at some very concrete scientific issues and then at some very abstract, almost philosophical ones. In chapter 16 we'll learn about our body's biological clock and the relationship between mood and the sleep cycle and about the seasonal cycles some persons with bipolar disorder have. In chapter 17 we'll explore an area of intense interest to bipolar patients and their family members: the genetics of bipolar disorder. Chapter 18 considers other aspects of bipolar biology: how mood disorders can be caused by medical illnesses, some of the ways we are able to literally look at bipolar disorder in the functioning brain, and, finally, the possible connections between bipolar disorder and viruses.

Then, after we've finished talking about DNA molecules and chromosomes and brain chemicals, we'll leave the laboratory and go into the artist's studio, to examine some of the intriguing connections between this terrible illness and artistic genius and creativity.

CHAPTER 13

Bipolar Disorder in Children and Adolescents

FOR MANY YEARS BIPOLAR DISORDER WAS THOUGHT TO BE EXTREMELY rare in young people, even though research data on adults indicated that the first appearance of the symptoms of the illness usually occurred before age twenty. (Emil Kraepelin found that the highest number of "first attacks" of manic-depressive illness occurred between the ages of fifteen and twenty.) Perhaps because of a reluctance to diagnose children with an illness known to be a lifelong problem and the unwillingness to prescribe for children the powerful medications used to treat its symptoms, bipolar disorder in young children received little attention from researchers until quite recently.

Recent research suggests that bipolar disorder is much more common in young people than previously recognized. In 2011 the World Health Organization estimated that pediatric bipolar disorder is the fourth leading cause of disability in adolescents aged fifteen to nineteen worldwide, accounting for a total of 5 percent of disability in this age range.

For a long time, the treatment of children and adolescents with bipolar symptoms consisted mostly of improvised variations on adult treatments. Fortunately, this too is changing; there is now quite a bit of research available to guide the clinician in crafting a treatment plan for young patients with bipolar disorder.

Even very young children can have bipolar symptoms. In one study that looked at such symptoms in the pediatric (under eighteen) age range, nearly one-third of the patients were younger than twelve, and the average age of onset for these young bipolar patients was eight and a half.[1] This same re-

TABLE 13-1 Comparison of adult and pediatric bipolar disorder

	Pediatric	Adult
Initial episode:	Major depression	Mania
Episode type:	Rapid cycling, mixed	Discrete episodes
Duration:	Chronic, continuous	Weeks
Functioning between episodes:	Poor (continuous cycling)	Improved

search is also shedding light on why psychiatrists used to think pediatric bipolar disorder was a rare diagnosis: although adolescents with bipolar disorder have symptoms similar to those of adults, bipolar disorder in young children can appear rather different (table 13-1).

It appears that when bipolar disorder occurs in young children (before puberty), it is a more severe form of the illness. Perhaps this is because children who develop symptoms of bipolar disorder at so young an age have a heavier genetic "loading" for mood disorders than do people whose symptoms begin later. Bipolar children often have more individuals with mood disorders in their families than adult-diagnosis bipolar patients; for many of these children, mood disorders exist on both sides of the family.[2] Another difference between childhood- and adult-onset bipolar disorder is that instead of mania or hypomania, a major depression is frequently the first sign of the disorder in children. Several studies indicate that 20 to 30 percent of young children with major depressions develop manic symptoms later in life.[3]

But the most striking difference between childhood-onset and later-onset bipolar disorder is the course of the illness. Pediatric bipolar disorder is a much more continuous illness than adult bipolar disorder. In most adults the illness appears in discrete episodes of depression or mania, and the symptoms go into remission for months or years at a time. Children, in contrast, often have long periods of continuous rapid cycling. These children sometimes cycle between depression and mania several times a day, having a laughing fit one moment and talking about wanting to shoot themselves the next.[4] One study of bipolar disorder in the pediatric age range described children who had more than one hundred minimanias in a year, mood episodes that lasted only a day or two. In this study, none of the research subjects under the age of nine had a single mood episode lasting two weeks or more as his only episode. For these children a complex pattern of frequent, short episodes was the rule, not the exception.[5]

Symptoms of Pediatric Bipolar Disorder

Depression is comparatively easy to spot in children: the weepy, listless, and lethargic child is quickly recognized as a sick child. But how do you distinguish hypomanic or manic behavior in a child from the boisterousness and high energy of normal children? An even more difficult task is to differentiate manic symptoms from the hyperactivity and "can't sit still" picture of attention-deficit hyperactivity disorder (ADHD).

The differentiation is possible if close attention is paid to changes in mood. Children with ADHD are hyperactive but don't have the expansive, grandiose mood of mania. The child with ADHD may disrupt a classroom with clowning around and restlessness, but a manic child may tell the teacher that the lessons are being taught incorrectly and try to take over the class. The manic child caught taking things that belong to someone else may say that it's wrong for other people to steal but not for her. The manic child may be convinced that he is destined for a brilliant career as a doctor or a lawyer despite failing nearly every subject in school. The child may believe that he is on the verge of becoming a rock star despite being unable to play a musical instrument.

Normal children, of course, fantasize in similar ways about their future, but they are able to separate their fantasies from reality and apply themselves to school work and follow the rules at home. Manic children, convinced of the reality of their grandiose ideas, speak and act based on the belief that the usual rules and requirements don't apply to them.

Manic children jump from topic to topic in their speech patterns, are difficult to interrupt, and complain that their thoughts are moving too fast. Hypersexuality is a symptom in older children, who may become sexually promiscuous or masturbate excessively; they may suddenly start using sexual profanity or say that a teacher or a famous person is in love with them. Spending sprees may take the form of ordering items over the phone using 1-800 and 1-900 numbers.

Very young children may have manic exaggerations of the normal magical thinking of childhood but will act on this thinking instead of using it as a basis for play. Normal children may imagine that they can fly and may run through the back yard "flapping" their arms like the wings of a bird or making airplane noises. A manic child under the influence of the delusion that she has become an angel or a superhero may jump out of a window or off the roof of a house. The symptoms of bipolar disorder in children can be every bit as deadly as they are in adults.

When a young person develops serious depression, how can we tell whether he might be having the first episode of what will turn out to be bipolar disorder? Although it's impossible to know for sure, there are some indicators that seem to be fairly reliable. In one study, researchers investigated a group of sixty adolescents, aged thirteen to sixteen years, who had been hospitalized for major depression over the course of three to four years; the purpose was to see whether any particular clinical variables might predict which of them would eventually develop a bipolar course of illness (20 percent of the group eventually did). Statistical analyses showed that bipolarity was predicted by a depressive symptom cluster that included rapid symptom onset, a slowed-down, "retarded" type of depression, and psychotic features (hallucinations or delusions). A family history of mood disorders (bipolar disorder or major depression) in many family members and through successive generations was also a predictor, as was a history of the adolescent developing hypomanic symptoms when she took antidepressant medications—a clinical indicator that turned out to be 100 percent accurate in predicting bipolar disorder in this group.[6]

Bipolar Disorder and Attention-Deficit Hyperactivity Disorder

Psychiatrists use the term *comorbidity* to describe two separate conditions or illnesses that frequently occur together in the same patient. There is a high degree of comorbidity between ADHD and mood disorders, in some studies as high as 75 percent.[7]

Children and young adolescents with bipolar disorder often do not have the discrete periods of elevated, usually euphoric mood seen in older adolescents and adults. Rather, extreme irritability and prolonged aggressive temper tantrums called "affective storms" are common, and the abnormal mood is ongoing and continuous rather than episodic as in older individuals. Distractibility, impulsivity, hyperactivity, and "mood swings" are symptoms of both ADHD and mania. For these reasons, the diagnosis of both mood disorders and ADHD is difficult in young people, and the relationships between the two diagnoses are, at this point, poorly understood.

It is possible to differentiate between the symptoms of ADHD and bipolar disorder in many young people, but there are some individuals who seem to have both disorders simultaneously. In one study of children who had already been diagnosed with ADHD, 21 percent were also found to meet the diagnostic criteria for bipolar disorder by age fifteen—that is, they seemed to have both disorders. This suggests that, in some youngsters at least, ADHD symptoms may in fact be early signs of bipolar disorder. The ADHD children who eventually developed bipolar symptoms had more severe symptoms and more disturbed behaviors than those who did not. Even more of these ADHD children with more severe symptoms met the criteria for a diagnosis of major depression: by age eleven, 29 percent had major depression; and by age fifteen, 45 percent had been diagnosed with major depressive disorder.[8]

How do we understand the children whose ADHD seems to develop into bipolar disorder? Did they really have ADHD symptoms in the first place, or does very-early-onset bipolar disorder mimic ADHD in its early stages? Are ADHD and early-onset bipolar disorder two separate illnesses that share similar symptom pictures but have different causes? Can ADHD develop into bipolar disorder? If so, how? And what do we make of the extremely high comorbidity between ADHD and mood disorder? These questions are, as yet, unanswered.

It has been suggested that the link between the two disorders may be genetic. When family members of ADHD children are studied, they are found to have high rates of mood disorders. Children of parents with mood disorders have high rates of ADHD. The researchers studying the group of young people with ADHD described above investigated the prevalence of mood disorders in family members. They found that relatives of children with both ADHD and bipolar disorder were five times as likely to have bipolar disorder themselves as family members of children with only ADHD. They also found high rates of major depression among the relatives of the children with ADHD and bipolar disorder. The researchers speculate that ADHD with bipolar disorder is a particular subtype of the illness.[9] Or perhaps these are two separate illnesses that happen to be inherited together frequently because the genes that cause them are located near one another on the chromosome and thus are usually inherited together. The only thing about this mysterious connection that we are really sure of is that much research in the area remains to be done.

Treatment and Prognosis

Some studies have indicated that lithium is effective in children, but it is fairly clear that it is not as effective in children as in adults. If complicated rapid-cycling bipolar disorder is indeed the rule in early-onset bipolar disorder, then lithium resistance should not be a big surprise: similar types of bipolar symptoms seem relatively lithium-resistant in adults, too. Pediatric lithium doses are, of course, lower than adult doses, but the effective therapeutic range for lithium in the bloodstream when it does work seems to be about the same in children as in adults. (Remember that the therapeutic range in the bloodstream is a measure of lithium concentration. Because children have a smaller total blood volume than adults, a lower dose of lithium for a child will result in the same concentration in the bloodstream.) Getting regular blood tests done is, of course, more challenging with children than with adults, but given the toxicity of lithium, blood-level tests are if anything even more important in children. Several studies have been done using methods that avoid the needles and determine lithium levels from saliva rather than from blood, but the results have been disappointing, and so for now these little patients must, unfortunately, have blood tests.

Several studies have indicated that valproate is effective for some young children with bipolar disorder, and some have suggested that it is more effective than lithium in this age range. There is now substantial research supporting the use of atypical antipsychotic medications for pediatric bipolar disorder. These agents appear to be more effective than lithium or anticonvulsant mood stabilizers in young patients. Because of these issues, a combination of medications is commonly required to keep pediatric bipolar-disorder symptoms under control.[10]

The combination of ADHD and bipolar disorder seems to be especially difficult to treat, and in those cases especially, combinations of medications are often necessary. In a study of adolescents being treated with lithium for a manic episode, a comparison was made between the treatment response in adolescents with and without a history of childhood-onset ADHD. The adolescents with the ADHD history took significantly longer to get better on lithium than the adolescents with no history of ADHD symptoms. This seems to be further evidence that the combination of ADHD and bipolar disorder may be a subtype of illness and that it is especially challenging to treat.[11]

Many clinicians recommend avoiding stimulant medications completely in young persons with bipolar disorder. The same goes for some other treatments for ADHD, most notably antidepressants. The problem here is the same as with stimulant medications: the possibility of precipitating mania in a predisposed youngster. Another medication used to treat ADHD, atomoxetine (Strattera), has also been reported to precipitate mania. When it was given to an eleven-year-old boy who had been diagnosed with ADHD, had a family history suggestive of bipolar disorder, and had experienced manic-type symptoms from antidepressants, he developed severe manic symptoms.[12]

Clonidine (Catapres) and guanfacine (Tenex), medications used to treat high blood pressure in adults, have been found to be helpful in ADHD. Whereas stimulant medications help with inattention but are not very helpful for impulsivity and hyperactivity, clonidine and guanfacine seem to be effective in reducing these symptoms. There is also very preliminary evidence that medications that affect the neurotransmitter acetylcholine may be helpful for the symptoms of ADHD. Tacrine (Cognex) and donepezil (Aricept), two medications with this therapeutic mechanism that are used to treat Alzheimer's disease in the elderly, have been reported to be helpful for the treatment of ADHD.[13] These alternatives may be safer for youngsters with bipolar disorder who need additional treatment for ADHD.

How is normal psychological development in children affected by bipolar disorder? Relationships with family members are often strained for these patients, as are relationships with their peers. Their educational development inevitably suffers as well. Clearly, attention to the psychological needs and the special educational requirements of these children is vitally important to minimize the effects of the illness on their psychological development. Thus, perhaps even more than in adults, counseling and therapy must be a high priority when developing treatment plans for children with bipolar disorder.

Does earlier onset of bipolar symptoms predict a stormier course of illness later on? As noted previously, children frequently have continuous rapid cycling and mixed symptoms. Does the illness take on the more usual adult pattern of discrete episodes as these children age? If so, are the episodes more frequent than in persons with later-onset illness? The jury is still out on this question; research results are lacking. But at least one small study shows that bipolar disorder in young persons can indeed be a difficult illness to manage. In this study, fifty-four adolescents who were admitted to a university hospital with a diagnosis of bipolar I disorder were followed for five years.[14] Of these youngsters, nearly half had a relapse, and about half of these had two or more episodes during the five years of the study. This study was done on patients who needed to be admitted to the hospital, and so it is biased toward sicker patients. This type of research problem is called *ascertainment bias:* the results of the study may be skewed because of the method used to gather patients for the study. In this case, since patients who were not ill enough to need hospitalization would not have made it into the study, the study group may not be representative of all pediatric bipolar I patients. Nevertheless, these results would seem to indicate that at least some of these young patients are especially prone to relapse and so need careful monitoring.

But as to the longer course of bipolar disorder that begins in childhood, there is practically no information. Is the course of illness different at age thirty or forty depending on whether it started at age ten or at twenty? There are no definitive answers to this sort of question for now.

Several tasks lie ahead for those researching bipolar disorder in children. First will be to improve upon the diagnostic process and find out how to better separate bipolar (especially manic) symptoms from other similar diagnostic pictures—especially attention-deficit hyperactivity disorder. Clarifying the relationship between bipolar disorder and ADHD will be a very instructive area of research for other reasons as well and will surely lead to better understanding of and treatments for both disorders. More research to determine which of the available treatments for bipolar disorder work best for children and adolescents is also needed, as are long-term follow-up studies to see if pediatric-onset bipolar disorder looks different from late-adolescent-onset bipolar disorder as the patient grows to adulthood.

Women with Bipolar Disorder: Special Considerations

ALTHOUGH WOMEN ARE NO MORE LIKELY THAN MEN TO SUFFER from bipolar disorder, the hormonal changes that accompany menstruation and pregnancy affect the course of bipolar disorder in women and deserve special attention, as do some patterns of symptoms more often experienced by women than men with bipolar disorder. In addition, medication use during pregnancy and while breast-feeding requires careful consideration.

Symptom Differences in Women

Of the various differences between the genders in the course of illness and symptoms of bipolar disorder, the greater incidence of rapid cycling in women is the best documented. A review article on bipolar disorder in women looked at ten studies involving several hundred persons with rapid-cycling bipolar disorder and found that 74 percent of the rapid-cycling patients were female.[1] Thus, the ratio of women to men with rapid-cycling disorder is 3:1.

Several reasons have been proposed for this difference. Since thyroid problems have been associated with rapid cycling in bipolar disorder, and since women are more likely than men to have certain types of thyroid problems, it was thought that a higher incidence of thyroid disease among women might explain the difference. But when women with rapid-cycling bipolar disorder were tested for thyroid problems, no greater incidence of thyroid disease was found. Theories implicating female hormones have also been suggested, but so far they are mostly speculative; no research data exist clearly proving that hormonal differences between men and women explain this difference.

Another intriguing idea about the increased incidence of rapid-cycling bipolar disorder in women is related to the finding that women with bipolar disorder have a slightly greater ratio of depressive to manic episodes than men have. Several studies have found that women with bipolar disorder tend to have more episodes of depression during the course of their illness than men have.[2] This being the case, it may be that women with bipolar disorder are more likely to be treated with antidepressants that can cause them to enter a rapid-cycling phase of the disorder. The types of clinical studies that could prove this theory have yet to be carried out.

The finding that women with bipolar disorder have more depressive episodes than their male counterparts seems to fit with the finding that women are more likely than men to suffer from nonbipolar depression. No one understands this greater tendency of women to suffer from depressive illnesses. Research on the levels of the female reproductive hormones in depressed women has generally been unrevealing.

It is now known that there are many differences in brain organization between women and men, differences that have little to do with sex and reproduction. Psychological testing profiles indicate that women are superior to men in their performance on certain tests of language and memory; men perform better on certain specialized tests of three-dimensional visualization. It is thought that there are subtle differences in the way the brains of men and women are "wired" during prenatal development, probably under the influence of hormones in the womb, especially testosterone. The differences between men and women in the incidence and symptom profile of mood disorders may be due to these differences in "wiring." Explaining the significantly higher incidence of serious depression, including bipolar depression, in women is perhaps the most important unanswered question before us in the field of women's mental health.

Postpartum Mood Disorders and Family Planning

Many clinical studies indicate that women with bipolar disorder are at very high risk for an episode of illness in the period after giving birth. One review article on bipolar disorder in women put it this way: "There is no other time in the life of any bipolar patient when the risk of an episode is higher than it is for a female bipolar patient in the post-partum period."[3] The numbers are indeed sobering: studies have shown that between 25 percent and 30 percent of women with bipolar disorder who become pregnant and deliver will have an episode of depression or mania either during pregnancy or following delivery. Between 80 percent and 100 percent of women with bipolar disorder who stop taking mood-stabilizer medication during pregnancy will experience relapse soon after discontinuing the medication.[4] Episodes are usually characterized by depressive or mixed symptoms; pure manic symptoms are less common. Thus, many women who experience a "postpartum depression" will turn out to have bipolar disorder, not "unipolar" depression, and the treating physician needs to carefully evaluate any patient who develops serious depression following childbirth for this possibility.

One can speculate on why the period after giving birth is such a high-risk period for women with bipolar disorder: there are the emotional and physical stress of labor and delivery, with the inevitable sleep deprivation; periods of physical pain; and the dramatic changes in the levels of reproductive and stress hormones that attend childbirth. Although the exact reasons remain unknown, it appears that these sorts of environmental issues are not as important as biological factors: younger age and first pregnancy are two, but the most significant appears to be a family history of postpartum mood disorders in relatives. In one study, having a relative who had suffered a postpartum episode more than doubled the risk for postpartum relapse in women with bipolar disorder.[5]

Women with bipolar disorder who want to have a child are thus faced with a challenging dilemma. On the one hand, physicians usually recommend that a woman not take any medications during pregnancy, to protect the unborn child from prenatal exposure to pharmaceuticals. On the other hand, it is clear that a woman with bipolar disorder is at high risk for relapse after giving birth and perhaps needs medication late in her pregnancy more than at any other time in her life. Another problem is that several commonly used mood-stabilizing medications have been associated with birth defects.

There are no easy solutions to these problems, but a few facts suggest some ways out. Taking lithium during pregnancy appears to be much safer than originally thought; although there is an increased risk of certain very serious heart malformations in the child, the absolute risk is still quite low—1 to 2 out of 1,000.[6] Among the anticonvulsants, valproate and carbamazepine have definitely been shown to cause birth defects. Lamotrigine appears to be much safer, as do the atypical antipsychotics.[7]

One fact, however, is very clear: simply stopping all medications while trying to get pregnant and for the duration of the pregnancy in order to eliminate all risk to the fetus is *very* risky for the mother. Some women will, of course, be willing to take this risk, and there are many arguments to support this approach. But the first weeks and months—and some say the first few moments—of mother-child contact are very important for mother-child bonding, and this process may be disrupted if the mother is depressed or hospitalized with bipolar symptoms. Another very risky scenario is the woman who unknowingly becomes pregnant while taking medication for bipolar disorder and then abruptly stops taking it. This is risky for the child because by the time a woman discovers she is pregnant, the fetus has already been exposed to any medications she is taking for several days to several weeks. Significant organ development has already occurred during this time. I've already mentioned the high risk of relapse in women who stop medication treatment suddenly during pregnancy. For both of these reasons, I can't stress enough that women with bipolar disorder should plan and prepare for pregnancy so as not to be faced with such difficult choices and decisions on short notice.

Many women with bipolar disorder have healthy babies and remain well in the weeks and months following delivery. Careful planning, conscientious symptom monitoring, and timely resumption of treatment will increase the chances of this happening. The woman with bipolar disorder owes it to herself and to her child to think and plan carefully about pregnancy. She should find an obstetrician and a psychiatrist who will support her decision to become pregnant and work closely with her and with each other toward the healthiest possible outcome for both mother and baby.

Is it safe to breast-feed while taking medication? Many medications are secreted in breast milk, including those used to treat bipolar disorder. Careful monitoring for infant exposure to pharmaceuticals by testing breast milk and the baby's blood and urine make it possible for some patients to breast-feed more safely while taking some medications.

Premenstrual Syndromes

There has been intense interest for many years in the mood symptoms that some women experience for several days before the monthly onset of menstruation. Although many women experience some unpleasant physical and psychological symptoms for a few days before their periods, a subgroup of women suffer clinically significant and impairing mood symptoms premenstrually and sometimes midcycle as well. Whether women with bipolar disorder as a group are more likely to have cycling of their mood with their menstrual cycle is not clear. However, bipolar women who do experience this cycling can have very significant and destabilizing mood fluctuations that can make their illness more difficult to control. It has been shown that women with such monthly mood cycling do not have abnormal reproductive hormone levels. Rather, it appears to be the completely normal but dramatic changes of hormonal levels during the menstrual cycle that are responsible for these mood fluctuations. One way to address these symptoms is to take a contraceptive. Such medications dampen down the normal cycling of hormones and essentially hold hormone levels to what is normally present at the beginning of the menstrual cycle (when the flow begins). To prevent hormonal cycling, the patient takes active medication all the time, skipping the placebo (inactive) pills that are supplied in most contraceptive dispensers. This also means that there is no monthly menstrual flow. Women who notice that menstrually related mood fluctuations consistently cause significant problems for them should consider discussing this approach with their psychiatrist and their gynecologist.

I can't leave the subject of premenstrual mood symptoms without mentioning an intriguing study published in the *American Journal of Psychiatry* by several researchers who had noticed a significant overlap between premenstrual syndrome (PMS) symptoms and the symptoms of seasonal affective disorder (SAD). In both syndromes depressed mood is accompanied by low energy, a tendency to sleep too much rather than too little, and an increase in appetite with carbohydrate craving. (We'll go into the details of the symptoms of SAD in chapter 16.) When the researchers asked patients referred to a PMS clinic if their PMS was worse during the winter, about two-thirds said that it was. Of the original group, 38 percent met the diagnostic criteria for full-blown seasonal affective disorder. These women, then, had a mood disorder that cycled in at least *two* ways: with the monthly menstrual cycle and with the twelve-month cycle of the seasons.[8] This study shows us once more that there are intricate and complex relationships between mood and bodily rhythms and cycles and that mood disorders are affected by many different factors in ways we are only beginning to understand.

CHAPTER 15

Alcoholism and Drug Abuse

OF ALL THE STATISTICS ASSOCIATED WITH BIPOLAR DISORDER, here is one of the most significant and most disturbing: according to one very important study, more than 60 percent of persons with bipolar disorder also suffer from alcoholism or drug-abuse problems.[1]

Does having bipolar disorder make individuals more likely to use and abuse drugs and alcohol? Can alcoholism or drug abuse trigger the development of bipolar disorder in someone who is genetically vulnerable? Do bipolar disorder and substance-abuse disorders have a common biochemical or genetic cause? There is evidence to support an answer of yes to all of these questions.

Bipolar Binges

Perhaps the easiest-to-understand model for the observed link between bipolar disorder and alcoholism and drug abuse is the idea that the mood changes of bipolar disorder propel people into situations they would otherwise be able to avoid and cause them to do things they otherwise wouldn't do.

Brad was a forty-two-year-old writer. He had a day job as a copywriter for a small advertising firm, but his creative juices really started flowing late at night when he worked on his "stories." In college Brad had won a writing contest and had seen his very first attempt at writing a short story published in a prestigious national publication. Since then he had published one or two stories a year, sometimes in little literary journals that paid him practically nothing, once in *Atlantic Monthly,* most often in something in between.

I first met Brad when he was starting to get treatment for alcoholism at the substance-abuse treatment facility affiliated with the hospital where I worked. A psychiatric consultation had been requested because Brad had told the staff he had been troubled by depression and thought it made his drinking problems worse.

"I know what you're thinking: another alcoholic writer. But I'm not."

"Slow down, Brad," I said. "I didn't even know you were a writer until you told me just now." He was a serious and intense man with dark, deep-set eyes. I had to admit he looked the part of the troubled writer. "But I'm interested in hearing your ideas about your drinking problem."

"Sorry, I shouldn't jump to conclusions. But people always think of writers as alcoholics. You know, Hemingway, Tennessee Williams, sitting at their typewriters with a glass of Scotch. Well, I don't drink when I write, I drink when I can't write."

This was beginning to sound interesting. "What do you mean?" I asked.

Brad drank when he couldn't write because it made him feel better. And it gradually became clear to me that when he couldn't write, it was because he was depressed. "My mind just goes blank for days at a time. I get behind at work, I sleep too much, and I don't even bother turning the computer on at home. I can get the car-wax and potato-chip commercials written at work, but I couldn't be really creative if my life depended on it. This 'what's the use?' feeling comes over me, and I find myself bringing home a fifth of vodka two or three times a week and just sipping the nights away."

"Have you ever used any other drugs? Marijuana? Cocaine?" I asked.

"Oh, yes," Brad said with a deep sigh. "About three years ago I drained my bank account over a summer—blew it all on cocaine. If I hadn't ended up in the hospital, I might never have stopped."

"What happened?"

"Well, this is really embarrassing. I don't know what got into me, but I got this inspiration to try writing for TV. I had never tried scriptwriting before, but I was sure I could do it. I got an idea for a script about a guy who falls in love with a woman with a cocaine problem. I thought I needed to do some research—you know, where you go to buy the stuff, what those areas of town are like, the people involved."

"Maybe you should have tried the library first."

Brad turned, looking at me intently. At first I thought I had offended him with my little attempt at humor. But I hadn't. "That's just it," he said. "That's what I usually *would* have done." He looked away again. "I'm not a particularly brave person, and certainly not a fool. But I was . . . I don't know quite how to put it . . . uninhibited, confident. I found myself walking down streets at midnight that I would have been nervous walking down in broad daylight. I bought the stuff and had no qualms about using it. And I was hooked in no time at all. I would get off work, go home, and write until it got dark. Then I'd make a run for the cocaine, kind of cruise around for a while, then come home and snort it. I'd get back to the writing and go at it until the sun came up."

"When did you sleep?" I asked.

"I didn't, not for days at a time. I didn't need to. I felt energized all the time."

"All the time?"

"Yes, I think cocaine must affect me differently than it does most people. I was feeling high even hours and hours after I had used. Once the high lasted three days."

This was sounding like more than just a drug and alcohol problem. People don't feel high from cocaine for three days. Something else had energized Brad that summer. His mood and behavioral changes had all the hallmarks of hypomania.

"So how did you end up in the hospital?"

"One morning my heart started beating real fast and my chest started to hurt. I left the office and got myself to the emergency room. They wanted to admit me right away, but I wouldn't let them."

"Why not?"

"It didn't seem necessary to me. I thought my heart was fine; I just wanted something for the pain. I know that sounds crazy now, but I think I *was* a little crazy by then. I don't remember much about what happened next, but they told me I started shouting and fighting. All I know is I got two shots in the butt and didn't wake up until eleven hours later."

Fortunately Brad's heart *was* fine, but he was discharged with a prescription for Risperdal to take for a few days for what was called a "cocaine-induced psychosis." His sleep patterns and energy level got back to normal.

"It's funny," he added, "I haven't had even the slightest temptation to use cocaine again. I didn't drink either for the whole next year. But then I found myself slipping into the pit again, and I didn't have the energy to say no anymore. But this time I knew I needed help. I think memories of that cocaine summer made me realize that the drinking might lead to something else again if I didn't get some serious treatment. That's why I checked in here."

I couldn't help asking one more question before telling Brad I thought he probably had bipolar disorder: "Did you finish the script?"

"Yes, I did. It turned out great. I've sent it to a producer, and she's interested. You know, I might even make back the money I spent on my, uh . . . research."

Not all stories like Brad's have such a happy ending. Some persons with bipolar disorder can indeed pull out of substance abuse when their mood episodes come to an end, either spontaneously or with treatment, but for others the substance-abuse problem takes on a life of its own. In the worst-case scenario, the mood disorder and the substance-abuse disorder start feeding on each other, and a vicious cycle of mood symptoms, increased substance abuse, and even more severe mood fluctuations takes over until it's impossible to separate one problem from the other.

Psychiatrists used to talk a great deal about "self-medication" in discussing the relationship between bipolar disorder and substance abuse. The idea was that bipolar patients sometimes started down the road to a full-blown substance-abuse problem by attempting to "treat" their mood symptoms with alcohol or drugs of abuse. Although this certainly occurs in some patients, it doesn't seem to be the most common scenario. Although some patients, like Brad, find themselves drinking while depressed because it deadens the psychic pain of depression, bipolar patients seem at greater risk for alcohol and drug abuse when they are hypomanic or manic. Brad's cocaine binge is actually the more typical story. The "self-medication" hypothesis might predict that bipolar patients would use stimulants like cocaine to alleviate their depressions. But studies show that, like Brad, bipolar patients are more likely to use cocaine—and to a lesser extent alcohol—to intensify and prolong their hypomanic and manic states.[2]

The link between mania and cocaine abuse has convinced many researchers that it is manic disinhibition and loss of judgment rather than a tendency to "self-medicate" that puts bipolar patients at such high risk for substance abuse.

Effect, Cause, or Association?

Another possible relationship between bipolar disorder and substance abuse works in the other direction—that is, alcohol and drug abuse may bring on episodes of abnormal mood in bipolar-disorder patients, perhaps by triggering episodes in persons who are vulnerable to the disorder because of genetic factors. Several studies have shown that bipolar patients who have a substance-abuse disorder have a stormier course to their mood disorder than patients who do not abuse alcohol or drugs. "Dual-diagnosis" patients, on average, first develop symptoms of their bipolar disorder at a younger age, and in some studies they have been shown to have more frequent hospitalizations. This has been interpreted to indicate that substance abuse may worsen the course of bipolar disorder, perhaps because of some direct effect on the brain caused by repeated use of drugs and alcohol.[3]

Finally, it may be that, like bipolar disorder, a vulnerability to addiction has a strong genetic component, and the two problems tend to occur together simply because the genes for both are located close to one another on the chromosomes and tend to be inherited together. I, for one, have seen too many patients like Brad—patients whose bipolar-disorder symptoms and substance abuse seem to trigger and reinforce each other—to believe that these so often tightly intertwined problems are randomly associated.

Use or Abuse?

At what point does substance use become "abuse" (table 15-1)? It would be easy for me to launch into a long and complex discussion of diagnostic criteria for substance abuse and chemical dependency, but that probably wouldn't be very helpful. I think the issue is quite clear for individuals with a mood disorder: with the possible exception of occasional alcohol use, I advise persons with a mood disorder to *scrupulously avoid any and all intoxicating substances in any quantity whatsoever.*

All abused substances appear to work by stimulating "reward" centers in the brain. You have probably heard that laboratory animals will push a lever that delivers an electrical stimulus to certain brain regions rather than another one that delivers food to their cage, and that they will continue doing so until they're practically dead from hunger. When a similar lever device is used to deliver an intravenous dose of alcohol or another drug to laboratory animals, the substances that animals will willingly and persistently self-administer in this way are almost exactly the same ones that humans use to get intoxicated: narcotics, cocaine, and certain stimulants and tranquilizers. These are the same substances that humans abuse and become addicted to. Some drugs, like cocaine, affect these centers quickly and powerfully; oth-

TABLE 15-1 Signs of alcoholism

Many medical and professional organizations endorse the **CAGE** questionnaire to identify problem drinking:

1. Have you ever felt you should **C**ut down on your drinking?
2. Have people **A**nnoyed you by criticizing your drinking?
3. Have you ever felt bad or **G**uilty about your drinking?
4. Have you ever had a drink first thing in the morning to steady your nerves or get rid of a hangover (an **E**ye opener)?

One *yes* suggests a possible alcohol problem. More than one *yes* means that an alcohol problem is highly likely.

Source: National Institute on Alcohol Abuse and Alcoholism, *Alcoholism: Getting the Facts,* 1996.

ers, like marijuana, work more slowly, but they all work the same way: by disrupting the normal operation of the brain's "feel-good" circuitry.

Now, you don't need to be a psychiatrist to realize that persons with bipolar disorder already have enough problems with the "feel-good" circuits of the brain, and that mucking things up further with "recreational" drugs is a *very* bad idea. There is some evidence to suggest that intoxicating substances actively interfere with the therapeutic effects of the medications used to treat mood disorders. It seems to me that *any* use of intoxicating substances by persons with bipolar disorder is unhealthy and extremely risky and for those reasons amounts to substance abuse.

The question that usually comes next is, Can't I even have an occasional glass of wine with dinner? Although I'm hard-pressed to forbid my patients ever to drink, it's clear that when it comes to alcohol, less is better. Given the known high risk of bipolar patients for serious substance-abuse problems, the best course is probably no alcohol at all.

A Deadly Combination

There is one well-established research finding that is much more significant than all the speculation about the nature of the association between bipolar disorder and substance abuse and even more disturbing than the extremely high rate of substance abuse among people with bipolar disorder. This is the finding that persons who have mood disorders and also abuse alcohol or drugs have a greatly increased risk of suicide. Severe depression complicated by alcoholism or drug abuse has been found to be one of the most frequent diagnostic pictures in study after study of the psychiatric diagnoses of suicide victims. In a 1993 study attempting to make psychiatric diagnoses of suicide victims, clinicians reviewed the medical records and interviewed the relatives of almost fourteen hundred persons who had committed suicide. This study, which found that most of the suicide victims had suffered from a mood disorder, also found that *nearly half* (48 percent) had suffered from alcoholism or drug abuse.[4]

Another point to emphasize here is that when bipolar disorder and a substance-abuse problem coexist, they *both* need treatment. Getting proper treatment for the mood disorder will certainly make the substance-abuse problem easier to treat, but it cannot be assumed that a substance-abuse problem will simply go away when a coexisting mood disorder is treated. An active substance-abuse problem will in fact make the mood disorder difficult to diagnose, let alone treat.

Substance abuse and addiction can best be understood as problem *behaviors.* A certain behavior becomes a problem when the individual engages in the behavior despite negative consequences that are so significant that continuing the behavior is literally self-destructive. A person who continues to drink alcohol or use some other intoxicating substance despite physical, psychological, or social problems that are caused or made worse by his use has a substance-abuse problem. Substance abuse is not defined by physical dependence (some substances, such as cocaine, don't even cause physical dependence) or by amount of use. Loss of control and continued use despite negative consequences define substance abuse.

Treating Substance Abuse and Addiction

The most important prerequisite for the successful treatment of substance abuse, or any problem behavior, is accepting the need to stop the disordered behavior—that is, recognizing that the behavior is causing problems, is out of control, and needs to be given up. This is often the most difficult step. Unless the person overcomes denial ("I don't have a problem; I can stop any time I want to") and accepts his need to change, treatment can't even get started.

One way to conceptualize the process of recognizing this need to change behavior is outlined in the *transtheoretical model,* more commonly called the *stages of change* model, which was initially developed specifically to define the thought patterns and process of behavioral change in smoking cessation.[5] It proposes that individuals who successfully change an unhealthy behavior pass through several stages in the process of change, in a highly predictable way (figure 15-1).

The first phase is called the *precontemplative stage.* In this phase, individuals simply don't consider that they may have a problem. They see no reasons for stopping or getting treatment, because they have little or no appreciation of the negative consequences and danger of their behavior. People with

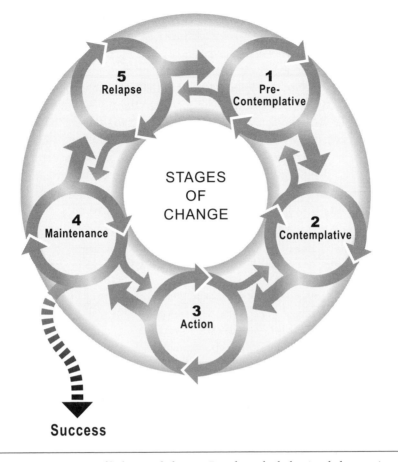

Success

FIGURE 15-1 Stages of behavioral change. People make behavioral changes in stages, moving clockwise through the cycle from *precontemplative* (not accepting the need to change) to *maintenance* (maintaining the behavioral change). Many slip backward (counterclockwise in the cycle) on their way to recovery, and many suffer a full relapse, moving from maintenance to the precontemplative phase and needing to go through the cycle another time, even multiple times, before achieving success.

problem behaviors engage in them because doing so benefits them in some way. Drinking alcohol makes you feel good. It is an expected part of many social situations. It decreases anxiety and boosts one's mood a bit, at least initially. In large amounts, it deadens the psychic pain of depression to some extent, at least for a few hours (although we know that alcohol and other intoxicating substances worsen depression when used regularly). During this stage, the individual is continuing the behavior because she judges that the benefits of the behavior are not outweighed by negative consequences.

It's important to emphasize here that whether *others* think that negatives outweigh positives is not important. Only the affected individual's judgment in this matter can lead him to change.

The next phase is known as the *contemplative stage*. At this point individuals begin to see that their behavior has at least some negative consequences—to themselves and their health, or to their loved ones. They are beginning to think there might be some advantages to stopping the behavior and may even take some steps to at least investigate what that might entail. They have made no commitment to stop, but they are at least somewhat open to the possibility of stopping. This is one of the most important phases in the cycle, because it is an important place to intervene. People can be stuck here for some time: they may fear the difficulty of stopping, feel uncertain about putting together a plan, or just be "waiting for the right time." This is sometimes as far as a person gets in the process of change, and it can be a torturous time in her life; she now sees the negative results of her actions but is still powerless to stop.

The third phase is known as the *action stage*. Individuals take steps to implement a plan to stop their negative behavior. This is also a crucial stage in the process—if the individual can't tolerate the loss of the behavior's positive effects, he may quickly give up on this plan and move back to the contemplation phase. During the action stage, individuals need support, empathy, and strong encouragement to keep on track and continue in treatment.

If the action individuals take leads to cessation of the behavior, they enter the *maintenance stage,* in which they continue to abstain from negative behaviors and have coping mechanisms and support in place to do so. As with the action phase, individuals may need a great deal of support to remain committed to abstinence. This can be particularly important as their situation improves and the previous negative consequences of the behavior recede. It is easy to see how seductive thoughts like "just one more time" or "I can handle it now" can sneak in.

One important and unique aspect of the stages-of-change model is that it incorporates the concept of relapse and sees it as a common next phase that many individuals move into. The *relapse stage* is seen not as a failure but simply as the next phase in the cycle. Many people, when initially trying to stop negative behaviors, will have one (or many) relapses. Seeing a relapse as failure encourages the person to give up, see the process as too hard, and go back to her old ways. The stages-of-change model sees it as a nearly inevitable consequence of having a behavioral disorder and understands that people are frequently seduced to revert back to their old ways when they become stressed, or, conversely, when they are quite happy and "let their guard down."

Many people cycle through the stages several times before they have distanced themselves enough from the problem behavior—for which they have substituted healthy coping mechanisms and now have broad and deep support systems—that even maintenance is no longer necessary, and they exit the cycle.

Psychiatrists and other mental-health professionals are well versed in the available treatment resources in their community for chemical-dependency problems. But perhaps more than most other types of mental-health problems, the treatment of alcohol- and drug-abuse problems requires a wide range of specialized services and support groups. Mental-health professionals will usually refer a patient to a chemical-dependency center or organization for evaluation and treatment of a chemical dependency. Treatment options might include inpatient rehabilitation, outpatient treatment, or a new type of treatment program wherein patients spend the day at the program and return home at night. There are even evening programs that allow people to return to work during the day.

The first step is admitting that there might be a problem. This is often the most difficult step. When in doubt, talking about these concerns with the psychiatrist or therapist is not just important; it can be literally lifesaving.

CHAPTER 16

The Science of Cycles: Chronobiology

CHRONOBIOLOGY (FROM *KHRONOS*, THE GREEK WORD FOR "TIME") is the science of bodily rhythms and biological clocks. Nearly every organism on the planet lives in rhythm with the astronomical cycles of the earth, the sun, and the moon. The activities of animals and the growth cycles of plants harmonize with the daily rising and setting of the sun, the monthly ebb and flow of ocean tides, and the annual cycle of the changing seasons.

Ancient peoples erected immense astronomical calculators and observatories to track these cycles at places like Stonehenge in England and the monuments at Carnac in France, where rows of more than a thousand stones stretch across the countryside. At these sacred places and others, including the pyramids of the Mayans and the Incas, ancient astronomers determined the dates and times of solstices, equinoxes, and eclipses. In festivals like the Roman Saturnalia, our forebears celebrated the lengthening of the daylight hours that heralds the arrival of spring and the return of the sun. Our modern midwinter holidays, Christmas and Hanukkah, recall these sentiments with traditions centered around candles, lights, and greenery.

Once we humans learned how to predict eclipses, we were no longer terrified by them. As we learned how to extend the daylight hours with fire and gaslight and electricity, we depended less on the cycles of the sun to structure our activities and felt more in control of time. We learned to warm ourselves in winter and cool ourselves in summer. The changes of seasons were still lovely to watch and interesting in the way they affected the plants and animals around us, but they didn't really affect us very much anymore—or so we thought.

But the changes of the seasons certainly *do* affect other creatures: we know about the migration of birds, salmon, and whales; Arctic rabbits that change color in winter; the astonishing changes in plant life that occur from fall to winter to spring; and, of course, those hibernating bears. But humans have evolved beyond all that, haven't we? Our cycles of activity, like our sleeping at night and being awake during the day, are just conventions set by our culture rather than expressions of our biology. We humans have severed our connections with the rhythms of the celestial bodies. Haven't we?

That's what many of us thought—until 1982, when a paper by researchers from the National Institute of Mental Health appeared in the *American Journal of Psychiatry*.[1] This paper, titled "Bright Artificial Light Treatment of a Manic-Depressive Patient with a Seasonal Mood Cycle," described a patient with bipolar disorder whose symptoms occurred in a pattern related to the seasons: depression in winter and mood elevation during the summer.

Seasonal patterns in bipolar disorder had been described previously by astute clinicians, including (as you might expect) Emil Kraepelin, who observed, "Repeatedly in these cases, I saw moodiness set in in autumn and pass over in spring 'when the sap shoots in the trees,' to excitement."[2] But there had been little organized research into the relationship between mood and the seasons. Then in the late 1970s, a group of researchers were drawn together at NIMH by a mutual interest in seasonal mood changes, and they started to look at these relationships. One of them, Norman Rosenthal, had for years noticed his own seasonal shifts of mood in his native South Africa, and he had seen these mood swings worsen when his psychiatric training brought him to New York—a city located much farther from the equator than his native Johannesburg had been. In New York the summer days are much longer and the winter days much shorter than in South Africa. Rosenthal recalled his first autumn in New York this way:

> Daylight-saving time was over and the clocks were put back an hour. I left that first Monday after the time change and found the world in darkness. A cold wind blowing off the Hudson River filled me with foreboding. Winter came. My energy declined, and I wondered how I could have undertaken so many tasks the previous summer. Had I been crazy? Now there seemed to be no alternative but to hang in and try to keep everything afloat. . . . Finally, spring arrived. My energy level surged again, and I wondered why I had worried so over my workload.[3]

Some mood-disorder patients with seasonal mood changes found out about the NIMH group and sought out Rosenthal and the other scientists working on seasonal mood disorders. One was a woman who experienced regular winter depressions characterized by low mood and the development of an intense craving for sweets and starches. She had made an important observation during the two winters before she came to NIMH: during both of those winters, she had taken vacations in the Virgin Islands. On both occasions, traveling south toward the equator—to a latitude where the winter days were significantly longer—resulted in a dramatic improvement in her mood. Furthermore, the improvement vanished abruptly when she returned to her colder—and darker—home up north. It was becoming obvious to the NIMH team that the crucial factor in seasonal mood changes was *light.*

The word *photoperiod* refers to the length of daylight hours in the twenty-four-hour day. It has been known for many years that photoperiod has a profound effect on many living things. If you've ever put a poinsettia plant or Christmas cactus in a dark closet to coax it into bloom for the holidays, you've used photoperiod manipulation to influence the plant's physiology. The shortened photoperiod causes the plant to produce hormones that cause its flower buds to be set.

One member of the NIMH team suggested trying to treat winter depressions by artificially lengthening the photoperiod. Several patients volunteered to sit in front of bright lights for several hours before dawn and several more after sunset. Within three days the first patient began to feel better. "The change was dramatic and unmistakable," Rosenthal later wrote.[4] Phototherapy had been born.

Circadian Rhythms

We need to pause here and review an important concept in chronobiology, *circadian rhythms.* The term comes from the Latin words "circa," meaning "around," and "diem," meaning "day." It refers to rhythms in the body that have an approximately twenty-four-hour cycle, that is, the day-night cycle. It turns out that many bodily functions follow a circadian rhythm. Body temperature cycles daily, with the lowest body temperature occurring about 4:00 a.m. and the highest around 7:00 p.m. Blood pressure drops while we are asleep and jumps up about 7:00 a.m. in response to a surge in the adrenal hormone cortisol, which itself rises and falls in a twenty-four-hour cycle. The hormone melatonin, which is secreted by the pineal gland, located deep within the brain, has a circadian cycle and appears to be very important in regulating sleep and wakefulness, as anyone who has used melatonin pills to help him sleep knows.

Humans, like most animals, have an internal biological clock. It has been demonstrated under experimental conditions that this clock has a natural cycle of about twenty-*five* hours, but it is reset every morning by environmental cues, primarily light, to stay in synch with the twenty-four-hour cycle of the day. Another fact about this internal clock, familiar to world travelers, is that this "reset" can shift by only about one or two hours per day. When we reset our watches for daylight saving time or travel to an adjacent time zone, we hardly notice the change. But when we travel across several time zones, it takes several days for our internal clock to become synchonized to the new time. During that time, we awaken and get sleepy at the wrong times for our new time zone and generally feel out of sorts, the phenomenon known as jet lag. Eventually, our internal clock adjusts, but the farther we've traveled, the longer it takes: about one day for each hour of time change. So what happens to people whose internal clocks are out of synch with their environment for prolonged periods of time?

English researchers set out to investigate this question in the late 1990s. They asked fourteen healthy young men and women to volunteer for a biological-clock experiment. Two or three at a time, the volunteers entered experimental living quarters where, for about a month, instead of a twenty-four-hour day, they lived on a thirty-hour day: twenty hours of wakefulness, ten hours of sleep. Every several hours while awake they took a ten-minute battery of psychological tests and rated their mood.

Since these individuals were forced to live on a thirty-hour cycle, their internal clocks could *never* catch up with their sleep-wake cycle. For them, this schedule was the equivalent of traveling through five time zones every day. During the experiment, the researchers had the volunteers take their temperature every few hours, and in this way they were able to determine what time it was for each person's biological clock. They found that the volunteers' internal clocks went in and out of synchronization with their artificially prolonged sleep-wake cycle and that the more out of synchronization the volunteers were, the worse their mood became. In fact, it was the *interaction* of the two cycles that seemed to make the most difference in their mood. They felt worst when their internal temperature clock was telling them it wasn't time to get up yet and their environmentally enforced sleep-wake cycle was telling them it was time to start winding down from a long day. The researchers proposed that "temporal alignment between the sleep-wake cycle and the [internal] circadian rhythms affects self-assessment of mood in healthy subjects."[5] Put more simply: when our sleep-wake cycle and our internal clock are out of synchronization, it has a very *negative* effect on our mood.

Seasonal Affective Disorder

Several theories for SAD involving circadian rhythms have been put forward, but none fit the experimental findings very well. It was proposed that people with SAD might have an abnormal delay in circadian rhythms. Early-morning bright light would be expected to correct this problem by advancing the cycle. Evening phototherapy would be expected to have the opposite effect and make things even worse. But research clearly shows that morning and evening phototherapy are equally helpful for SAD. It has also been suggested that SAD patients have lazy circadian rhythms and even that they are abnormally sensitive to light. But tests of these hypotheses have led to more confusion than clarity, and no one has come up with a theory that ties SAD to a particular circadian rhythm disturbance.

A research group from Columbia University attempted to discover the factors that predicted who would have a good response to photoperiod manipulation. They gave a course of phototherapy to 103 people who reported seasonal mood changes. Some of these individuals met diagnostic criteria for bipolar I, some for bipolar II, and some had unipolar depressions—that is, they had never been manic or hypomanic.

The researchers found that it was not diagnosis (as bipolar I or II or nonbipolar depression) but a particular *pattern* of depressive symptoms that predicted a good response to phototherapy. The people helped by phototherapy tended to sleep more rather than less when they were depressed (hypersomnia) and to complain of low energy and fatigue. They noticed increased appetite during depressions, especially for sweets and starches ("carbohydrate craving"), and an accompanying weight gain. Finally, they had a striking diurnal variation in mood (a consistent pattern of change in mood through the day), but in a pattern that was the opposite of that usually seen in severe depression: instead of waking up early in the morning with the worst mood of the day and then feeling better as the day went on, these people felt better in the early part of the day but had an afternoon or evening "slump," a pattern called *reverse diurnal variation.*[6]

I've been talking about SAD as if it were a diagnostic category of its own, but it's not. SAD can refer to a bipolar I, bipolar II, or nonbipolar depressive illness that shows a seasonal pattern in its symptoms. But a lot of what we know about mood disorders suggests that bipolar I, bipolar II, and nonbipolar depressive illnesses are very *different* illnesses in course and causation. What does it mean that *each* can have a seasonal pattern? The study I described earlier showed that it was not diagnosis but rather symptom pattern that predicted who gets better with light therapy. Does this mean that our whole diagnostic classification system is called into question?

Don't throw out your *DSM* just yet. The bipolar-nonbipolar and bipolar

I–bipolar II diagnostic divisions are still very useful in choosing treatments, and so is the "with seasonal pattern–without seasonal pattern" designation. It may just be a few more years before we figure out how all the classifications fit together.

In the meantime, patients with bipolar symptoms who notice a seasonal pattern should talk with their physician about phototherapy, especially if they have the typical SAD depressive symptom pattern: low energy, hypersomnia, carbohydrate craving, weight gain, and reverse diurnal variation of mood (afternoon or evening "slump").

Several years of research have found that bright blue-tinged light is the most effective for treating SAD, and there are now relatively inexpensive lights with this wavelength specifically designed to treat SAD. The usual recommendation is that the patient use the light in the morning and start with an exposure of thirty minutes daily. A recent study suggests that reading while in front of the light is especially beneficial, because the light reflected from the page increases the total light exposure. The therapeutic effect of light therapy is sometimes evident within days, but as with antidepressants, several weeks of therapy may be needed to obtain good remission of symptoms. Side effects are minor: headaches and eyestrain, for example.[7] Too much light exposure can sometimes precipitate mild hypomanic symptoms: irritability, insomnia, feeling "hyper." Fortunately, this problem seems to respond quickly to decreased light exposure, and phototherapy doesn't seem to have the risks of mood destabilization that taking antidepressant medication does. Light therapy can be thought of as an adjunctive therapy for bipolar disorder with seasonal variation, an add-on treatment that works with medication and psychotherapy to regulate mood through a natural cycle of the body. There's another cycle that's also extremely important to pay attention to: the sleep-wake cycle.

The Sleep Cycle and Bipolar Disorder

We're not finished with circadian rhythms yet. One of our most prominent circadian rhythms, the sleep-wake cycle, turns out to be very significant in bipolar disorder. The study with our English volunteers demonstrated how important the sleep-wake cycle is in the regulation of mood in persons who do *not* have mood disorders. So it should come as no surprise that sleep-wake cycle manipulation has dramatic effects on persons with bipolar disorder. Clinical observations confirm this: sleep deprivation can be used therapeutically to treat the symptoms of depression, and it can also cause a switch into the manic state. To understand these observations, we need to take a closer look at normal sleep.

For quite a long time, sleep wasn't of much interest to experimental

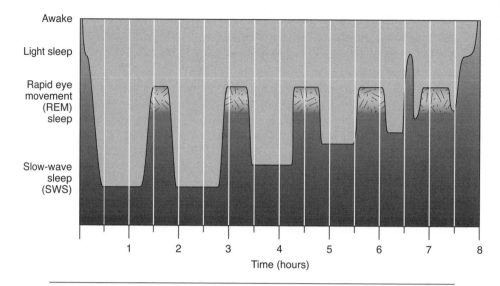

FIGURE 16-1 Normal sleep architecture.

psychologists and psychiatrists. This may seem odd, especially considering Freud's and others' intense interest in dreams. Possibly because of a lack of investigative tools, interest in dreams never extended to interest in the process of dreaming, and so the physiology of sleep was a neglected area of research for many decades.

The change came in 1953, when a group of researchers used an electro-encephalogram (EEG) machine on sleeping volunteers in a clinical laboratory to investigate the long-standing observation that people move their eyes beneath closed lids during some periods of sleep. When the researchers awakened the subjects during what came to be called *rapid eye movement sleep* (REM sleep), 90 percent of them reported that they had been dreaming. Further studies revealed that sleep is a complex process, with several different stages and rhythms of activity that together are now called *sleep architecture*.

As figure 16-1 indicates, after falling asleep, a person passes through lighter and then progressively deeper stages of sleep. Brain activity slows, and the heartbeat and blood pressure drop to the lowest levels of the twenty-four-hour day. The process is like a submarine descending into darker, quieter, deeper water. The very deepest stage is called *slow-wave sleep* (SWS), because the EEG shows slow synchronized rhythms in the electrical activity of the brain. SWS is thought to be the physically restorative part of sleep; experimental subjects who are awakened whenever they enter SWS but are allowed to experience the other stages complain of muscle aches and other symptoms of physical discomfort.

About ninety minutes after a person falls asleep, the sleep "submarine" begins to rise again. The EEG indicates a brain-activity pattern not very different from that seen in awake individuals. The EEG electrodes that track eye movements measure intense activity, and individuals awakened during this stage report dreaming: the sleeper has entered a period of REM sleep. After fifteen to twenty minutes of REM sleep, eye movement ceases, and the sleeper drifts back down into the deeper stages again and has another period of SWS, which predominates during the first part of the night. As the night progresses, the sleeper spends more time in REM sleep and less in SWS. Toward dawn, sleep becomes lighter and REM periods become longer, until finally the person wakes up. It is thought that REM sleep and body temperature are both tightly linked to the body's main circadian clock (often called the *strong oscillator*), because the lowest point of the body's temperature cycle coincides with the most intensive period of REM sleep.

When we look at EEG sleep studies done on depressed persons, the REM cycle seems to have shifted. Depressed individuals go into REM almost immediately after falling asleep, a phenomenon called *decreased REM latency*. Some slow-wave sleep still occurs in the later part of the night, but the overall amount of SWS is reduced. Some researchers have interpreted these findings as indicating that depressed individuals suffer from a *phase advance* of the REM cycle and that the rhythm of the strong oscillator has gotten out of phase with other bodily rhythms. We saw from the study on the English volunteers that when the strong oscillator (as measured by their temperature cycle) is out of synchronization with the sleep-wake cycle, dips in mood occur. In the few patients with bipolar disorder who have been studied, striking shifts of the REM and temperature cycles were observed as the patients cycled in and out of depression and mania.[8]

These findings bring together a lot of what we know about the symptoms of depression and about circadian rhythms. The decreased amounts of SWS may explain the fatigue and bodily discomfort typical of depression. The shifting of the usual period of REM from the early-morning hours to the early part of the sleep cycle may explain the early-morning awakening typically seen in depression.

These findings may also explain the therapeutic effects of sleep deprivation on symptoms of depression. Patients with the typical diurnal variation of mood seen in depression often report that they have their best mood of the day during the late evening, before they go to sleep, and feel their worst in the morning after they've slept. This and other observations led some researchers in the 1950s to experiment with sleep deprivation as a therapeutic technique for the treatment of depression. With the introduction of antidepressant medications, interest in sleep deprivation faded, but recently it has been growing again. This work shows that if patients are totally deprived of sleep—kept up all night—about 60 percent of them report a sometimes dramatic improvement in their mood. Unfortunately, the effect is temporary; in most patients the benefits disappear after even a brief nap, making this interesting technique a not terribly useful one. But experiments with partial sleep deprivation indicate that waking patients up at about 2:00 a.m. and making sure that they do not sleep during the second half of the night is nearly as effective as total sleep deprivation. Advancing the sleep cycle by six hours, so that patients go to sleep at 6:00 p.m. and get up at 2:00 a.m., has also been found to have antidepressant effects.

Although the technique has not caught on in the United States, sleep deprivation and phase advance are popular in Europe as adjuncts to medication in the treatment of bipolar and nonbipolar depression. An Italian study published in 1997 compared the recovery time from depression in ten bipolar patients. All of them were treated with fluoxetine (Prozac), but five were also given several cycles of total sleep deprivation. The patients who had sleep deprivation got better faster on the medication than those who did not.[9]

The other relevant clinical observation about sleep in persons with bipolar disorder is that sleep deprivation can precipitate mania. This is a very well-documented finding, and for this reason my discussion of sleep deprivation as a treatment for depression comes with a "don't try this at home" warning: even one night of sleep deprivation can precipitate mania. There have been numerous reports of individuals with bipolar disorder becoming manic after transatlantic flights or after sleep deprivation caused by medical emergencies or family crises. Emotional upsets can, of course, lead to insomnia and poor sleep because of anxiety. It has been proposed that lack of sleep for *any* reason may be what tips the balance for many bipolar patients and brings on an episode of mania.[10]

All of the work on chronobiology and biological clocks indicates that there are important links between bodily rhythms and mood, and we've barely scratched the surface of this fascinating area of study. So far we have only tantalizing hints about these links rather than clearly understood mechanisms and relationships. Nevertheless, studies of sleep and SAD point the way toward new and safer treatments for certain mood disorders—techniques like phototherapy and sleep phase advance. This work also indicates the importance of lifestyle regularity in controlling the symptoms of bipolar disorder, a topic we'll explore in more detail in chapter 20.

CHAPTER 17

The Genetics of Bipolar Disorder

IT HAS LONG BEEN RECOGNIZED THAT BIPOLAR DISORDER EXISTS in clusters within families. In *Manic-Depressive Insanity,* Emil Kraepelin wrote of one family in which "of the ten children of the same parents who were both probably manic-depressive by predisposition, no fewer than seven fell ill the same way; of the five descendants of the second generation, four have already fallen ill."[1]

For many years research on the genetics of bipolar disorder was hampered by foggy diagnostic criteria and a lack of laboratory methods to identify genes. But this state of affairs has changed dramatically. Not only have psychiatrists become more skilled in the diagnosis of bipolar disorder, but the biochemical methods available to locate and identify genes on the human chromosome have become tremendously more sophisticated. These developments will, sooner or later, lead to a better understanding of the genetic mechanisms of bipolar disorder, which will in turn lead to better diagnosis and treatment of the disorder.

Genes, Chromosomes, and DNA

The patterns and rules of inheritance in living things were first described by Gregor Mendel, an Austrian monk who over many years performed elegantly planned and executed experiments with plants, mostly garden peas, in his monastery garden. Mendel discovered that traits are transmitted from parent to child in discrete bits of information, bits that we now call *genes,* the units of inheritance.

We now understand that genes are sets of instructions for building proteins. All plants and animals, from seaweed to snapdragons and from earthworms to elephants, are constructed of and operate by means of proteins. Myosin (muscle protein), hemoglobin (the oxygen-carrying protein of red blood cells), and collagen (the structural protein of skin and cartilage) are just a few examples. Even the nonprotein structural materials of the body, such as the calcium salts in our bones, depend on proteins. Proteins called enzymes direct the manufacture of bone from calcium salts by expediting certain chemical reactions. Many hormones are proteins (insulin, for example), and those that are not (for example, testosterone and cortisol) are manufactured by protein enzymes. All proteins are built according to specifications contained in genes.

For many years what genes were made of and exactly how they were transmitted from parent to offspring was a complete mystery. But by the mid-1940s, experiments with bacteria had shown that a family of biochemical compounds found in cells, called *nucleic acids,* contained genetic information. In 1953 James Watson and Francis Crick published a paper in the British scientific journal *Nature,* describing the structure of the most important of these compounds, deoxyribonucleic acid (DNA), and the modern age of genetics had begun.

DNA molecules are long spiral chains whose links consist of four simpler compounds called nucleotides. The four DNA nucleotides, adenine, cytosine, guanine, and thymine (usually abbreviated as A, C, G, and T), are the elements of an elegantly simple code. Just as you can write out a Morse code version of *Hamlet* using only dots and dashes, you can write out instructions for building hemoglobin, myosin, collagen, or any other protein using A's, C's, G's, and T's. That's what DNA does. You can think of the physical structure of a gene as the section on the DNA molecule that contains the code for one protein.

When the DNA molecule is doing its work in the cell, it is unraveled and stretched out, surrounded by a whole retinue of ultramicroscopic attendants busily reading the coded instructions and making proteins. When it's time for the cell to divide, another set of attendants carefully coil the DNA molecule into a compact cylinder and surround it with protective proteins to form the threadlike structures you may have looked at under the microscope in high school biology: the chromosomes.

Genetic Diseases

For some disorders, the links from a certain gene to a certain protein to a certain trait or disease are easy to follow. Sickle-cell anemia is one such disease. When the blood of sickle-cell patients is examined under the microscope, instead of seeing the normal saucer- or disk-shaped red blood cells, one sees abnormal crescent- or sickle-shaped cells. Once scientists had the biochemical methods that allowed them to look at the components of blood cells, they discovered that sickle-cell patients had an abnormally shaped hemoglobin molecule (hemoglobin is the protein in red blood cells that transports oxygen). This abnormal hemoglobin tends to form abnormal chains within the cell, stretching the normally disk-shaped cells into the sickle shape characteristic of the disease.

Because hemoglobin is easily purified, it was one of the first proteins whose structure was completely described (a feat that earned Cambridge University biochemist Max Ferdinand Perutz the Nobel Prize in 1962). Researchers discovered that sickle-cell hemoglobin (now called hemoglobin S) differs from normal hemoglobin by only one molecular element that is caused by a single misprint in the hemoglobin gene of persons with the disease. At one particular spot on the DNA molecule of persons with sickle-cell anemia, there is an A instead of a T. An abnormal hemoglobin molecule results from the reading of these incorrect instructions, and the abnormal hemoglobin molecules cause the abnormally shaped red blood cells, which block blood vessels and result in the symptoms of the disease. The pathway from abnormal gene to abnormal protein to abnormal cells to symptoms has been completely described.

Genes have been identified and located in several other human diseases whose inheritance pattern indicates that they are single-gene illnesses, including cystic fibrosis, many forms of hemophilia, and Duchenne's muscular dystrophy.

What We Know

In the absence of specific identified genes or any knowledge about what proteins these genes code for, we can talk about the inheritance of bipolar disorder in only a very general way. Children of individuals with bipolar disorder have an increased risk of developing bipolar disorder. Assigning a number to that risk is very difficult, for some of the same reasons that the search for a bipolar gene has been so difficult, especially problems of diagnosis. But the risk seems to be several times that of the general population, on the order of 10 percent. However, children of persons with bipolar disorder are also at a higher risk for unipolar (depression-only) illness, and when you add in this risk, the percentages go up into the high twenties. This means that the children of persons with bipolar disorder have about a one-in-four chance of developing some kind of mood disorder and about a one-in-ten chance of developing bipolar disorder.[2]

Individuals with bipolar disorder need to be alert to signs and symptoms of mood disorders in their children and to get them into treatment if such symptoms occur. Although we may be uncertain about the details of the inheritance of bipolar disorder, we are not at all uncertain about the importance of early diagnosis and treatment.

The Search Continues

Several factors make scientists optimistic about eventually discovering genes for bipolar disorder. The explosive growth of technologies available to geneticists is perhaps the primary reason for optimism. The Human Genome Project was able to tackle the sequencing of the DNA in all 46 human chromosomes only after automated technology to perform DNA sequencing became available in the 1990s and when supercomputers were developed that could analyze the literally astronomical amount of data that was generated. This technology has advanced even further in the intervening years, and it is now possible to test for 1 *million* genetic markers in an individual using a silicone "chip" called a "DNA microarray" that costs only a few hundred dollars to manufacture. It will soon be possible to sequence the entire genome of an individual for less than one thousand dollars, a possibility all the more amazing when one learns that the budget of the investigation that resulted in the first whole-genome sequencing was in the tens of millions of dollars.

Even when genes are identified, however, and tests are developed that can look for these genes in individuals, predictions about who will develop symptoms will still be imprecise. This is because several genes are likely involved and also because genetics is almost certainly not the whole story in bipolar disorder. Environmental factors are undoubtedly important (perhaps equally important) in determining who will and will not be affected; psychological and perhaps physical stresses and traumas are probably very important. So even when a gene or genes are identified and can be tested for, finding that a person has a bipolar gene will probably mean that he or she has a higher chance of developing symptoms than someone who does not have the gene—but not a 100 percent chance. This will raise a lot of questions about who should and should not be tested and who is entitled to know genetic test results.

But finding responsible genes may lead to new treatment approaches that will benefit everyone with mood disorders. Gene identification, as well as identification of the function of these genes or the gene products, will undoubtedly shed light on the biochemical basis of bipolar disorder. It may then be possible to design medications or other treatments based on knowledge about the causes of bipolar symptoms on a cellular or biochemical level—rather than stumbling upon treatments by accident, as has been the case so far. Genetics research is one of the most challenging but most promising areas of investigation of bipolar disorder, and it holds the promise of truly revolutionizing the treatment of this disease.

CHAPTER 18

Bipolar Biology

THERE ARE SEVERAL MORE TOPICS IN THE REALM OF BIOLOGY that tell us a lot about bipolar disorder. A common theme in them, it seems, is to show that staying well with bipolar disorder depends quite a lot on taking care of one's general health. In part IV of the book (chapters 20–23), I will discuss some of the lifestyle changes that are vital in helping persons with bipolar disorder stay well. Many of these changes are such things as getting a good night's sleep, exercising regularly, and eating a healthful diet. Now I know some readers (surely not you) will read through that list and say to themselves, "Right, a good night's sleep, exercising, blah, blah, blah. I know all that stuff. Tell me something *important*." Well, this next section, on stress, explains exactly why these things are important and why stress is *not* good for your brain.

How the Body Handles Stress

The most dramatic bodily response to stress is the familiar "fight or flight" response. If you are hiking along the Appalachian Trail and suddenly encounter a bear twice your size, some dramatic physical changes take place in the body, changes that prepare you to face combat with the creature ("fight") or, perhaps more likely, run as fast and as far as you can ("flight"). There is a hormonally triggered flood of energy-containing glucose, fat molecules, and proteins into your bloodstream; your heart rate and blood pressure go up, to get these energy molecules to the muscles as quickly as possible; and your breathing becomes faster and deeper to provide the oxygen needed to turn the energy molecules into power. Simultaneously, body systems that are not involved in fighting or fleeing shift down: digestion slows down, cellular growth and tissue repair grind to a halt, and even the immune system temporarily goes into hibernation. The stress response is really a brilliantly orchestrated symphony of physiological responses in many organ systems that prepares the body for intense physical exertion. All of this is terrific in a physical emergency, but if this hyperactive physiology goes on for too long, bad things begin to happen.

In other animals, the stress response is either active or inactive; the system is either "on" or "off." But in humans (and the animals most closely related to them), elements of the stress response can be active for much longer periods of time. Neuroscientist Robert Sapolsky highlighted this difference between humans and other animals in a book about the role of stress in health and disease that he called *Why Zebras Don't Get Ulcers.* The title refers to the fact that when a grazing zebra spots a lion on the edge of the jungle, its stress response kicks in at full force and the animal bounds off at breakneck speed, but then, if it's been fast enough and lucky enough, the zebra escapes the hungry lion and simply resumes eating, as calm and placid as if nothing had happened, with bodily functions quickly returning to baseline. Other than the sight of a lion, there isn't much that brings on the stress response in zebras, because zebras don't have the cognitive capacity to worry. But we are quite different: "We humans can be stressed by things that simply make no sense to zebras. . . . It is not a general mammalian trait to become anxious about mortgages or the Internal Revenue Service, about public speaking or fears of what you say in a job interview, about the inevitability of death."[1] Nevertheless, these very un-zebralike sources of stress activate many of the same physiological responses in the human body as our zebra's sighting of the lion or our hiker's encounter with the bear.

The main hormones responsible for the stress response are the *glucocorticoids,* a group of hormones that are produced by the adrenal glands, and the most important of these is *cortisol.* You can think of cortisol as responsible for controlling the changes to the energy economy of the body that are part of the stress response: the release of glucose into the bloodstream, the damping down of the immune system, and the suppression of cellular growth. It is this last feature of cortisol that is most relevant to persons with bipolar disorder.

As you may remember from chapter 5, our mood-regulation system depends on the constant active remodeling of networks of neurons in the brain, especially in an area of the brain called the hippocampus. The cells in the hippocampus are very busy, sprouting new connections and disconnecting and reconnecting with other neurons, and new neurons are constantly

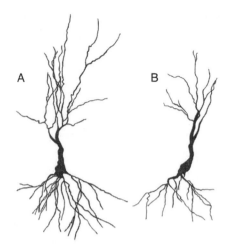

FIGURE 18-1 The effects of chronic stress on hippocampal neurons. *A* is a representative neuron from a control animal, and *B* is from an animal that was subjected to chronic stress for several hours daily for ten consecutive days.

Source: A. Vyas, R. Mitra, B. Rao, and S. Chattarji, "Chronic Stress Induces Contrasting Patterns of Dedritic Remodeling in Hippocampal and Amygdaloid Neurons," *Journal of Neuroscience* 22 (2002): 6810–18.

needed to replenish the ones that simply wear out from all this work. It's easy to see, then, how too much cortisol damping down cellular growth over too long a time can have a very deleterious effect on the mood system.

The damaging effect of high levels of cortisol on the brain has been abundantly demonstrated in animal studies. Mice are timid little creatures. They scurry around their environment, not being still for very long except to eat, and they prefer darkness. A relatively humane way to subject mice to stress, then, is to confine them to a Lucite tube in a well-lit environment for several hours. If you do this day after day, an experimental technique known as "chronic immobilization stress," the mice will exhibit changes in their behavior that resemble depression in humans: They don't eat as much and they lose weight. Sleep is disrupted and sexual activity reduced. They are less active; they spend less time running on the wheels that have been put in their cages. Tests of object recognition and memory show that their cognitive functioning suffers as well. When the blood level of corticosterone, the mouse equivalent of cortisol, is measured, it is found to be elevated. But the most striking findings involve changes in neurons in the hippocampus. As Figure 18-1 shows, when the hippocampal neurons of mice subjected to chronic stress are compared to those of control mice, the difference is unmistakable.

The neurons of the stressed animals look shrunken and stunted, compared to those of the nonstressed animals. Most importantly, research has shown that it is cortisol that is responsible for these changes. Injecting the rodent equivalent of cortisol (corticosterone) into animals that are not subjected to chronic stress produces exactly the same effect: shrunken brain cells in the hippocampus, the area of the brain thought to be the most important in mood regulation.[2]

But here's the most impressive thing of all: stress-caused damage to brain cells in the hippocampus can be *prevented* by lithium. Scientists at Rockefeller University, along with colleagues in other institutions, designed an experiment to investigate whether lithium might protect neurons in the hippocampus from the effects of stress. Some experimental mice were divided into two groups. One group was given lithium for two weeks and the other was not; then both groups were subjected to chronic stress. Figure 18-2 is one of those pictures worth a thousand words.

The first cell is from a control animal that was not subjected to stress; it shows a normally developed cell (*A*). Cell *B* is a representative neuron from a stressed mouse, showing, as expected, a stunted and shrunken cell. *C* is a cell from the hippocampus of a mouse that received lithium for two weeks

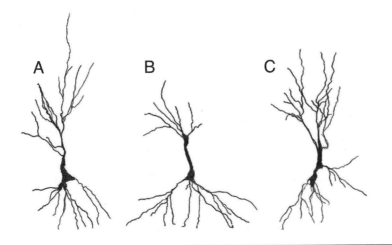

FIGURE 18-2 Protecting hippocampal neurons from the damaging effects of chronic stress with lithium. *A* is a representative hippocampal neuron from a control animal, *B* is from an animal subjected to twenty-one days of immobilization stress, and *C* is from a stressed animal that had been pretreated with lithium for two weeks before experiencing the stress.

Source: G. Wood, L. Young, L. Reagan, B. Chen, and B. McEwan, "Stress-Induced Structural Remodeling in the Hippocampus: Prevention by Lithium Treatment," *Proceedings of the National Academy of Sciences* 101 (2004): 3973–78.

before being subjected to stress and continued on lithium through the period of stress. You don't need to be a neuroscientist to see that the cell from the lithium-treated mouse (C) was protected from the effects of stress and looks just as healthy as the one from the control animal (A).

So what should we conclude from all this? First of all, stress is *not* good for your brain. Stress raises the levels of steroid hormones in the bloodstream, and cortisol, the most important of these hormones, is practically toxic to neurons in the most important mood-regulation center of the brain, the hippocampus. So it follows rather obviously that persons with bipolar disorder should avoid the kinds of stress that increase their cortisol levels. And what are those stresses? They are all those things that your doctor (and probably your mother) told you to avoid: an unhealthful diet, not exercising, smoking, drinking alcohol, not getting a good night's sleep—well, you get the idea. And although zebras don't worry about financial problems, deadlines, or relationship conflicts, humans do. Those things increase cortisol levels as well. In the chapters of part IV, I'll talk about how to put this knowledge into practice.

Bipolar Disorder and Hormonal Systems

By far the most important hormone systems in the regulation of mood are the thyroid hormones and the adrenal hormones. We've already discussed both of these systems a bit, but a brief review will help.

The thyroid gland, located just below the larynx (the "voice box") at the base of the neck, secretes several hormones into the blood. These hormones are very important in the body's regulation of energy. Thyroid hormones help control the rate of calorie consumption by the body, known as *metabolism,* and the rate at which calories are converted to and stored as fat. If the thyroid gland secretes an excess of its hormones (*hyper*thyroidism), the person's metabolism speeds up; if not enough is secreted (*hypo*thyroidism), the metabolism slows down. This "speeding up" or "slowing down" affects emotions and behavior as well and can cause symptoms mimicking a mood disorder even in persons who otherwise don't seem to have mood problems (table 18-1).

When a person is suffering from *severe* hyper- or hypothyroidism, the clinical picture is pretty unmistakable. But in mild thyroid problems, changes in mood and activity level can be the *only* symptoms of the thyroid troubles. Not only can thyroid disease cause mood symptoms directly; it can also make the symptoms of a preexisting mood disorder more difficult to treat. We have already discussed the link between rapid-cycling bipolar disorder and thyroid disease. Mood disorders can be very resistant to treatment if there is even the slightest thyroid problem. These are more reasons why

TABLE 18-1 Psychiatric symptoms of thyroid disease

Hyperthyroidism	Hypothyroidism
Irritability	Depressed mood
Insomnia	Drowsiness
Restlessness	Lethargy
Hyperactivity	Poor concentration
Paranoia	Slowed thinking
Poor concentration	Apathy and social withdrawal
Delusional thinking	Hallucinations

it is very important to pay attention to this hormonal system and to test for thyroid hormone levels in persons with mood disorders.

The adrenal glands sit atop the kidneys in the lower back and secrete many hormones, the most important of which are the corticosteroids. We've discussed one of these, cortisol, in some detail. In addition to their role in the stress response, the corticosteroid hormones are very important in the regulation of metabolism.

Corticosteroids are potent anti-inflammatory agents, and many pharmaceutical products, such as cortisone, prednisone, and others are artificial versions of these adrenal hormones. These drugs are a component in some creams used to treat allergic skin reactions, but corticosteroids are also given orally and intravenously to treat inflammatory conditions such as rheumatoid arthritis, asthma, and inflammatory bowel disease, and they are often given as a treatment for acute pain, especially back pain.

On one hand, excessive corticosteroids from adrenal tumors can cause symptoms of agitated depression with suicidal thinking. On the other hand, hypomanic symptoms seem to be more common in patients being treated with artificial corticosteroids for medical conditions. Persons with bipolar disorder need to be very careful about taking these drugs for medical conditions and should ask about alternatives when such treatment is being considered. (Steroid creams do not cause psychiatric symptoms. The creams are formulated so that the medication affects only the tissue it comes into direct contact with. Only minute amounts of the active ingredient are absorbed into the bloodstream.)

Picturing Bipolar Disorder in the Brain

For decades clinical scientists have searched for a way to test for bipolar disorder. As we have developed more sophisticated ways of probing the workings of the brain, we have been able to measure subtle differences in brain functioning in mood-disorder patients, and although none of these observations have led to the development of reliable tests yet, we are nevertheless learning a great deal about the disorder with these techniques.

As we saw in chapter 4, early researchers who dissected the brains of deceased people who had had bipolar disorder or examined their brain tissues under a microscope found no abnormalities of brain structure and questioned whether bipolar disorder was really a brain disease at all. We now know that it is—but that's because we have learned how to look for and measure abnormalities of brain *chemistry*. Looking at the *structure* of the brain, whether with the naked eye, the microscope, or the x-ray machine, has been unrevealing until quite recently. But now two new imaging techniques are beginning to allow us to picture bipolar disorder in the brain.

The first of these techniques is *magnetic resonance imaging,* or *MRI*. MRI is based on the discovery that the atoms of objects placed in a powerful magnetic field absorb energy or "resonate" at characteristic frequencies that can be measured with the proper equipment. In medical MRI scans, the patient lies encircled by a large doughnut-shaped instrument that generates a powerful magnetic field. Sensitive instrumentation measures the different resonances of different tissues: bone, muscle, fat, blood, and so forth, and the signals from each are assembled by computer into a picture. MRI is a very sensitive technique, and even small and subtle tissue differences show up with astonishing clarity.

A number of studies have shown that the brains of persons with bipolar disorder show an increased number of unusual MRI findings called T_2 *hyperintensities.* These are small areas of high MRI signal intensity thought to indicate changes of water content in brain tissue. MRI scans of persons with blood-vessel diseases of the brain and several other brain diseases also indicate T_2 hyperintensities, and T_2 hyperintensities seem to increase with the normal aging process. But although T_2 hyperintensities are not unique findings in bipolar disorder, they are found in higher numbers in people with bipolar disorder than in control subjects matched for age. In one study, hyperintensities were found 1.6 times as often in bipolar I as in bipolar II patients and twice as often in bipolar I patients as in comparison subjects who did not have bipolar disorder.[3]

It's not clear exactly what is represented by these signal differences on the MRI images of persons with bipolar disorder. Most of the other conditions in which T_2 hyperintensities are found involve loss of neurons and other brain cells and also the pathological process called demyelination, the loss of the fatty insulating material of nerve fibers. Perhaps T_2 hyperintensities are a result rather than the cause of bipolar disorder; perhaps permanent brain changes occur after many years and many episodes of bipolar disorder symptoms, and T_2 hyperintensities are the tiny "scars" of these episodes. Much work remains to be done to explain the significance of these intriguing findings.

More recently, another form of MRI imaging has been developed that has revolutionized the field of brain imaging. *Functional* MRI (fMRI) is a technique in which the MRI instrument is adjusted so that it can measure the amount of oxygen in areas of the brain in exquisite detail. In this way, not only is the structure of the brain revealed, but variations in the level of metabolic activity of brain areas can be visualized. Functional MRI scans can pinpoint changes in activity in brain areas only a few cubic millimeters in size that last only a second or two.

While these are early days in using this approach to understand bipolar disorder, various basic facts are emerging. As might be expected, several centers deep in the oldest part of the brain that are already known to be important in strong emotions such as fear and anger (a set of structures known collectively as the *limbic system*) show differences in activity in bipolar patients compared to healthy controls. In addition, however, it has been found that areas of the prefrontal lobes also show patterns of activity that are different in individuals with bipolar disorder; these are areas of the brain where advanced intellectual processing take place. One of the most consistent findings in fMRI studies of mood disorders is a decrease in metabolic rate in an area of the left prefrontal lobe in depressed patients, a finding that led to the development of transcranial magnetic stimulation (TMS), one of the brain-stimulation treatments discussed previously. Some neuroimaging studies of bipolar disorder have found a similar pattern of underactivity in this area, but others have not, suggesting that "unipolar" depression and bipolar disorder have different biological bases.[4]

Yet another new form of MRI neuroimaging is called *diffusion* magnetic resonance imaging (dMRI). This technique visualizes water molecules as they move along brain connections and can reveal variation in the connections between different brain areas. Studies using this approach have found differences in the size of connecting bundles of fibers connecting different centers of the limbic system in persons with bipolar disorder.

Neuroimaging in psychiatric illness is a relatively new field, but research in this area is booming. It's difficult to keep up with the development of new imaging techniques, let alone the new findings that emerge from their use. Unfortunately, the metabolic patterns seen in these studies are apparent only when groups of individuals are compared; most of the studies compare a dozen or so individuals with bipolar disorder to a similar number of healthy controls to detect differences. The differences are too small and the range of normal results too large for these approaches to be helpful for clinical purposes such as forming the basis for a reliable test for bipolar disorder—so far, at least. But these findings show conclusively that bipolar disorder is a brain disease with real physical changes in the function of brain areas that can be visualized and measured with the right equipment.

CHAPTER 19

Bipolar Disorder and Creativity

ARISTOTLE SAID, "NO GREAT GENIUS HAS EVER EXISTED WITHOUT some touch of madness."[1] Most truisms contain a kernel of truth, and that of the "mad genius" seems to as well. Scholars who have studied the lives of highly creative people have discovered that among them there are unexpectedly high numbers of individuals with severe psychiatric illness. Clinicians involved in this work have concluded that bipolar disorder is by far the most common of these illnesses. It doesn't require extensive research to come up with a long list of writers, artists, and composers whose biographies indicate that they probably had a mood disorder. Let's take a glimpse into the lives of several of them.

George Gordon, Lord Byron (1788–1824) (figure 19-1), had periods of fiery expansiveness and hollow despair throughout his life. The recorded observations of his friends and his physicians make a diagnosis of bipolar disorder all but certain in the great English poet. Lord Byron's family history is entirely consistent with the diagnosis of bipolar disorder—suicide, "madness," and murder can be traced back for several generations on both sides of his family tree.

Medical biographers of Vincent van Gogh (1853–1890) have speculated for decades about the illness that drove him to self-mutilation and repeatedly confined him to the Asylum of Saint Paul at Saint-Rémy. The episodic nature of van Gogh's illness and the acceleration of its course toward the end of his life are highly suggestive of bipolar disorder. Van Gogh described his dreadful depressions in his letters and was diagnosed with mania by sev-

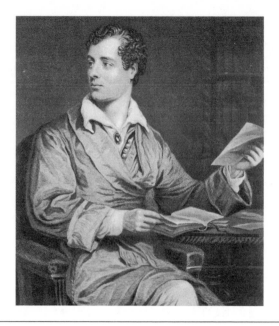

FIGURE 19-1 George Gordon, the English poet usually known as Lord Byron, suffered from severe mood symptoms throughout his life (as did several members of his family). "I must think less wildly," he wrote in his epic *Childe Harold's Pilgrimage*. "I have thought too long and darkly, till my brain became . . . a whirling gulf of phantasy and flame."

Source: Culver Pictures, Inc.

eral of his physicians. Van Gogh's family history, like Lord Byron's, seems to confirm the diagnosis of bipolar disorder: Vincent's brother Théo described his own struggles with depression in letters to Vincent, and a third brother, Cor, committed suicide. A person needs only to imagine the brilliant, swirling, sometimes frenzied colors and shapes of van Gogh's paintings as visual representations of his moods to understand what psychiatric illness best explains the artist's episodes of psychosis.

The Romantic composer Robert Schumann (1810–1856) wrote of suicide at age eighteen, but only a year later reported, "I am so full of music, and so overflowing with melody that I find it simply impossible to write down anything." Schumann suffered his first major episode of psychiatric illness in 1844 at the age of thirty-four, but he had written a description of his depressions several years earlier in a letter to his future wife, Clara: "No one knows the suffering, the sickness, the despair, except those so crushed. In my terrible agitation I went to a doctor and told him everything—how my senses failed me so that I did not know which way to turn in my fright, how I could not be certain of not taking my own life when in this helpless condition."

Schumann recovered from this episode to write some of his greatest musical works, including three of his four symphonies, but ten years later he suffered another collapse. In February 1854 Clara recorded, "In the night, not long after we had gone to bed, Robert got up and wrote down a melody which, he said, the angels had sung to him. Then he lay down again and talked deliriously the whole night. When morning came, the angels transformed themselves into devils and sang horrible music, telling him he was a sinner and that they were going to cast him into Hell."[2]

A few weeks later, probably in the grip of an episode of psychotic depression, Schumann ran out of their home and threw himself off a bridge into the icy waters of the Rhine. He was rescued by fishermen and placed in the asylum in Endenich, where he died a year later, possibly of self-starvation. As with van Gogh, biographers have quarreled at times about Schumann's diagnosis, but a glance at the opus numbers of his works grouped by year of composition (figure 19-2) leaves little doubt that he suffered from bipolar disorder. What other illness could better explain these intense fluctuations of productivity, periods of intense creative energy that gave way to psychosis and despair?

The fact that many great artists have suffered from bipolar disorder does not in itself indicate a special link between bipolar disorder and creativity. There have certainly been many other great artists, writers, and composers who as far as we can tell did *not* suffer from major psychiatric illnesses. Johannes Brahms, Schumann's musical protégé, who arguably went on to surpass his mentor's accomplishments as a composer, was as staid and steady a man as ever lived. Brahms ate dinner at the same restaurant in Vienna nearly every day for the last several *decades* of his life, often sitting at the same table and ordering the same items from the menu.

Nevertheless, several researchers who have performed psychobiographical surveys of groups of creative individuals have found that a striking and inordinate number of accomplished artists, writers, and musicians have suffered from bipolar disorder. Most studies have come up with prevalence rates of between 30 and 50 percent—nearly ten times the rate of mood disorders in the general population. Perhaps the most careful of these studies has been done by Kay Redfield Jamison, who examined autobiographical and biographical materials and, when available, the medical records of all major British and Irish poets born between 1705 and 1805. Jamison concluded that over half of these writers suffered from a mood disorder, more than one-third of them from bipolar disorder. These numbers are so high that one can't help but wonder if there might be some bias in the research method: do the more tumultuous biographies of psychiatrically ill artists result in more biographical material being available, thus skewing the results? To avoid such a bias, researchers have made studies of living writers,

FIGURE 19-2 data — Robert Schumann's musical works (by opus number) arranged by year of composition:

1829	007
'30	001
'31	124, 004, 003, 002
'32	010, 005
'33	011, 099
'34	014, 009
'35	012, 013
'36	022, 016, 006
'38	032, 021, 017, 025, 015
'40	142, 127, 077, 057, 053, 051, 049, 048, 045, 043, 042, 040, 039, 036, 035, 034, 033, 031, 030, 029, 027, 018, 038, 024
'41	120, 064, 054, 026, 044
'42	052, 050, 041
'43	047, 046
'44	072, 060, 058
'45	065, 055
'46	080, 061, 059
'47	081, 071, 063, 062
'48	084, 073, 070, 068, 066
'49	146, 145, 141, 138, 137, 108, 106, 102, 101, 098, 095, 094, 093, 092, 091, 086, 085, 082, 079, 078, 076, 075, 115, 089, 088, 069, 067
'50	136, 128, 121, 119, 117, 144, 130, 129, 125, 097, 096, 074, 105, 104, 087, 083
'51	116, 113, 112, 111, 110, 109, 090, 140, 139, 103, 100
'52	143, 134, 133, 148, 107, 126, 123, 034, 122
'53	132, 147, 131, 118, 114
'54	

Axis years: 1829 '30 '31 '32 '33 '34 '35 '36 '38 '40 '41 '42 '43 '44 '45 '46 '47 '48 '49 '50 '51 '52 '53 '54

Annotations along the timeline:
- Suicide attempt (1833)
- Hypomanic throughout 1840
- Severely depressed throughout 1844
- Hypomanic throughout 1849
- Suicide attempt (1854)

FIGURE 19-2 The severe fluctuations of the German Romantic composer Robert Schumann's musical productivity become strikingly apparent when his musical works (identified here by opus number) are arranged according to the year of their composition. Schumann died in an asylum a little more than a year after his suicide attempt in 1854.

Source: Adapted from Eliot Slater and Alfred Meyer, "Contributions to a Pathology of the Musician Robert Schumann," Confinia Psychiatrica 2 (1959): 65–94. Reproduced with the permission of S. Karger, AG, Basel.

TABLE 19-1 Artists, writers, and composers with bipolar disorders

Artists
   Paul Gauguin
   Vincent van Gogh*
   Mark Rothko*
Writers
   William Blake
   Lord Byron
   Ernest Hemingway*
   Robert Lowell*
   Sylvia Plath*
   Anne Sexton*
   Virginia Woolf*
Composers
   Hector Berlioz
   George Frederick Handel
   Robert Schumann*
   Hugo Wolf*

*Attempted or committed suicide.

musicians, and artists who were selected because they had won literary and artistic prizes. Those studies have come up with virtually the same numbers. The prevalence of bipolar disorder is simply much higher in groups of accomplished artists than in the general population (table 19-1).[3]

How can this striking finding be explained? Emil Kraepelin thought that manic-depressive illness could free a person from the inhibitions that might otherwise stifle creativity: "The volitional excitement which accompanies the disease may . . . set free powers which are otherwise constrained by all kinds of inhibition[s]."[4] Fear of failure, sensitivity to criticism, worry that one has nothing important to contribute—these kinds of inhibitions, of course, vanish during periods of hypomania and mania.

One can argue that the extraordinary mental states experienced by persons with bipolar disorder provide them with rich raw materials for the production of works of great creativity. As I tried to make clear in chapter 1 of this book, the clinical states of mania and major depression often bear little resemblance to normal mood states. They are not simply exaggerations of normal happiness and sadness but rather are normal moods transcended and transformed. Is it any wonder, then, that those who endure them have put such great effort into chronicling and communicating these remarkable experiences? Because of the relapsing and remitting course of the illness, a person who has recovered from mania or major depression can record what it was like. Individuals in the midst of an episode will usually be too disorganized or too lethargic to be very productive, but later, when their mood state returns to normal, they can express these almost inexpressible feelings and experiences in art, music, and poetry.

It has been suggested that the changes in thinking patterns that occur during the hypomanic and manic states are especially conducive to creative endeavor. When the thinking processes of highly creative individuals (with or without mood disorders) have been studied, it has been found that their thinking tends to be very fluid and divergent. Ideas spring from and give rise to other ideas only loosely connected by logic and convention. Unrelated ideas are merged and mingled in novel ways. The loss of logical progression in thinking and a rapid flow of loosely connected ideas are, of course, a fundamental aspect of the hypomanic state.

It has also been suggested that it is not any one mood state, normal or abnormal, that gives rise to the creative powers of these artists, but rather the flux and tensions between the different mood states. Constant changes in mood and temperament give the individual with cyclothymic mood changes a kaleidoscopic view of the world, always changing, always new. Perhaps bipolar disorder stimulates creativity in part because its sufferers experience the world through the emotional prisms of its many and shifting moods, some of them extreme, even violent. As the English poet John Keats observed, "What shocks the virtuous philosopher delights the chameleon poet."[5]

Individuals with bipolar disorder may be drawn to creative endeavors out of a need to understand and heal themselves through art and the act of creation. The French author and filmmaker Jean Cocteau said, "Art is science made clear."[6] When medicine and psychiatry fail to explain the inner experiences of the disease, when lithium and antidepressants and therapy all flounder and the terrible moods return again and again, people can find ways of understanding and transforming their suffering through poetry, music, and painting.

All these reasons help us to understand why this dreadful and often destructive illness can also generate such intense creativity and artistic accomplishment. If creative work requires unique experiences, fluid imagination, confidence in one's abilities, and energetic excitement about the act of creation, bipolar disorder would seem to fit the bill.

But reading the biographies of these bipolar artists reveals the high price they often paid. Bipolar disorder was a mighty but malignant muse for Vincent van Gogh and Ernest Hemingway and Sylvia Plath, all of whom committed suicide. How many more symphonies would Robert Schumann have composed if, like his quiet, steady friend Brahms, he had lived into his sixties?

Perhaps the most intriguing question about the connection between bipolar disorder and creativity is whether or not the illness was somehow *essential* to the creative powers of these individuals. Van Gogh might have lived to paint many more paintings if he had not suffered from bipolar disorder, but would they have been great paintings? Would he have been a painter at all? Or would he have acquiesced to his father's wishes and contentedly applied himself to becoming a member of the clergy? This is, of course, an unanswerable question when historical figures are involved, but a related question poses a very real dilemma for many individuals with bipolar disorder and their physicians. Does the treatment of bipolar disorder with mood-stabilizing medication suppress creativity and dull the artistic spirit?

Several studies attempting to answer this question were done just after the introduction of lithium as a treatment for bipolar disorder in the 1970s (one of them by Morgans Schou, who, as you may remember from chapter 4, was a pioneer in the use of lithium as a mood stabilizer). Artists and writers were asked whether they thought treatment with lithium had increased, decreased, or had no effect on their productivity. The results are fairly unequivocal and perhaps a little surprising. Over half (57 percent) reported that treatment of their mood disorder with lithium had *increased* their artistic productivity, and another 20 percent thought it had not affected their artistic output. Only one-quarter of these artists and writers felt that lithium had adversely affected their work.[7] Since one of the side effects of lithium in some persons is a dulling of thinking, it is also possible that these individuals were reporting the impact of a medication side effect rather than the impact of mood stabilization. Would artists treated with valproate or carbamazepine have reported the same results?

Over the years a very few of my patients have resisted taking mood stabilizers because they felt that their creative powers would be or actually were adversely affected by these medications. I have usually thought that these individuals were reluctant to take medications for other reasons: unwillingness to accept a diagnosis of bipolar disorder, ambivalence about taking a medication that they felt would "control" them, and other understandable concerns that can usually be resolved with therapy and counseling (see chapter 20 for more discussion of these issues). People seize upon all kinds of reasons not to take medication; my impression is that this particular plausible-sounding reason is usually a substitute for facing and working through understandably conflicted feelings about taking medication.

The mysterious link between bipolar disorder and creativity, though unexplained by either psychiatrists or philosophers, is real. It poses challenges for patients and dilemmas for clinicians and offers opportunities for researchers. Better understanding of this connection will not only expand our understandings of mood disorders but will perhaps lead us to new insights into the magic of artistry and the creative process.

PART IV

GETTING BETTER
AND STAYING WELL

There are millions of people living with bipolar disorder today. Many are living healthy, happy, and productive lives, but many others are not. This section of the book is intended to help you to maximize your chances of getting into and staying in the first category and staying out of the second.

If you're looking for a simple list of dos and don'ts, I'm afraid you will be disappointed. Instead, in chapter 20, "Living with Bipolar Disorder," I've tried to lay out general principles that underlie the sorts of advice and recommendations that are usually given to patients in the doctor's office or clinic. I hope that after reading this chapter, you'll have a better understanding of why some of the recommendations that you hear from your doctor and therapist are so important.

Chapter 21 offers some principles for dealing with emergencies and highlights the types of emergency situations that patients and their families often fail to prepare for. We're always tempted to put off thinking about and planning for things we hope won't happen. But it is important not to give in to this temptation. I explain here how easy it is to be prepared for emergencies.

Bipolar disorder doesn't affect only the individual with the diagnosis of the illness. Inevitably, family and friends are affected in countless ways, both directly and indirectly. Chapter 22, "The Role of the Family," addresses this aspect of the illness. I talk about what family members can do—and, just as important, what family members cannot and should not try to do—to help their loved one who has bipolar disorder.

A short final chapter looks into the future at some of the exciting possibilities that we hope will help us to better understand bipolar disorder, to better diagnose and treat it, and, yes, perhaps one day to *cure* this illness.

CHAPTER 20

Living with Bipolar Disorder

THERE IS NO ONE MEDICATION OR TREATMENT APPROACH FOR bipolar disorder that works for everyone. The symptoms of the illness in a specific person are often as unique as the individual, and treatment must be carefully individualized to each patient and his particular symptom pattern. This said, there are some approaches and pieces of advice that I think are always going to be helpful. In fact, the principles I lay out in this chapter are, in my experience, indispensable to staying well and having the best possible control of symptoms.

Confront and Accept the Illness

There is no cure for bipolar disorder, only treatment and management. It is a relentless illness whose symptoms inevitably and repeatedly return to torment its sufferers. The only way to keep it at bay is for the patient to be relentless as well—relentless about getting needed treatment and sticking to it. No other piece of advice I can give is as important as this one.

Human beings have an almost unlimited capacity to explain away the obvious. People who don't want to confront serious physical illnesses can ignore and explain away even the most alarming symptoms: for example, the middle-aged man with a history of high blood pressure who doesn't pay attention to his repeated episodes of chest pain ("Oh, it's just heartburn; must have been something I ate") and the woman who feels a lump in her breast and tells herself, "It's probably just a cyst, I'm sure it will go away." Confronting a possibly life-threatening illness is perhaps the most frightening experience we can face. Small wonder that we sometimes put ourselves through some impressive mental gymnastics to avoid the confrontation.

When there are no *physical* signs of illness, no pains or lumps or dizzy spells, it may be all the easier to convince oneself that the symptoms of illness are something else. I don't know how many times I've had a patient ask if I thought she really needed to continue on a mood stabilizer after a manic episode had resolved: "After all, I was under a lot of stress, and I hadn't slept for weeks. Maybe I just need to take it easy." As we'll see, stress can indeed play a role in precipitating an episode of a mood disorder, *but it's not the cause*. Stress doesn't make people manic or send them into a major depression unless they have bipolar disorder. Neither does drinking too much or sleep deprivation or the loss of a job or the end of a love affair or the hundred other things that you can convince yourself explain your symptoms better than a diagnosis of bipolar disorder.

People with bipolar disorder can go through years of denial and anger about their illness. I have seen patients repeatedly stop taking medication and drop out of treatment and explain their repeated hospitalizations, shattered relationships, and ruined finances in all sorts of ways: "My wife has it in for me, she put me in the hospital again." "If my boss wouldn't put so much pressure on me, this wouldn't happen." "I think you need to check my thyroid again; I know that's the real problem." Or in its simplest form: "I don't need this medicine, because I'm not crazy."

If you have been diagnosed with bipolar disorder and you have read to this point in the book, you have almost certainly gotten past a great deal of this understandable denial and anger. This is a tremendous accomplishment and signals a turning point in your recovery. (If you're reading this book to better understand another person with bipolar disorder who hasn't yet made it past denial, chapter 22 is especially for you.) But there's a gap between complete denial and complete ability to confront and accept this illness. Unfortunately, people sometimes try to hold on to the notion that nothing is seriously wrong by refusing to take the problem seriously. It is especially easy and especially problematic to take this view in bipolar disorder.

In bipolar disorder the patient ultimately determines how well *any* treatment is going to work—because it is the *patient* who puts treatment recommendations into action. It is the patient who will determine whether he takes *every* dose of medication, or just 90 percent of the doses, or 50 percent, or even less. The patient will determine whether the blood for her lithium or valproate blood-level test is drawn exactly twelve hours after the last dose, or whether she gets to the lab ten hours or fifteen hours after the last dose, throwing the results and the doctor's calculations off by 10 percent or 20 percent. The patient will determine how many appointments are kept with the doctor and the therapist and how many are missed, and how many are shorter than scheduled because of tardiness. It's so easy to let your guard down, let treatment lapse in little ways, and convince yourself that missing a dose of medication here or there, having that second beer, ignoring a string of sleepless nights, isn't really important. To do so is to turn away from rather than to confront this disease, and often the turning away springs from ambivalence about the need for treatment: *less than complete acceptance of the diagnosis.* Not to accept this illness, not to confront it, puts treatment success in jeopardy, because in bipolar disorder perhaps more than in any other serious illness, it is the patient who administers the treatment most of the time.

Imagine that a surgeon is evaluating a patient with recurrent abdominal pain. He has done a physical examination and has ordered some lab tests and x-rays. All the evidence points to gall bladder problems, and the surgeon decides that the best treatment among several possibilities is gall bladder removal. Now imagine that the surgeon is in the middle of the operation and suddenly says to the operating room nurse, "You know, this operating room's getting awfully hot, and besides, I'm hungry. I think we'll cancel the operation. I'll give our patient here the antibiotics for another week or so. Maybe we didn't stick with the medication approach long enough after all. Isn't there some new medication that's supposed to dissolve gallstones? Maybe I'll ask Dr. What's-his-name about that. But I just don't think I want to go on with this operation right now."

Sound far-fetched? (I certainly hope so!) Well, here's another scenario: A man with bipolar disorder has driven off with the family for their three-week vacation. The family has already traveled fifty miles when the wife says, "Honey, I packed Timmy's asthma medicine, but I didn't see your medication bottle in the cabinet; did you remember to bring your lithium?" The man realizes that he didn't. "Ah . . . sure I did," he tells his wife, and then says to himself, "Three weeks won't make any difference. Besides, I haven't felt depressed or anything in a long time. This is a vacation, after all. And if I get just a little high, it would be OK; I'm sure I could handle it."

Now, what do these scenarios have in common? In both cases, a treatment plan had been decided upon, presumably after much consideration and discussion as to the best course of action. In both cases, something comes up that makes continuing with the treatment a bit inconvenient. In both cases, rather than make a rational decision about the best course of action, the person in charge of the treatment uses flimsy logic—accompanied perhaps by a large measure of preexisting ambivalence about the treatment being the correct one in the first place—to justify doing what's easiest. Add in some misinformation—there *is* no medication that dissolves gallstones; three weeks without lithium *can* make a difference, and nobody can just "handle" evolving mania—and you have a recipe for disaster. No one would go back to a physician who treated him this way, and no one should treat himself this way, either.

I am suggesting that making a commitment to treatment means (1) being active, not passive, in formulating a treatment plan with your providers, (2) taking charge of treatment implementation 100 percent of the time, and (3) making the decision that you will do everything possible to take control of this illness rather than be controlled by it.

But can a person be "on guard" all the time? In fact, who would *want* to be? What kind of life is it to be constantly worrying about one's mental health? A terrible one, of course. But worrying all the time is certainly not what I'm suggesting. Rather, accepting and confronting this illness means deciding to do whatever you need to do to be as healthy as you can possibly be. This means sticking with treatment and being frank and open with the treatment professionals. It also means more self-discipline and restraint than you may be used to; it means making some lifestyle changes that I'll call *mood hygiene*.

Practice Mood Hygiene

Hygiene is a word that we might not use in medicine as much as we should, and we certainly don't use it as much as we used to. Hygeia was the Greek goddess of health, the daughter—or in some versions of the story, the wife—of Asclepias, the god of medicine. Hygiene, or hygienics, is the science of *the establishment and maintenance of health*—as opposed to the treatment of disease—and has to do with conditions and practices that are conducive to health. The hygienic conditions and practices we think of today usually relate to cleanliness, but the word has a much broader meaning. At the beginning of the twentieth century, institutions such as the Johns Hopkins University School of Hygiene and Public Health (now the Bloomberg School) and the London University School of Hygiene and Tropical Diseases were founded to study methods for *preventing* disease and for promoting and improving the health of whole communities. Predating them both was the Mental Hygiene Association, founded in 1909 by former asylum inmate Clifford Beers (who probably had bipolar disorder). Now called the Mental Health Association, its purpose is to promote emotional health and well-being and to lobby for better and more readily available treatment for psychiatric illnesses.

So, what do I mean by *mood hygiene*? Simply put, practices and habits that promote good control of mood symptoms in persons with bipolar disorder. Several areas of research on bipolar disorder show how important preventive measures can be for improving symptom control in bipolar disorder. Things like stress management and lifestyle regularity make a big difference.

Emil Kraepelin noticed that early in the course of his manic-depressive patients' illnesses, their mood episodes often came on after a stressful event in their lives: "In especial, the attacks begin not infrequently after the illness or death of near relatives. . . . Among other circumstances there are occasionally mentioned quarrels with neighbors or relatives, disputes with lovers . . . excitement about infidelity, financial difficulties. . . . We must regard all alleged injuries as possible sparks for the discharge of individual attacks." Kraepelin was quick to point out that these events were triggers, not causes, and that "the real course of the malady must be sought in permanent internal changes which . . . are innate." Kraepelin noticed, however, that later in the course of the illness, attacks occurred "wholly without external influences," and he proposed that for patients at that stage of the illness, "external influence[s] . . . must not be regarded as a necessary presupposition for the appearance of an attack."[1]

The accuracy of these observations has been borne out in later studies: initial and early mood episodes in patients with bipolar disorder are often related to psychological stressors, but after several episodes, the illness can take on a life of its own, such that later episodes are more likely to arise spontaneously.

An interesting parallel in animals can be demonstrated by repeatedly giving animals small doses of stimulants such as cocaine. Over time, animals become *more* rather than less sensitive to the stimulant, and repeatedly giving the same small dose causes *increasing* amounts of behavioral stimulation in the animal. When these animals' brain cells are closely examined, it is found that a certain gene that had not been active previously had been turned on by the repeated stimulant exposure. This same gene can be made to turn on by stressing the animals—by depriving them of water, for example. This work with animals, showing that chemical stimulation as well as stress can bring about long-term changes in behavior—possibly through alterations in gene function—is thought by many experts to be highly relevant to the study of bipolar disorder.[2]

Several direct observations of patients indicate that a similar phenomenon may occur in individuals with bipolar disorder: (1) Patients sometimes show more environmentally triggered mood episodes at first in the course of their illness and more spontaneously occurring episodes later. (2) They sometimes show an acceleration in their illness as they age, with episodes occurring more and more frequently as time goes on. (3) Mood episodes make patients more sensitive to stress and more likely to relapse than they might otherwise be. In a study of fifty-two patients with bipolar disorder followed for two years, those who relapsed during the time of the study were much more likely to have experienced some stressful event. In this group of patients, those with a greater number of prior episodes were *more* sensitive to these stresses: they were more likely to relapse under stress, and they relapsed more quickly.[3]

The converse, however, may be true as well: as time in remission gets longer, people seem to develop a resiliency that helps them stay well. I previously repeated a colleague's comment that "the second year on lithium" was better than the first. Here's a corollary: several years ago, I was leading a seminar for psychiatry residents at Johns Hopkins on the treatment of bipolar disorder with lithium. We were lucky enough to have my colleague Hopkins professor Kay Jamison drop by and join us that afternoon. As we were finishing up, I repeated my other colleague's maxim for the residents, "The second year on lithium is better than the first." Smiling, Dr. Jamison added, "That's right . . . and the *twenty*-second year on lithium is just terrific!" Her point was that longer periods of mood stability confer a kind of resilience on persons with bipolar disorder and lessen the probability that stresses will trigger an episode. Several studies have demonstrated that treatment and the prevention of mood episodes improve the long-term outcome in bipolar disorder. Treatment intervention during the first ten years after diagnosis appears to be especially important; the prevention of manic episodes is very important, too.[4] Working hard to stay well, especially in the first years after diagnosis, makes it easier to stay well over the longer term; put another way, "stability begets stability." This means that one of the foundations of mood hygiene needs to be *relapse prevention*. And there should be no doubt in your mind at this point that the most effective relapse-prevention tool is medication.

Persons with bipolar disorder should make peace with the idea of taking medication every day for the foreseeable future. That is an especially hard thing to do in this disease. The symptoms and the need for medication often start when people are in their twenties or even younger, when none of their peers have to bother with medication—when the only people they know who take medication are "old people" and "sick people." It's very difficult for a young, physically healthy person who's feeling well to take medication every day.

The idea of taking medication to control one's moods and mental processes is also a daunting one. An early study asked forty-seven persons who were attending a clinic about their attitudes toward taking lithium.[5] Of those who had stopped taking lithium at some point during the course of their treatment, the most frequently given reason was that they were "bothered by the idea of moods being controlled by a medication." On the face of it, this is quite understandable, perhaps even reasonable. Remember, however, that in bipolar disorder the medication allows the patient to be in control of her moods rather than the other way around.

Each individual needs to work out for himself a method for making sure that every single dose of every medication is taken. Pharmacies sell a variety of clever devices to help make this happen. There are pillboxes with built-in clocks and timers, with alarms that can be set to go off when it's time for the next dose. There are boxes that hold a whole week's worth of medication in little compartments, one for every dose, so that the answer to "Did I take my dose this morning?" is always clear and certain: if the little compartment is empty, the dose was taken. Ask your treating physician if your medication can be taken just once a day, or twice rather than three times a day. Ask about controlled-release forms of medications; several are available, often making it possible to eliminate midday doses, which are inevitably the most difficult ones to fit into a busy life.

The body of evidence showing that medication prevents relapse cannot be argued with; it is simply overwhelming. But there is some evidence that persons who stop medication for bipolar disorder may run more than just the risk of a relapse. There have been several case reports of persons who stopped taking lithium for bipolar disorder, had a relapse, *and then did not respond to lithium when it was restarted.* Once the lithium had been stopped, it did not work very well for these patients when they started back on it, a phenomenon that has been called "lithium-discontinuation-induced re-fractoriness." Out of fifty-four patients who stopped lithium, ten of them—nearly 20 percent—had a poor response when they restarted it. For these patients, lithium had lost some of its effectiveness.[6] The results of this study provide even more proof of the importance of relapse prevention for the long-term course of bipolar disorder. I already mentioned the work showing a better prognosis for persons whose illness is well controlled from the beginning. Lithium-discontinuation-induced refractoriness illustrates the converse of the adage "stability begets stability": *instability begets instability,* at least in some persons.

Next on the list of mood-hygiene practices is *stress and conflict management.* Most of us have very little control over when and how stress and conflict come into our lives. But we can learn how to manage stress and conflict better—and here I'll put in another plug for counseling and therapy. This is because I am talking about serious, *vigorous* attention to whatever ongoing sources of serious stress there may be: primary relationship and marital conflicts, job and career problems, and chronic financial or legal problems are good examples. Immediately after diagnosis with bipolar disorder may not be the time to deal with ongoing and chronic problems of these sorts. But several months later, after mood symptoms have been under good control for a while, would be a good time for some very serious stocktaking, and professional help is highly recommended.

By *stocktaking* I do not mean some process that can be described in a few paragraphs or distilled into the kinds of "helpful hints" and "do and don't" lists that you might find in a magazine article. Rather, I mean *serious examination and fundamental change*. This may involve changing jobs or even careers; selling a house you can't afford, or declaring bankruptcy instead of struggling with an austerity budget; postponing or reconsidering marriage (or divorce); not going back to school. Just as a person who has had a heart attack would do some serious investigation and hard thinking before taking a job as, say, a high-level manager of a big company, the bipolar patient needs to go through the same process before making big decisions. The stress and strain involved in whatever is being considered should be seriously weighed in the decision-making process.

But serious attention to the "big stuff" doesn't mean that the details of everyday life will just take care of themselves. *Structuring your life* is a very important aspect of mood hygiene as well. In chapter 16 we reviewed the data and studies on the relationship between sleep and bipolar disorder. Remember that a properly synchronized sleep-wake cycle is important to the regulation of mood and that periods of sleep deprivation precipitate hypomanic and manic symptoms. *Establishing and sticking to a personal schedule* is very important. This means establishing regular times for going to bed and getting up in the morning—seven days a week, if possible.

Research on sleep shows that many other lifestyle factors contribute to or detract from good sleep. Consider cutting caffeinated beverages out of your diet completely, or at least make a rule for yourself not to drink coffee, tea (including iced tea), or soft drinks containing caffeine after noon. Heavy meals late in the day should be avoided. Regular exercise has been shown to benefit sleep and has many other benefits as well; it helps to stabilize blood pressure, for example, most likely because of the cortisol-lowering effect that regular exercise provides. *Schedule* your daily walk and your Monday-Wednesday-Friday swim or visit to the gym. Don't exercise only when you "have the time" or "feel like it." Make it part of your regular week, not a luxury.

Don't allow yourself to procrastinate. Putting things off until the last moment invariably increases stress levels. Waiting until the eleventh hour to work on your income tax return and then staying up late tanked up on coffee, searching for receipts and W-2 forms, is not something people with bipolar disorder should let happen to themselves. It's no fun for anybody, but for the bipolar individual, it's downright dangerous. File your taxes early, renew your driver's license early, get your car inspected early—you get the idea. Eliminate procrastination as a way of dealing with things, and you've gone a long way toward eliminating a lot of stress. This advice holds true for putting off dealing with interpersonal problems, too. Smoldering tensions in a relationship, chronic conflicts with a co-worker, a neighbor, or a landlord—these are chronic stresses that will inevitably take their toll on *anyone's* mental health and can exact a higher price on the individual with a mood disorder. Don't put off dealing with these problems, and if you don't know how to approach them, get the professional help you need, whether that means consulting a counselor or a therapist or an attorney.

Alcohol? As I've already said, *the less, the better.*

As I explained in a previous chapter, the stress hormone cortisol has a direct injurious effect on neurons in the hippocampus, an area of the brain that is at the center of mood control. Psychological stress, sleep deprivation, lack of exercise, alcohol and drugs, and even an unhealthy diet are all environmental factors that have been shown to raise cortisol levels in the blood. Whatever you can do to keep cortisol levels down is going to make it easier for your medication to work to keep you well.

Some people find it helpful to keep a record of their moods, a *mood chart.* This can be a journal or diary if you're so inclined, but simpler and less time-consuming techniques can work just as well. If you need to keep an appointment calendar anyway, it's a simple matter to make a notation of your mood every day using a numerical scale. Clinicians commonly ask patients to rate their mood on a 1 to 10 scale, with 1 being the most depressed they've ever felt, 10 the best mood they've ever had, and 5 a normal, neutral, everyday mood. If 1 to 10 seems too confining, use a scale of 1 to 100. It's important to rate your mood at the same time every day to control for diurnal mood variations. Simply record your mood ratings every day by jotting down a number in your appointment book, recording it in your computer time-management program, or marking it on a calendar you keep on your bedside table. One of the first things I ask my patients to do when we're having trouble with persistent mood cycling is to keep a more detailed mood chart that also captures changes in their sleep pattern, levels of anxiety, and medication changes.

A quick Internet search is all it takes to find any number of blank mood charts you can easily print out. You will also find several websites that allow you to set up an account and track your symptoms online, and mood-tracker apps for smart phones are available, too. Keeping this kind of record will provide you and your clinical team with invaluable information that can help show what medications are or are not working, determine whether there is a premenstrual or seasonal component to mood changes, and, of course, detect evolving depressive or hypomanic episodes early.

All of this is much easier said than done for persons with bipolar disorder. Regularizing your life in these ways may seem quite foreign and strange, not to mention boring. If throughout your life you've learned to wait for the good moods to get things done and just put off thinking about things during the inevitable return of the bad ones, such planning and regularity won't come easily. But a growing body of research supports the notion that external regulators like regular sleep and activity schedules help with mood stability.

Build Your Support System

Everyone should have a team of supporters and well-wishers to help her get through difficult times. Persons with bipolar disorder are no exception. All of the advice I've given you so far will be much easier to put into practice if you've got a team behind you.

The most important members of the team are likely to be your family and friends. A trusted family member or friend can be extremely helpful by acting as an objective observer of mood changes. One problem that persons with bipolar disorder all struggle with at one time or another is difficulty figuring out which mood changes are normal and which are not. I have seen patients go from one extreme to another in this regard. They may explain away severe and obviously pathological mood changes as "normal ups and downs" while they are in denial about the illness. Then they may overreact and worry that every low mood after a disappointment, every enthusiasm over a new project or relationship, means that their medication isn't working. The physician and the therapist can help with this, of course, but someone who is concerned and caring and closer to home can be an invaluable ally in this regard. An astute friend or family member who knows how to communicate observations in a caring, nonprovocative way upon noticing sustained changes in mood is one of the best supports you can have. You may need to give the person you choose permission to be blunt with you. The best person for this task might not be someone who lives in the same house with you; that person may be too close to the situation to be objective. Look around you and choose carefully.

This topic leads to the question, To whom should you disclose your diagnosis? Two good rules are that the disclosure should be made only to those who *need to know* and to those who *can help and want to help*. The "need to know" category includes, of course, the family doctor, all treating physicians, and any health professional who might be in a position to prescribe medication—even dentists, for example. If you have an attorney or accountant who handles your affairs on an ongoing basis, that person probably needs to know, too.

With employers, things get a bit trickier. If you are asked to disclose conditions you are being treated for as part of receiving medical insurance or other benefits, then you need to disclose your diagnosis. Failure to do so can result in benefits being denied at a later date and claims for reimbursement of treatment costs not being paid. Disclosure up front can avoid a lot of problems down the line, whether this means sharing facts about diagnosis with a new employer or with the current employer at the time of diagnosis. Letting an employer know that shift changes, frequent long business trips, and late hours are things you will not be able to take on because of a medical condition is not only a reasonable request but also a workplace right protected by the Americans with Disabilities Act. I routinely write letters for my patients who are nurses or others who work night shifts, requesting that they not be assigned shift work—and reminding them that the ADA requires them to provide "reasonable accommodations" to employees to keep them healthy. Your provider will be able to supply documentation to support such a request, too. Basing the employer-employee relationship on openness and honesty is always good policy. (The same is true for all other relationships, of course.)

Although employers are legally prohibited from discriminating against individuals with medical problems in hiring and firing decisions, they can make life difficult for employees they want to get rid of. "Choose your battles" would seem to be good advice here. If you sense hostility at your workplace toward persons receiving psychiatric treatment, you might be doing yourself a favor to look for a different employer rather than for an employment-law attorney.

As for peers and co-workers, the "helping" criterion would seem to be the applicable one, and careful consideration is necessary here. But if you find that you're telling co-workers about your diagnosis to get sympathy, to get special consideration, or to get out of unpleasant assignments, you're headed for trouble. There's no better way to breed resentment and conflict on the job. You don't want to develop a reputation as one of those people who use some factor beyond their control to get co-workers to cover for them in various ways. That's not building a support system; it's manipulation, and it will make things worse, not better.

I cannot speak too highly of *support groups* for persons with mood disorders. Under the auspices of several different national support organizations, hundreds of groups provide support to thousands of individuals with bipolar disorder. (See "Resources" at the end of this book for information on these organizations.) Support groups organized by and for individuals with mood disorders and their families not only provide peer support but also are sources of accurate information about the resources available in a particular community.

I sometimes hear a patient say that he doesn't want to attend a support group because he "doesn't want to sit and listen to other people's problems." Certainly, sitting through an hour of whining is no fun and probably not helpful, but that's not what a support group should be (if the one you find yourself in is, think about starting to look for another group). A good support group brings together individuals who share a common problem and want to learn from each other about coping with it better. It's one thing to ask your doctor about the side effects of a medication that you're contemplating starting, but talking to someone who is actually taking it for the same problem you have provides a different and a very valuable perspective. Within a support group, you may have an opportunity to ask other persons with bipolar disorder how *they* told their boss or their children about their diagnosis, what *they* do to remember a complicated medication schedule, and a thousand other questions.

Another advantage of attending a support group is the reassurance you'll get when you meet other persons with bipolar disorder who are doing well and leading healthy, happy, and productive lives. Don't be surprised, however, if these folks seem to be in the minority in your group. It's not that doing well is a rare outcome, not at all. Rather, many persons simply "outgrow" support groups as they do better and better. You can think of these folks as having gotten what they needed from a support group and having moved on.

Don't Be a "Bipolar Victim"

Individuals with any incurable but treatable medical problem must learn how to walk the fine line between not taking their illness seriously enough and taking it *too* seriously. We psychiatrists see the consequences of not taking bipolar disorder seriously enough every day in our offices and clinics—and, more often than not, in hospitals and emergency rooms. Individuals who stop taking medication, who won't get the treatment they need for a substance-abuse problem, who ignore ongoing environmental stresses and interpersonal problems until they are overwhelmed by them—these individuals are truly victims of bipolar disorder who abdicate to the whims and erratic rhythms of their illness rather than do what they can to control their symptoms. But there's another kind of victim as well: the person who worries about her symptoms and illness all the time, who avoids challenges and withdraws from work and the community into a world of medications, blood tests, doctor's visits, and support-group meetings. I think most people with bipolar disorder spend some time on both sides of this fine line as they sort out the impact of the illness on their view of themselves and figure out how to integrate what they need to do about the illness into their lifestyle.

Neither extreme is healthy, and it takes time, good advice, and hard work to find the proper balance.

Perhaps the biggest obstacle to finding this balance is *stigma*. Sociologist Erving Goffman explained the grisly origins of that word in the introduction to his 1963 book on the subject, *Stigma: Notes on the Management of Spoiled Identity:* "The Greeks, who were apparently strong on visual aids, originated the term *stigma* to refer to bodily signs designed to expose something unusual and bad about the moral status of the signifier. The signs were cut or burnt into the body and advertised that the bearer was . . . a blemished person, ritually polluted, to be avoided, especially in public places." Goffman originally became interested in the issues of stigma, prejudice, and discrimination against physically handicapped individuals who had some immediately visible sign of being different: persons who were blind or disfigured or who had had a limb amputated. He soon came to realize, however, that the same issues were relevant, but became much more complicated, when there was no outward sign of the stigmatized condition, as in "the blemishes of individual character . . . mental disorder, imprisonment, addiction."[7]

Fortunately, psychiatric conditions such as bipolar disorder are not often considered "blemishes of individual character" anymore, but they are stigmatized just the same. Persons with psychiatric conditions are too often regarded as untreatable and thus unpredictable and dangerous, or at the least unreliable and incompetent. Too many films and television programs still ridicule or demonize individuals with psychiatric illnesses, and words like *crazy* and *insane* are generalized terms of contempt that you can hear in any schoolyard during recess. People with bipolar disorder have usually incorporated these prejudiced and negative views into their own way of thinking from a very young age—a process psychologists refer to as the "internalization" of stigma. Therefore, when they are diagnosed with bipolar disorder, they have to deal not only with the prejudices and unfair biases others may have toward them, but also with their *own* internalized negative ideas and feelings about persons with a psychiatric illness. People can react to this in opposite ways, either not accepting the diagnosis and remaining in denial about it, or giving in to their negative thinking and feelings and becoming "a bipolar" rather than "a person who has bipolar illness," telling everyone and anyone about their illness and using it as an excuse to avoid responsibilities and challenges. In either case, the individual has become a victim of the illness.

How can you avoid becoming a victim? You've taken a big step by reading this book. Accurate information about what bipolar disorder is and is not provides an excellent defense against prejudiced thinking and bad decisions based on misinformation. A close second to getting accurate information is getting the support, feedback, and advice—and the opportunity to ask questions and just vent your fears and frustrations—that counseling, therapy, and support groups provide. No one needs to confront this problem and sort through all the conflicting emotions and feelings alone—and no one should.

CHAPTER 21

Planning for Emergencies

THE DECISIONS WE ARE FORCED TO MAKE IN A CRISIS ARE FREQUENTLY not the decisions we would have made under other circumstances. When an emergency arises for which we are unprepared, we usually have to improvise a response as we go along. In this chapter I identify several potential emergencies that may face the individual with bipolar disorder and his family and discuss how to prepare for and deal with them. One of the best ways to prepare for an emergency is to have a crisis plan ready beforehand.

Because we have such effective treatments available for bipolar disorder, we sometimes forget that it is a potentially lethal illness. And when you are dealing with a disease that can become life-threatening, the last thing you want is an improvised response to an emergency situation.

People usually enjoy making plans—vacation plans, wedding plans, retirement plans. Planning for a psychiatric emergency is much less enjoyable but, unfortunately, much more important. Unlike vacation plans, these are plans that no one would be disappointed about not getting to use. But if you do need them, odds are you'll be very glad you made them.

I could sense the frustration in Lisa's voice as I listened to her speaking into the emergency-room phone. She was a psychiatric nurse and we were both at the ER.

"I hear you, ma'am, but the magistrate won't approve a petition for involuntary treatment just because your husband isn't taking his medication. I need more information before we can—"

Suddenly she stopped and put the phone down. "I can't believe it; she hung up on me." Lisa looked down at her notepad, then turned to me. "Does the name Stanley Winters mean anything to you? That was his wife. She wanted someone to come out to their house and bring him in to the emergency room. She said he's very depressed."

"The name doesn't ring any bells with me," I replied. "Let's try the computer to see if he's ever had any treatment here before. Then we can try calling her back." As Lisa stepped over to the emergency room's computer terminal, I glanced at my watch. "Lisa, I'm going to go grab some lunch. You know how to reach me."

Twenty minutes later, a text from Lisa arrived, a message to call the emergency room.

"Frank, this is Lisa. Mr. and Mrs. Winters are here in the ER. Well, that's not exactly true. Mrs. Winters is here, but Mr. Winters won't get out of the car. Do you think you could come down?"

I hadn't done any parking-lot therapy for a while, and as I walked past the "Authorized Personnel Only Please" sign that marked the door to the emergency department, I wondered who and what would be waiting for me. At the nursing station, I asked the secretary where the psychiatric nurse was. I had no sooner asked the question than Lisa walked in. "I went out and persuaded him to come in. They're in room 5. He's not doing too well; I think he'll need to be admitted. I'll call the unit and see if we have any beds."

"Has he been here before? Were you able to get a chart?" I asked.

"The last time he was here was about ten years ago, so he only has a paper chart and it's in off-site storage. We might get it in 48 hours, but . . ." She turned the computer screen so I could see it. "The computer says he was admitted to the mood disorders unit for 11 days and the discharge diagnosis was bipolar disorder, manic episode."

"Well, that's some help. Let's go see them."

As soon as I opened the door to the interview room, I could see that (as usual) Lisa had sized up the situation pretty accurately. Mr. and Mrs. Winters looked to be in their early fifties. He was sitting in a corner, staring at the floor, and he looked as if he hadn't shaved in about a week. Mrs. Winters was sitting next to him but got up as I entered the room. "I practically had to carry him to get him into the car to come here," she said. "I've been desperate. He hasn't eaten anything in four days. We've only been married for a year, and I didn't realize—I mean, I didn't know how bad . . . I called his psychiatrist's office, but they said she wasn't practicing anymore."

It took a while to get Mrs. Winters calmed down, and even longer to get the whole story. Mr. Winters was obviously in the grip of serious depression and was barely able to talk, let alone give any kind of history of his problems.

Mrs. Winters showed me an empty bottle of lithium capsules with a "filled" date three months old and "NO REFILLS" clearly indicated. I recognized the name of the prescribing psychiatrist as a colleague who had retired about six months before. I knew for a fact that she had sent letters announcing her retirement almost a year before she quit her practice group.

I was getting the more recent history from Stan's wife when I heard a knock on the door. Lisa peeked in. "Dr. Mondimore, can I see you for a moment?"

"Excuse me," I said and stepped outside. Lisa was holding the "preferred-provider" and HMO list that was posted on the ER bulletin board. "His insurance doesn't pay here. If he needs to be admitted, he'll have to go to Harris Memorial."

"Great," I grumbled. "He definitely needs to be in the hospital, but his wife had a terrible time getting him here. I don't think we should let her transport him. Can you have the secretary call the hospital transportation people?"

Lisa frowned. "Our transportation won't take patients to a hospital outside our system. We'll need to call an ambulance."

"That will cost these folks several hundred dollars. We can't use our people for a three-mile ride?" Lisa gave me her very best "I don't make the rules, I just follow them" look and said nothing. I took a deep breath and prepared to go tell the Winterses that it would probably be several more hours before Stan would be in the hospital.

Mr. Winters appeared to be operating under the assumption that his bipolar disorder had gone away for good (mistake number 1). So when the letter came from the office of his psychiatrist announcing her retirement, he put off making arrangements to get hooked up with a new one (mistake number 2). When the emergency came along, he had no treating physician familiar with his situation. He and his wife had obviously not had a very detailed discussion about bipolar disorder, about what she should do if symptoms flared up leaving Stan unable to make good decisions about treatment (mistake number 3). Mrs. Winters was not familiar with the law and the procedures in their community regarding involuntary commitment of persons with psychiatric illness (mistake number 4). And last but not least, the Winterses were unfamiliar with the requirements of their medical insurance plan and went to a hospital where their insurance would not approve hospitalization (mistake number 5).

How long would it have taken to prevent all these mistakes? An hour or two? Maybe three? Obviously this would have been time well spent. Let's review some of the things it is important to know about in planning for this type of emergency.

Know Whom to Call for Help

I've always thought that the people who can handle almost anything are those who know when they need help and whom to call for it. Persons with bipolar disorder owe it to themselves to be under the care of a psychiatrist who is familiar with their symptoms and the course of their illness. That means establishing yourself with a new physician when you move to a new community or if any other factor, such as the retirement of your psychiatrist, leaves you "uncovered." Changes in insurance plans sometimes force a change in psychiatrists. Don't put off making an appointment to get established as a patient in a new community or with a new practice. Because administrative hassles and delays can prolong the time it takes for records to be transferred from one office to another, ask your providers if you can be given a copy of your records or a letter of introduction that you can take to your new doctor at the first appointment.

Don't hesitate to ask the psychiatrist how her practice is covered after hours. And how easy is it to get a routine office appointment? Are some appointment slots set aside so that urgent appointments can be set up within a day or two? Every psychiatrist or mental-health clinic should have some means of seeing patients within twenty-four hours in cases of true emergency. One that does not is one to steer clear of.

Be sure you know how to contact the psychiatrist or his office at any time of the day or night and what arrangements are in place to handle emergencies. Does the psychiatrist see his own emergencies, or does everyone in the practice take emergency "on-call" duty on a rotating basis? The on-call system, though not ideal, is often the standard in a practice; it means that you may well see a doctor other than your regular one if you have an acute emergency. Are you prepared for such an arrangement in order to be under the care of a psychiatrist who comes highly recommended?

What hospitals does your psychiatrist or her practice have a relationship with? Does she admit to the hospital you prefer? To the hospital where your insurance covers inpatient psychiatric treatment?

If the answers to these questions are not satisfactory, consider your options. Ask your family doctor, family members, friends, or members of your support group for recommendations. Call the local chapter of the National

Mental Health Association, the Depression and Bipolar Support Alliance, or some other advocacy group for a referral. (These groups are listed in "Resources" at the end of this book.) Sometimes your options are limited by medical insurance coverage—which brings us to another important aspect of being prepared.

Insurance Issues

Be familiar with the details of your medical insurance coverage for psychiatric illness. Although the situation is changing, many plans treat psychiatric illnesses differently from nonpsychiatric illnesses. For example, they may have different and stricter limits on hospitalization coverage, the number of outpatient visits they will pay for, and the percentage or amounts that patients must pay out of pocket (copayments) for certain services. Do you have a lifetime "cap" on psychiatric services? This might be a limit on days of hospitalization or on the number of outpatient visits per year, or there might be a dollar-amount limit to coverage. Are you limited to certain hospitals or practice groups or covered at a lower rate if you don't go to certain hospitals or psychiatrists? If your insurance company denies coverage for a hospitalization or for several days of hospitalization, what are the procedures by which you can appeal the decision?

Hospital stays of all types have become shorter, and psychiatric hospitalization is no exception. Hospitalization is now reserved almost exclusively for life-threatening emergencies, and patients are discharged as soon as possible. Patients are no longer hospitalized in a psychiatric unit or a psychiatric hospital for weeks or months. Does your psychiatrist have access to a *partial hospitalization* program (sometimes also referred to as a *day hospital*)? This alternative to traditional hospital treatment provides hospital-like monitoring and treatment during the day, or sometimes for only part of the day, but allows patients to return home in the evening and spend the night there. It is a very useful treatment option for bipolar disorder because it offers a way to provide daily monitoring of mood symptoms and treatment response without the disruption to personal and family life that staying in a hospital causes. Some insurers cover a partial hospitalization—even insist on it—but others do not. Know where your insurance company and your psychiatrist stand on partial hospitalization.

Nearly all insurers have some form of *utilization review* for their policyholders. Most contract this role to a *managed care organization* (MCO) that supervises or manages how much medical care you receive. The utilization review is accomplished in a variety of ways, some of which may be visible to you, some not. The main purpose is to minimize your use of the more expensive types of medical care, usually meaning hospitalization and treatment by specialists. In an HMO you may have to be referred by a primary physician to any specialists—including psychiatrists—in order to be covered. Lab tests may be covered only if your primary physician approves them (this can make it inconvenient to get the blood tests needed to monitor therapy with lithium and some other psychiatric drugs). If you are admitted to a hospital, your doctor is likely be called every few days by someone from the MCO asking why you still need to be in the hospital. If the reviewer (usually a nurse) thinks you should be discharged, he will tell your doctor (and you) that coverage will be denied after a certain date and that you will be financially responsible for any additional inpatient treatment. (A variety of appeals procedures usually kick in at this point if your doctor disagrees.) Managed care, which was once usually limited to inpatient treatment, is now applied to outpatient treatment as well, and psychiatrists are being asked to fill out forms specifying a treatment plan and requesting a certain number of office visits.

If the insurance plan includes coverage for pharmacy charges, you may not have a choice of brands of medication but will need to take a generic equivalent instead of the exact medication your psychiatrist prescribes. Some plans cover only certain drugs in a broadly defined class of medications, thus limiting the doctor's prescribing options. Your insurance company may allow you to receive only thirty days of medication at a time, or may impose such a limit unless you use a mail-order pharmacy. Your doctor may need to justify prescriptions and ask permission to prescribe a higher dose of a medication than usual, or to use a medication "off-label" to treat you. Taking your prescription to the pharmacy is often only the first step in getting your medication; if a "pre-authorization" is needed, there will be a series of phone calls and faxes back and forth between pharmacy, doctor's office, and benefits manager, a process that often takes several days. If some sort of appeals process is necessary, it can take weeks. All of this means that you should scrupulously avoid waiting until the last minute to call for a refill.

Even then, some medications simply will not be covered under any circumstances. I once wrote a letter to a pharmacy benefits manager for permission to prescribe a medication "off-label" to treat a patient. I included a dozen or so research references supporting the request. We were denied because there had been no "large placebo-controlled clinical trial" testing the particular situation that this patient was in. This was an impossibly high standard to set: if a particular clinical situation doesn't arise very often, no one will invest in a multimillion-dollar clinical trial to test that situation.

Managed-care methods save millions upon millions of health-care dollars. Some people argue that as a result more people have access to better medical care because the system is more efficient and effective. Others argue that "managed care" is an oxymoron. But the fact is that managed-care methods are used in all types of insurance coverage now. Your type of medical insurance will almost certainly determine which hospital you can be admitted to, and it may determine which doctor you can see. Your insurance company will probably supervise the length of your hospitalizations and possibly control the number of office visits you can have, which medications can be prescribed for you, and likely what doses can be prescribed. Therefore, you should closely scrutinize all aspects of your insurance coverage for psychiatric illness, your existing policy and any new policies that you may have to choose from because of job changes. Don't be beguiled by the smiling faces on glossy brochures from insurance companies when it comes to picking a plan. Ask colleagues and co-workers and persons in your support group about their experiences with different plans and companies. Don't put yourself in the position of getting an emergency-room surprise.

Safety Issues and Hospitalization

The most dangerous emergency situation for persons with bipolar disorder, and one that frequently leads to hospitalization, is the development of suicidal thoughts and behaviors. In studies from the 1940s, suicide rates of 30 and even 60 percent were reported in groups of bipolar patients. Thankfully, the availability of modern treatments for bipolar disorder has greatly changed these grim numbers. Nevertheless, the rate of suicide deaths in persons with bipolar disorder has been estimated to be at least 15 times higher than that seen in the general population.[1] It may seem obvious to say that the most effective way of minimizing the risk of suicide in bipolar disorder is relapse prevention. But if I had said "*relapse* prevention is *suicide* prevention" in the previous chapter, you might have thought I was just being dramatic. Do not *ever* lose sight of the fact that bipolar disorder is a potentially fatal disease: relapse prevention *is* suicide prevention.

Individuals with bipolar disorder should not have firearms in the home. There are numerous scientific studies showing that having a firearm in a home increases the chances of a violent death occurring in that home, either by suicide or by homicide.[2] Where an illness whose symptoms can include suicidal depression and heightened irritability with loss of inhibitions is concerned, there is never, *ever,* any justification whatsoever for having a firearm of any type in the home. Period.

The emergence of self-destructive thoughts and impulses is frightening both to the patient and to those around her. The tremendous stigma and disgrace that have been associated with suicide for centuries still make people reluctant to discuss these thoughts when they occur. That context and notions such as "only crazy people kill themselves" complicate what is really a much simpler clinical issue: suicidal thinking is a serious symptom of this illness, which must be evaluated quickly by a professional and managed swiftly and effectively. Patients can be intensely ashamed of suicidal thoughts and feel that the development of self-destructive impulses is a kind of failure. Of course it is not a failing in any way; it is a symptom of an illness. It is important to understand the development of suicidal feelings in a bipolar patient as a very dangerous symptom of serious illness, as dangerous as the onset of chest pains in a heart patient. When they occur, it's not a time to wonder about what they mean. *It's time to call for help.* And like chest pains in a heart patient, suicidal feelings in a mood-disorder patient are often a reason for hospitalization.

Psychiatric hospitalization can be experienced as a terrible failure. Again, the clinical perspective tells us otherwise. Although we have become much better at treating bipolar disorder, our treatment methods are by no means perfect. Sometimes, despite everyone's best efforts, relapses occur and serious symptoms like suicidal feelings emerge and require hospitalization. Such an occurrence is not time for self-blame or questions like, What did I do wrong? Rather, it's time for healing.

Remember that the word we often used in the past for psychiatric hospitals was *asylum,* a term defined as "a place offering protection and safety."[3] Individuals whose will has been temporarily seized by this terrible illness and who are on the verge of terrible and desperate action deserve a place of protection and safety. No apologies are *ever* necessary, no reproach ever justified.

One more reminder: bipolar disorder can raise issues of personal safety. These issues need to be anticipated, discussed, planned for, and promptly addressed if and when they arise. Because family members are often a crucial part of dealing with these emergencies, I'll discuss their role further in the next chapter.

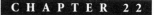

The Role of the Family

THE CHALLENGES OF LIVING WITH BIPOLAR DISORDER ARE NOT limited to those who have the disease. Family and friends face the challenges as well. It's intensely painful to see a loved one suffer from the desperate bleakness of major depression, and just as painful and frightening to see him in the frenzied grip of mania. As in any illness, the role of the family includes support, understanding, and encouragement of the person who is ill. The first step in being able to provide this kind of support is understanding some very important facts about the illness.

Recognizing Symptoms

Never forget that the person with bipolar disorder does not have control of her mood state. Those of us who do not suffer from a mood disorder sometimes expect mood-disorder patients to be able to exert the same control over their emotions and behavior that we ourselves are able to. When we sense that we are letting our emotions get the better of us and want to subdue them, we tell ourselves things like "Snap out of it," "Get hold of yourself," "Try and pull yourself out of it." We are taught that self-control is a sign of maturity and self-discipline. We are indoctrinated to think of people who don't control their emotions very well as being immature, lazy, self-indulgent, or foolish. But you can only exert self-control if the control mechanisms are working properly, and in people with mood disorders, they are not.

People with mood disorders cannot "snap out of it," much as they would like to (and it's important to remember that they want *desperately* to be able to). Telling a depressed person things like "Pull yourself out of it" is cruel and may reinforce the feelings of worthlessness, guilt, and failure already present as symptoms of the illness. Telling a manic person, "Slow down and get hold of yourself" is simply wishful thinking; that person is like a tractor trailer careening down a mountain highway with no brakes.

So the first challenge facing family and friends is to change the way they look at behaviors that might be symptoms of the illness—behaviors like not wanting to get out of bed, being irritable and short-tempered, being "hyper" and reckless or overly critical and pessimistic. Our first reaction to these sorts of behaviors and attitudes is to regard them as laziness, meanness, or immaturity and to be critical of them. In a person with bipolar disorder, criticism almost always makes things worse: it reinforces the depressed patient's feelings of worthlessness and failure, and it alienates and angers the hypomanic or manic patient.

This is a hard lesson to learn. Don't always take behaviors and statements at face value. Learn to ask yourself, "Could this be a symptom?" before you react. Little children frequently say "I hate you" when they are angry at their parents, but good parents know that it's just the anger of the moment talking; this is not the child's true feeling. Manic patients will say "I hate you" too, and it's the illness talking, an illness that has hijacked the patient's emotions. The depressed patient will say, "It's hopeless; I don't want your help." Again, it's the illness and not your loved one rejecting your concern.

I'm now going to make things really difficult by warning against the other extreme: interpreting *every* strong emotion in a person with a mood disorder as a symptom. This other extreme is just as important to guard against. I have seen many couples in which one partner has a bipolar disorder and the healthy partner wields the diagnosis as a weapon to emotionally subdue the other. (Come to think of it, that doesn't sound very "healthy," does it?)

"Vicky's medication needs an adjustment. I'm sure of it."

Vicky stared down at the floor angrily as Peter went on. "She won't give up on this crazy idea about going back to college." I winced a little at Peter's use of the word *crazy*, a word that can make a person with a psychiatric illness feel like they've just been slapped in the face. I made a mental note to bring it to his attention later, but to do so now might make it look as if I was "taking sides."

"Peter," I said, "I'd like to hear from Vicky about this. She's been doing well for over two years now; I think it may be time to have a serious discussion about her idea."

Vicky looked up. "I was six months away from graduating from Bryn Mawr when I got sick the first time. I've called State, St. James College, and Everett, and I could get my degree with only a year of study at any of them."

Vicky was in her mid-thirties, an intense, vibrant woman who I suspected was probably brilliant as well. Peter had been transferred to town by his company a month after Vicky had gotten out of the hospital following a nearly lethal suicide attempt. It had taken three hospitalizations for her to be properly diagnosed as having bipolar disorder—after nearly ten years of roller-coaster moods. She had been treated for a depressive disorder, for a personality disorder, even for schizophrenia before she started on valproate and had a big turn-around. She had done so well, in fact, that I had seen her only half a dozen times over the past two years. About half the time her husband came along to her appointments. Every couple of months I noticed a book review she had written in the local newspaper, and on one visit she had mentioned working on a biography of Mary Todd Lincoln. Going back to college seemed well within her capabilities.

Peter sighed, then went on. "It makes me really nervous to see her up late at night looking at college entrance requirements over the Internet. And we've gotten dozens of college catalogs through the mail that she's called or written for. I'm afraid she's getting manic, and I just can't go through that again."

Vicky's eyes flashed, and she drew in her breath, then slowly released it. "Peter's not used to me being this confident and energized about anything. We've only been married for four years, and for nearly two of those I was more or less depressed. This is me, not mania." Her voice became just the slightest bit louder. "But he's treating me like a child, an incompetent." She looked over at her husband. "A lunatic, right? I'm finally getting back to *my* goals and career after ten years, and what did you call it? 'Crazy'?"

Now it was Peter's turn to look angry. "You see, Doctor? Do you see what I mean, how angry she gets? She's not usually like this. Before we came here today, she—"

"Oh, God, stop it." Vicky said quietly, through clenched teeth. Tears were flowing now.

"OK, you two, let's cool down for a moment," I said. I could sense that this was a continuation of a power struggle between Peter and Vicky that had probably been going on for weeks, maybe even months.

But I also had the sense that Vicky was assessing herself accurately and that Peter was overreacting. Vicky was not being carried away by her feelings—not at the moment, at least; if anything, she was showing a lot of restraint. Peter *was* treating her like a child.

"Vicky," I said, "perhaps Peter doesn't understand your reasons for wanting to go back to college."

"I admit it might seem like a waste of time," she said. "But that degree means a lot to me. I was devastated when I had to withdraw from college. I felt like a complete failure. Maybe I just need to prove to myself that I can do it. That I'm not . . ." She hesitated before spitting it out: "Not crazy."

Peter was calmer, too. "It's not that we can't afford it," he said. "I just worry that it will be too much for her, that she'll get sick again. And she gets so angry when we talk about it; she seems obsessed with this idea. That's not normal, is it?"

"I don't think trying to decide how much obsessiveness is normal or abnormal is going to help us here, Peter," I said. "It seems to me that the problem is that Vicky is investing a lot of time and emotional energy in a project that you don't think is worthwhile."

"That's right," Peter said decisively.

"But *I* think it's worthwhile," Vicky said. "Just because I have a psychiatric illness doesn't invalidate me as a person. It doesn't mean I need someone to make all my decisions for me."

"Honey, I'm just trying to help you, to protect you—"

Vicky snapped back, "I don't want to be protected, I want to have a real life."

"Wait a minute, wait a minute," I said. "I think we were getting somewhere. Let's go back to Vicky's reasons for wanting to go back to school."

This struggle between Peter and Vicky illustrates a very common problem that can come up in families in which an individual has been diagnosed with a bipolar illness. It's possible to jump to the conclusion that everything the ill person does that might be foolish or risky is a symptom of illness, even to the point of hauling the person in to the psychiatrist's office for a "medication adjustment" every time he disagrees with spouse, partner, or parents. As with Peter and Vicky, a vicious cycle can take over: some bold idea or enthusiasm, or even plain old foolishness or stubbornness, is labeled as "getting manic," and feelings of anger and resentment are stirred up in the person with the diagnosis. When these angry feelings are expressed, they seem to confirm the family's suspicion that the person is "getting sick again," so more criticism ensues, followed by more anger, and so on. "He's getting sick again" sometimes becomes a self-fulfilling prophecy: so much anger and emotional stress are generated that a relapse *does* occur, because the person with the illness stops taking the medication that controls his symptoms, out of frustration and anger and shame: "Why bother staying well, if I'm *always* treated as if I were sick?"

So how does one walk this fine line between not taking every feeling and behavior at face value in a person with bipolar disorder, on the one hand, and not invalidating "real" feelings by calling them symptoms, on the other? I think communication is the key: honest and open communication. Ask the person with the illness about her moods, make observations about behaviors, express concerns in a caring, supportive way. Go along with your family member to doctors' appointments, and share your observations and concerns during the visit in the family member's presence. Above all, do not call the therapist or psychiatrist and say, "I don't want my _____ [husband, wife, son, daughter; fill in the blank] to know that I called you, but I think it's important to tell you that . . ." There's nothing more infuriating or demeaning than to have someone reporting on you behind your back.

But it's also possible to err on the side of not being involved enough in treatment for fear of being a "tattletale," assuming that the clinicians will notice the same things you've noticed about changes in moods or behaviors. One of the most valuable ways a family member can help is to provide a clear, undistorted view of the situation to the clinical team treating the illness. In my experience, family members are frequently the first to pick up on subtle changes in behaviors and attitudes that signal the beginning of a relapse. I don't know how many times I have seen patients in the clinic or even in the emergency room who reassured me that they were feeling fine; their behavior and mood seemed normal, so I sent them on their way with a note in the chart that they were doing well. Then I received a panicked phone call from a spouse or other relative a few hours later: "Didn't he tell you that he's lost ten pounds?" ". . . that she hasn't slept in three nights?" ". . . that he got fired from his job?" Contrary to popular belief, psychiatrists cannot read minds! Become involved with treatment, and communicate your concerns openly, sincerely, and supportively—almost anything that might otherwise seem intrusive can be forgiven.

Remember that your goal is to have your family member trust you when she feels most vulnerable and fragile. She is already dealing with feelings of deep shame, failure, and loss of control related to having a psychiatric illness. Be supportive, and yes, be constructively critical when criticism is warranted. But above all, be open, honest, and sincere.

Involuntary Treatment and Other Legal Issues

In every community there are laws and procedures to safeguard individuals who are unable to care for themselves. Laws that allow the removal of children from the care of parents who are abusing them are the most obvious example. Another set of laws allow individuals to be treated for psychiatric illnesses against their will in certain circumstances. One of the most difficult things a person might be called on to do for a family member with bipolar disorder is to initiate involuntary treatment or commitment. But given the power of this illness (especially bipolar I) to cloud judgment and create dangerous situations, there is sometimes no choice but to force the treatment issue in this way. It is always a last resort, but it can literally be lifesaving.

Commitment laws are usually state laws and so vary from one state to another; in addition to these state-by-state variations, local procedures can vary from community to community. Therefore, I can't provide a step-by-step procedure here, only general principles. But in my experience, it's not the procedures that confuse people; it's the general principles, so I think a brief discussion will be worthwhile.

Laws and legal procedures governing the provision of psychiatric treatment—or any kind of medical treatment, for that matter—against a person's stated wishes are based on the knowledge that an individual whose judgment is clouded by the symptoms of an illness often does not make the same decisions about treatment that he would make otherwise. The delirious motor-vehicle-accident victim who has suffered massive blood loss may moan "I want to go home" as she loses consciousness on the stretcher, but the ER team will ignore such a statement and proceed to do what they have to do to save the person's life. It is presumed that if the person were alert and thinking clearly and understood the implications of "going home," she would not make such a request. Similar principles underlie psychiatric commitment laws: treatment is given to persons against their will if clouded judgment prevents them from making good decisions about their treatment. Depressed individuals may be so hopeless that they feel treatment has no chance of helping. Thinking processes in mania can be so disorganized and scattered that seeking out and cooperating with treatment is not possible. In either case there are mechanisms to get needed treatment for persons whose psychiatric symptoms blind them to the need for it.

Fortunately, these laws also have safeguards built in to prevent confinement in a psychiatric hospital for the wrong reasons. Decades ago it was very easy to invoke commitment law, and it often required only the signature of a relative or family physician to hospitalize a person for weeks or months, or even years. People were hospitalized for all kinds of bogus reasons, and serious abuses of individual rights occurred. Laws became much stricter in the

1960s and 1970s to prevent such abuses. The main change was the addition of *dangerousness* as a commitment criterion. Unless an individual's behavior endangers himself—usually meaning suicidal behavior—or others, the person cannot be committed for involuntary psychiatric treatment.

Requests or petitions for involuntary commitment do not necessarily mean that the person who is alleged to be psychiatrically ill will be hospitalized. Friends and relatives cannot admit a patient in to a hospital; only a doctor can do so. The family's request for involuntary commitment usually will allow the patient to be transported to an emergency room, where a physician will make a decision about hospitalization. The patient may be released if she does not meet legal criteria for commitment.

Involuntary commitment is a legal procedure in which an individual is confined against his will and temporarily loses some rights of self-determination. For this reason the law and the courts take involuntary psychiatric treatment very seriously, and many safeguards against abuses are built in to the procedures. The person requesting the involuntary commitment must usually appear in person at the local courthouse or police station to give information and, in some jurisdictions, make a sworn statement before a judge or magistrate. Family or friends will be asked for very specific and detailed information about the behaviors they have observed. This is often frustrating for those trying to get help for their loved one. They may feel that it's uncaring for them to be asked such a lot of questions or that their judgment or motives are being questioned. It's important to remember that in the days when individuals could be confined to psychiatric hospitals simply because a relative or doctor "thought it was best" for them, there were significant abuses of civil rights. When there is serious attention on the part of the issuing magistrate or judge to documenting the facts and questioning the need for involuntary treatment, it means that the system is working.

There is a judicial review (a "commitment hearing") at some point (usually a few days after admission to a hospital), wherein a judge or hearing officer determines that the commitment procedure was done properly and legally. Although this is a legal proceeding, it is not a big courtroom scene. Usually a conference room in the hospital is used, only a few people are present, and the proceedings are kept confidential (they are not a matter of public record). The patient is allowed legal representation; in fact an attorney will be appointed to represent the patient if she cannot afford to hire one.

Involuntary commitment for psychiatric treatment does not usually affect a person's other legal rights. Wills or other legal instruments he has executed are not invalidated, and patients do not become legally "incompetent" in other areas. Hospitalization and treatment are the only issues that are addressed in commitment hearings.

Occasionally individuals with severe, poorly controlled bipolar disorder and their families make legal arrangements to safeguard the individuals' financial assets in case another severe episode of the illness comes upon them. This can involve actually having a legally appointed guardian who might control access to bank accounts, prevent the sale of property or other assets, and so forth. Although rarely necessary, this is a valuable option that can go a long way toward preventing financial ruin caused by manic spending sprees. A document called a *power of attorney* can convey certain specific responsibilities and powers—and not others—and does not constitute guardianship. Careful consideration and consultation with an attorney are, of course, necessary so that legally binding documents with safeguards appropriate to the situation can be drafted.

I am aware that the topic of this section of the chapter is a very frightening one, especially to persons with bipolar disorder, to whom it might seem that liberty and the right of self-determination can be taken away all too easily. At the risk of sounding glib, however, I want to reassure you that involuntary commitment of an individual is *not* a quick and easy procedure. On the contrary, in my experience most people are surprised at how difficult it is to invoke these laws, how many safeguards are built in to the procedures, and how seriously the strict interpretation of the laws is taken by everyone involved. The laws covering involuntary commitment have been carefully written in the interest of helping, not simply confining, people with severe psychiatric illnesses. In my experience they are effective at doing just that.

More on Safety

Never forget that bipolar disorder can occasionally precipitate truly dangerous behavior. Kay Jamison writes of the "dark, fierce and damaging energy" of mania and the even darker specter of suicidal violence that haunts those with serious depression.[1] Violence is often a difficult subject to deal with because the idea is deeply embedded in us from an early age that violence is primitive and uncivilized and represents a kind of failure or breakdown in character. Of course we recognize that the person in the grip of psychiatric illness is not violent because of some personal failing, and perhaps because of this there is sometimes a hesitation to admit the need for a proper response to a situation that is getting out of control: when there is some threat of violence, toward either self or others.

I've already talked a bit about suicidal thinking, and it bears repeating that people with bipolar disorder are at much higher risk for suicidal behavior than the general population. Although family members cannot and should not be expected to take the place of psychiatric professionals in evaluating suicide risk, it is important to have some familiarity with the issue. Again, patients who are starting to have suicidal thoughts are often intensely ashamed of them. They will often hint about "feeling desperate," about "not being able to go on," but they may not verbalize actual self-destructive thoughts. It's important not to ignore these statements but rather to clarify them. Don't be afraid to ask, "Are you having thoughts of hurting yourself?" People are usually relieved to be able to talk about these feelings and get them out into the open where they can be dealt with. But they may need permission and support to do so.

Remember that the period of recovery from a depressive episode can be a time of especially high risk for suicidal behavior. People who have been immobilized by depression sometimes develop a higher risk for hurting themselves as they begin to get better and their energy level and ability to act improve. Patients having mixed symptoms—depressed mood and agitated, restless, hyperactive behavior—may also be at higher risk for self-harm. In fact, there is some evidence that mixed or dysphoric mania is the most dangerous mood state in this regard.[2]

Another factor that increases the risk of suicide is substance abuse, especially alcohol abuse. Alcohol not only worsens a person's mood, but it lowers inhibitions. People will do things when they are drunk that they wouldn't do otherwise. Increased use of alcohol increases the risk of suicidal behaviors and is definitely a worrisome development that needs to be confronted and acted upon.

The development of serious suicidal risk calls for action. Have an emergency plan, and be prepared to use it. Don't hesitate to invoke involuntary commitment procedures if you are really worried and the patient is disputing the need for evaluation.

A less frequent but nevertheless very real risk of violence is the violence toward others that can occur in mania. Friends and family members should not hesitate to call for police help if they feel threatened. "What will the neighbors think?" should not be an issue where safety is concerned. If the situation is becoming dangerous, don't call the psychiatrist's office or the local emergency room; dial 911. Police officers are accustomed to dealing with psychiatrically ill individuals. They know safe physical restraint techniques, and they will be familiar with psychiatric emergency services in the community. Police officers can be expected to have the same goals you have in the situation: transporting the patient quickly and safely to the appropriate health-care facility so that she can receive proper treatment.

Getting Support

It's important for family members to recognize their own need for support, encouragement, and understanding in dealing with this illness. Mental-health professionals go home every day and leave their work of dealing with psychiatric illnesses behind, an option that family members often do not have. It can be exhausting to live with a hypomanic person and frustrating to deal with a seriously depressed person day after day. The changes and unpredictability of the moods of someone with bipolar disorder intrude into home life and can be the source of severe stress in relationships, straining them to the breaking point.

Perhaps the most difficult challenge is that posed by a family member with bipolar disorder who is resistant to obtaining treatment. The most astonishing learning experience that medical students and interns have is with their first patient who repeatedly refuses to continue with a treatment that will keep him well and out of the hospital. I remember as a resident reading the chart of a bipolar patient who had been admitted to the hospital dozens of times after stopping lithium. Why on earth, I wondered, would a person make such a foolish decision again and again? I remember thinking that taking three capsules of lithium a day seemed a very small inconvenience compared with spending what added up to several years of this patient's life in a psychiatric hospital. I've since learned that making peace with the illness and with the idea of staying in treatment is much more difficult than healthy people realize (see chapter 20). But the harder lesson is that there is no way anyone can *force* a person to take responsibility for her treatment. Unless the patient makes the commitment to do so, no amount of love and support, sympathy and understanding, cajoling or even threatening can make someone take this step. Even family members who understand this at some level may feel guilty, inadequate, and angry at times dealing with this situation. These are very normal feelings. Family members should not be ashamed of these feelings of frustration and anger but rather get help with them.

Even when the patient does take responsibility and is trying to stay well, relapses can occur. Family members might then wonder what *they* did wrong. Did I put too much pressure on him? Could I have been more supportive? Why didn't I notice the symptoms coming on sooner and get her to the doctor? A hundred questions, a thousand "if only's," another round of guilt, frustration, and anger.

On the other side of this issue is another set of questions: How much understanding and support for the bipolar person might be too much? What is protective, and what is overprotective? Should you call your loved one's boss with excuses regarding why he isn't at work? Should you pay off credit card debts from hypomanic spending sprees caused by dropping out of treatment? What actions constitute helping a sick person, and what actions are helping a person to be sick? These are thorny, complex questions that have no easy answers.

For all these reasons, it's vital that family members go along with the patient to support groups—and go to support groups themselves even if the patient will not go—and consider getting counseling or therapy for themselves to deal with the stresses caused by this illness. Comprehensive programs for the treatment of persons with bipolar disorder are increasingly emphasizing family involvement.

Like many other chronic illnesses, bipolar disorder afflicts one but affects many in the family. It's important that *all* those affected get the help, support, and encouragement they need.

CHAPTER 23

Looking Ahead

WE ARE MAKING ENORMOUS PROGRESS IN THE FIELD OF PSYCHIATRY. The diagnosis of bipolar disorder and other psychiatric illnesses is becoming more accurate all the time. The available treatments for these illnesses are more effective, and there are more of them. But these advances have come about largely through trial and error, not through a better scientific understanding of the causes of the diseases. The situation is changing, however. Thousands of scientists in two different disciplines are conducting research that will eventually lead to a fuller understanding of psychiatric illnesses and to new and more effective treatment approaches.

The first of these is the field of *neuroscience,* the study of the biology and chemistry of the brain and nervous system. At the beginning of the twentieth century, the physical and psychiatric examination of patients with brain disorders and the microscopic study of brain tissue obtained from them after death were the only available methods to investigate the diseases of the brain. Animal experiments complemented these studies, but this work resulted in only the vaguest outline of the organization of brain function. The location of brain areas important for speech, movement, vision, and so forth were discovered, but psychiatric illnesses remained so mysterious that ideas having nothing to do with biology, theories such as psychoanalysis, were the only ones that seemed to offer any hope of understanding these problems.

By the end of the century, however, breakthrough followed upon breakthrough, mostly in the field of the chemistry of brain functioning, as neurotransmitters were discovered, more powerful electron microscopes allowed the visualization of synapses and other cellular structures, and sophisticated chemical probes allowed scientists to work out the mechanisms by which neurons grow and communicate with each other. Understanding continues to grow concerning the fine details of how neurons develop and link to and communicate with each other through complex networks, and how brain cells and their networks adapt and change in the living organism in response to experience.

Now, new technologies for brain imaging permit scientists to see the brain at work in living persons for the first time. These imaging techniques can trace changes in blood flow within the brain, locate areas that are hyperactive or abnormally low in activity, and detect abnormally high or abnormally low levels of brain chemicals such as serotonin and dopamine. This information is revealing how the interplay of activity between different brain areas is important in the regulation of mood and is making it possible to identify the responsible circuitry. With the new techniques, we can see how the brain of a person with a mood disorder functions differently from that of a person who does not have the disorder. Perhaps an even greater benefit will result because we can see the changes that occur in the brain when a person receives treatment and is beginning to feel well again. Transcranial magnetic stimulation and deep brain stimulation for the treatment of mood disorders came about because of advances in neuroscience. One can argue that these new brain-stimulation techniques are a direct result of neuroscience research; they represent the very first psychiatric treatments that were developed based on science and research rather than stumbled upon accidentally.

The second scientific discipline is the field of *genetics*. Here again, it is the development of new biochemical methods and molecular probes that has made the new research possible. With the announcement that the Human Genome Project had mapped all of the genetic material in the human chromosomes, a new era in the understanding of genetics began. The discovery of new genes is announced every day, and it is only a matter of time before the genetic mechanisms of mood disorders are unraveled. But the identification of the genes responsible for mood disorders is only one of the goals of work in this field. Just as important will be understanding the epigenetic mechanisms by which genes turn on and off and other mechanisms that regulate the expression and work of the instructions encoded in the DNA molecule.

The first genetic approach to pay off in changing treatment is likely to be *pharmacogenomics*, the field within genetics that investigates genetic factors associated with responses to particular pharmaceuticals rather than with risk of disease. The promise of pharmacogenomics is that therapeutic agents can be rationally selected, based on a person's genetic profile rather than the trial-and-error process patients must now endure. In the not-too-distant future, a blood test will show whether lithium or valproate or lamotrigine or some as yet undiscovered drug will be the best treatment for a particular individual with bipolar disorder. A blood test may be able to identify the bipolar patients who can safely take an antidepressant.

As the genetic basis of the mood disorders is discovered, it may turn out that our classification system for these disorders is all wrong and a whole new diagnostic system will be needed for psychiatric illnesses, perhaps one based on the genes that are involved in individual patients. Instead of "bipolar disorder II" we may be diagnosing patients with something like "DISC I disorder," a diagnostic label derived from the name of a gene.[1]

The two fields of neuroscience and psychiatric genetics are closing in on the causes and mechanisms of mood disorders from different directions. As these two enterprises advance, they will begin to inform each other—that is, advances in one field will lead to advances in the other. The discovery that a gene for a particular protein is linked to a mood disorder will tell neuroscientists that that protein is important in the regulation of mood. The discovery of an enzyme in neurons that is important in neuroplasticity, the process of neuronal retuning that appears to go awry in mood disorders, will tell geneticists to focus on the gene for that enzyme in their association studies. Little by little the whole picture will become increasingly clear.

As our understanding of the biology of mood disorders improves, we get closer to better diagnostic methods and safer and more effective treatments. The number of new medications continues to grow, and many more new pharmaceuticals are "in the pipeline," some of them based on clues about the biological causes of these illnesses. The era of finding new medications essentially by accident may be coming to a close; soon we will be able to design treatments more effectively and more rationally. More sophisticated use of nonpharmaceutical treatments such as transcranial magnetic stimulation may make it possible to use lower doses of medications or may help medications work more quickly.

As we take the step from isolating genes to determining the function of those genes, there is the possibility of *gene therapy*: repairing the code in the DNA that causes mood disorders. The obstacles to be overcome before we can look for this type of cure can only be called monumental, even daunting. But scientists are learning more and more about these illnesses, and with enough time and enough hard work, a cure might be possible.

As the mechanisms of illness development become known and the genetic vulnerabilities are identified, another exciting possibility emerges: *prevention*. Genetic data and a better understanding of what triggers the illness may allow the development of programs aimed at preventing the development of illness in individuals known to be at higher risk for a particular disorder.

So, there is much reason to expect great strides in our ability to diagnose and effectively treat bipolar disorder. But we have *already* made great strides—individuals with bipolar disorder must not let denial or fear stand in the way of taking advantage of the very good treatments that are now available. Ignorance is no excuse, either. Support organizations provide up-to-date information about bipolar disorder through newsletters, brochures, websites, and, most importantly, in the support groups they sponsor (see the list of resources that follows this chapter). With the ever-growing online resources now available, anyone with access to a computer can, with the click of a mouse, get the very latest information on new pharmaceuticals and other treatments.

Like many other serious illnesses, bipolar disorder can be life-threatening. Unlike some others, however, it has a unique capacity to rob individuals of their spirit, to take over their humanity. And yet, some of its sufferers have taken inspiration from their struggle with this illness to produce music and art and literature that have inspired and exhilarated the world.

People with bipolar disorder frequently ask me, Will I have to take medication for the rest of my life? I always tell them that no one knows the answer to that question because no one knows exactly what the treatment of mood disorders might be in the future. Pediatricians practicing in the 1930s probably could not have imagined that vaccines would one day practically eliminate diphtheria, polio, measles, and other childhood diseases, the common, frequently crippling, and sometimes fatal illnesses they diagnosed so frequently in their patients but were so helpless to treat. The astonishing developments in neuroscience and genetics hold just this much promise for people afflicted with mood disorders. There is every reason to expect that the time is not too far off when treatments for bipolar disorder will be more effective than *we* can now imagine.

Resources

SUGGESTED READING

Barondes, Samuel H. *Mood Genes: Hunting for the Origins of Mania and Depression.* New York: Oxford University Press, 1999.
> A clearly written and engrossing account of the tough science involved in the search for the genetic basis of mood disorders. An excellent introduction to the science of genetics.

Cheney, Terry. *Manic: A Memoir.* New York: William Morrow, 2009.
> This is not an easy read. Words like "brutal" and "unflinching" capture the author's no-holds-barred descriptions of the terrifying journey that she traveled with her illness before achieving acceptance and the cautious but persistent optimism and steely determination that now sustain her. Not for the faint of heart but truly inspirational.

Goodwin, Frederick K., and Kay Redfield Jamison. *Manic-Depressive Illness and Recurrent Depression*, 2nd ed. New York: Oxford University Press, 2007.
> Comprehensive. Encyclopedic. Maybe more than a little overwhelming but a great resource. This 1,200-plus page tome probably doesn't need to be on your bookshelf unless you're a clinician, but it may be nice to know where you can get your hands on a copy to borrow to find the answer to that obscure question about mood disorders that no one else seems to have.

Jamison, Kay Redfield. *Touched with Fire: Manic-Depressive Illness and the Artistic Temperament.* New York: Free Press, 1993.
> A thorough survey of creative individuals who suffered from bipolar disorder,

and an excellent discussion of the connections between creativity and mood disorders.

Jamison, Kay Redfield. *An Unquiet Mind: A Memoir of Moods and Madness*. New York: Vintage Books, 1996.
> A powerful and moving narrative written with grace and wit by an international expert on the illness who suffers from it herself. This treasure of a book contains some of the most engrossing and vivid descriptions of the experience of bipolar disorder ever written. A "must read" for anyone touched by bipolar disorder.

Kraepelin, Emil. *Manic-Depressive Insanity and Paranoia*. Trans. R. M. Barclay, ed. G. M. Robertson. 1921; reprint, New York: Arno Press, 1976.
> Many college and university libraries have a copy of this book. Arguably the very first textbook on the illness ever written, it is definitely worth reading.

Miklowitz, David. *The Bipolar Disorder Survival Guide: What You and Your Family Need to Know*, 2nd ed. New York: Guilford Press, 2010.
> This book emphasizes the patient's role in managing bipolar disorder symptoms, in simple and easy-to-understand terms. A good introduction.

Mondimore, Francis Mark. *Adolescent Depression: A Guide for Parents*. Baltimore: Johns Hopkins University Press, 2002.
> OK, I'm biased in favor of this one. But if you're looking for a book that focuses on the diagnosis and treatment of mood disorders and coping with them (including bipolar disorder) in young people, I think this is the one to buy!

Noonan, Susan J. *Managing Your Depression: What You Can Do to Feel Better*. Baltimore: Johns Hopkins University Press, 2013.
> This slim volume is packed with truly helpful advice about managing the symptoms of depression, informed by the author's own struggle with a depressive illness as well as her expertise as a physician and background in public health. Dr. Noonan doesn't just offer suggestions but lays out exercises and lifestyle recommendations that are concise and eminently practical. All are presented simply, compassionately, and in small, realistic steps that recognize how difficult it is for a depressed person to get things done.

Rosenthal, Norman E. *Winter Blues: Seasonal Affective Disorder, What It Is and How to Overcome It*. New York: Guilford Press, 1993.
> A comprehensive and highly readable discussion of seasonal affective disorder.

Sapolsky, Robert M. *Why Zebras Don't Get Ulcers*. New York: Holt, 2004.
> A very accessible overview of the biology of stress, the impact stress has on physical and mental health, and what you can do about it.

Styron, William. *Darkness Visible: A Memoir of Madness*. New York: Random House, 1990.
> I recommend this book to medical students as one of the best accounts of the symptoms of depression available. A good book for family members to read to better understand the experience of serious depression.

The Lancet *Series on Bipolar Disorder*

In the spring of 2013, this three-part series of review articles appeared in one of the world's oldest and most prestigious medical journals, *The Lancet*. These three articles by a team of leading international experts are written for physicians and scientists, but anyone and everyone with an interest in this illness will learn something by glancing through them. This is a comprehensive resource covering nearly every aspect of the illness in about thirty pages. You can access the articles through most university libraries and many public libraries as well.

Cradock, Neil, and Pamela Sklar. "Genetics of Bipolar Disorder," *Lancet*, 381, no. 9878 (2013): 1654–62.

> A comprehensive update of the research into the genetic underpinnings of the illness. Although this article requires at least a working knowledge of genetics to fully understand and appreciate it, its optimistic conclusion is crystal clear: "the ongoing major investments of time and money in molecular genetic studies of psychiatric disorders have the potential to . . . help psychiatry move towards approaches to diagnosis and treatment that are grounded in a better understanding. . . . Such progress would help to revolutionize clinical psychiatry, and would be of great benefit to patients."

Phillips, Mary, and David Kupfer. "Bipolar Disorder Diagnosis: Challenges and Future Directions," *Lancet*, 381, no. 9878 (2013): 1663–71.

> This is perhaps the most thought-provoking of the three articles. It calls for an entirely new way of classifying mood disorders by using the "biosignatures" of illness types that neuroscience and imaging research are beginning to reveal rather than symptoms to come up with completely new categories.

Geddes, John, and David Miklowitz. "Treatment of Bipolar Disorder," *Lancet*, 381, no. 9878 (2013): 1672–82.

> An overview of treatment issues with an emphasis on treatments that are usually not emphasized enough: psychotherapy and counseling. An excellent overview of the studies showing the benefits of different types of psychotherapy, including CBT, as well as treatments that focus on family issues, education about the illness, and individualized case management.

SUPPORT AND ADVOCACY ORGANIZATIONS

All of the following organizations provide information and resources, and some offer referrals to support groups as well as to clinicians in your community who are skilled in treating mood disorders. Contact them all and become a member of each! In addition to the direct services they provide to consumers, they are active in combating the stigmatization of psychiatric illnesses, in lobbying for better medical insurance coverage for psychiatric disorders, and in supporting research.

Depression and Bipolar Support Alliance (DBSA)
730 North Franklin Street
Chicago, IL 60610
800-82-NDMDA
www.dbsalliance.org

National Alliance for the Mentally Ill (NAMI)
Colonial Place 3
2107 Wilson Blvd., Suite 300
Arlington, VA 22201
800-950-6264
www.nami.org

National Mental Health Association (NMHA)
2001 N. Beauregard Street
12th Floor
Alexandria, VA 22311
800-969-NMHA
www.nmha.org

INTERNET RESOURCES

All of the support and advocacy groups listed in the previous section have websites, and the astonishing range of resources on the Internet continues to grow. Remember, however, that inaccurate information, bias, and just plain nonsense can also be found on the Internet. It is important to consider information sources very carefully.

Here are some excellent resources:

International Society for Bipolar Disorders
www.isbd.org
> For scientists and clinicians specializing in bipolar disorders, the site also lists the latest research articles on bipolar disorder research from around the world.

Medscape
www.medscape.com
> This is primarily a news site for medical professionals, but it also has a "patient information" section with many useful articles and links to other resources.

PubMed
www.ncbi.nlm.nih.gov/entrez/query.fcgi
> Free access to the most comprehensive medical database in the world, maintained by the U.S. National Library of Medicine. Anyone can use PubMed to search through 15 million scientific journal citations on any medical topic. The vast majority of the citations include an abstract (short summary) of the article, and your local public library can often help you obtain a copy of the complete text.

WebMD
www.webmd.com

One of the best sources of information on just about any medical problem. Organized into "Condition Centers," including centers for bipolar disorder and depression, that pull together many resources for common illnesses.

Notes

PREFACE

1. For a discussion of the diagnosis of bipolar disorder in these historical personalities, see Kay Redfield Jamison, *Touched with Fire: Manic-Depressive Illness and the Artistic Temperament* (New York: Free Press, 1993).

2. Gabor Keitner, Ivan Miller, M. Tracie Shea, and Martin Keller, "Course of Illness and Maintenance Treatments for Patients with Bipolar Disorder," *Journal of Clinical Psychiatry* 56, no. 1 (1995): 5–13.

3. "National Survey of NDMDA Members Finds Long Delay in Diagnosis of Manic-Depressive Illness," in "News and Notes," *Hospital and Community Psychiatry* 44, no. 8 (1993): 800–801.

4. Frederick K. Goodwin and Kay Redfield Jamison, *Manic-Depressive Illness* (New York: Oxford University Press, 1990), 228.

CHAPTER 1. NORMAL AND ABNORMAL MOOD

1. *Webster's Third New International Dictionary, Unabridged,* s.v. "mood," http:// unabridged.merriam-webster.com.

2. Although I have made these clinical vignettes as realistic as possible by using symptom details culled from many patients, they are fictitious and do not portray any person, living or dead.

3. The word *mania* has ancient origins, deriving from the Greek word *mainesthai,* which means simply "to be insane." Very early English physicians sometimes used the word *madness* to describe the syndrome of disorganized hyperactivity that we now call mania. But during the eighteenth and nineteenth centuries, European physicians writing about mental disorders increasingly employed *mania* (in French

la manie and in German *die Manie*). When Emil Kraepelin used *manic-depressive insanity* in his groundbreaking work on bipolar disorder, the term *mania* for the excited phase of the disorder became firmly established.

4. Henry J. Berkley, *A Treatise on Mental Diseases* (1900; reprint, New York: Arno Press, 1980), 143.

5. Kay Redfield Jamison, *An Unquiet Mind: A Memoir of Moods and Madness* (New York: Vintage Books, 1996), 36.

6. Frederick K. Goodwin and Kay Redfield Jamison, *Manic-Depressive Illness* (New York: Oxford University Press, 1990), 23.

7. Quoted in ibid., 26–27.

8. Emil Kraepelin, *Manic-Depressive Insanity and Paranoia,* trans. R. M. Barclay, ed. G. M. Robertson (1921; reprint, New York: Arno Press, 1976), 31. This is a translation of volumes 3 and 4 of the 8th edition (1913) of Kraepelin's textbook *Psychiatrie*, which originally appeared in 1896.

9. Goodwin and Jamison, *Manic-Depressive Illness,* 29.

10. Kraepelin, *Manic-Depressive Insanity,* 31.

11. For a discussion of the concept of motivated behaviors in psychiatry, see Paul McHugh and Philip Slavney, *The Perspectives of Psychiatry* (Baltimore: Johns Hopkins University Press, 1998), 151–238.

12. Kraepelin, *Manic-Depressive Insanity,* 62.

13. Ibid., 56, 64.

14. J. D. Campbell, *Manic-Depressive Disease: Clinical and Psychiatric Significance* (Philadelphia: J. D. Lippincott, 1953), 159–60, quoted in Goodwin and Jamison, *Manic-Depressive Illness,* 24.

15. Jamison, *Unquiet Mind,* 83.

16. Kraepelin, *Manic-Depressive Insanity,* 70.

17. Berkley, *Treatise on Mental Diseases,* 160.

18. Gabrielle Carlson and Frederick Goodwin, "The Stages of Mania," *Archives of General Psychiatry* 28 (1973): 221–28.

19. Quoted in Edward Hare, "The Two Manias: Study of the Evolution of the Modern Concept of Mania," *British Journal of Psychiatry* 138 (1981): 89–99.

20. Norman Endler, *Holiday of Darkness: A Psychologist's Personal Journey out of His Depression* (New York: John Wiley and Sons, 1982), 4.

21. Ibid., 86.

22. William Styron, *Darkness Visible: A Memoir of Madness* (New York: Random House, 1990), 19.

23. Endler, *Holiday of Darkness,* 48–49.

24. Johann Wolfgang von Goethe, *The Sorrows of Young Werther,* trans. Elizabeth Mayer and Louise Bogan (New York: Random House, 1971), 114.

25. Quoted in Kay Redfield Jamison, *Touched with Fire: Manic-Depressive Illness and the Artistic Temperament* (New York: Free Press, 1993), 21.

26. Styron, *Darkness Visible,* 17.

27. Endler, *Holiday of Darkness,* 29.

28. Kraepelin, *Manic-Depressive Insanity,* 75.

29. F. Scott Fitzgerald, *The Crackup* (New York: New Directions, 1956), 75.

30. Styron, *Darkness Visible,* 17.

31. Endler, *Holiday of Darkness,* 54.

32. Styron, *Darkness Visible,* 44.

33. Endler, *Holiday of Darkness,* 46.

34. Kraepelin, *Manic-Depressive Insanity,* 84.

35. Ibid., 89.

36. Styron, *Darkness Visible,* 58.

37. Kraepelin, *Manic-Depressive Insanity,* 97.

38. Jamison, *Unquiet Mind,* 45.

39. Kraepelin, *Manic-Depressive Insanity,* 104.

40. Because some patients in an otherwise typical manic episode develop desperate, anxious, distraught symptoms as they become sicker, some researchers have made the case that mixed states can be thought of as a very severe stage of mania ("Stage III mania" as described in the section "Mania").

41. Kraepelin, *Manic-Depressive Insanity,* 99.

CHAPTER 2. THE DIAGNOSIS OF BIPOLAR DISORDER

1. Frederick K. Goodwin and Kay Redfield Jamison, *Manic-Depressive Illness* (New York: Oxford University Press, 1990), 132.

2. Modern diagnostic classifications are usually different from those that were used when these older studies were done. In most cases, however, patients with "manic-depressive illness" in these studies had full-blown manic episodes and severe depressions and thus would today probably be diagnosed with bipolar I. Nevertheless, cases that would today be diagnosed differently (as bipolar II, for example) may have been mixed in. Thus, the findings and statistics must be interpreted with some caution.

3. Thomas A. C. Rennie, "Prognosis in Manic-Depressive Psychosis," *American Journal of Psychiatry* 98 (1942): 801–14, quoted in Goodwin and Jamison, *Manic-Depressive Illness,* 133.

4. Emil Kraepelin, *Manic-Depressive Insanity and Paranoia,* trans. R. M. Barclay, ed. G. M. Robertson (1921; reprint, New York: Arno Press, 1976), 136.

5. Ibid., 3, 137.

6. G. Winokur, P. Clayton, and T. Reich, *Manic-Depressive Illness* (St. Louis: C. V. Mosby, 1969), quoted in Goodwin and Jamison, *Manic-Depressive Illness,* 141.

7. Athansio Koukopoulas, Daniela Reginaldi, Giampolo Minnai, Gino Serre, Luca Pani, and Neil Johnson, "The Long Term Prophylaxis of Affective Disorders," in *Depression and Mania: From Neurobiology to Treatment,* ed. G. Gessa, W. Fratta, L. Pina, and G. Serre (New York: Raven Press, 1995), 127–47.

8. William Coryell, Nancy Andreasen, Jean Endicott, and Martin Keller, "The Significance of Past Mania or Hypomania in the Course and Outcome of Major Depression," *American Journal of Psychiatry* 144 (1987): 309–15.

9. Sylvia Simpson, Susan Folstein, Deborah Meyers, Francis McMahon, Diane Brusco, and J. Raymond DePaulo, "Bipolar II: The Most Common Bipolar Phenotype?" *American Journal of Psychiatry* 150 (1993): 901–3.

10. J. H. Baek, D. Y. Park, J. Choi, J. S. Kim, J. S. Choi, K. Ha, J. S. Kwon, and

K. S. Hong, "Differences between Bipolar I and Bipolar II Disorders in Clinical Features, Comorbidity and Family History," *Journal of Affective Disorders* 131 (2011): 59–67.

11. Ibid.

12. Hagop Akiskal, Jack Maser, Pamela Zeller, Jean Endicott, William Coryell, Martin Keller, Meredith Warshaw, Paula Clayton, and Frederick Goodwin, "Switching from 'Unipolar' to Bipolar II: An Eleven-Year Prospective Study of Clinical and Temperamental Predictors in 559 Patients," *Archives of General Psychiatry* 52 (1995): 114–23.

13. Eduard Vieta and Trisha Suppes, "Bipolar II Disorder: Arguments for and against a Distinct Pathological Entity," *Bipolar Disorders* 10 (2008): 163–78.

14. Kraepelin, *Manic-Depressive Insanity,* 131.

15. Hagop S. Akiskal, "The Prevalent Clinical Spectrum of Bipolar Disorders: Beyond DSM-IV," *Journal of Clinical Psychopharmacology* 16, suppl. (1996): 4S–14S.

16. Kraepelin, *Manic-Depressive Insanity,* 132.

17. H. Akiskal, M. K. Khani, and A. Scott-Strauss, "Cyclothymic Temperamental Disorders," *Psychiatric Clinics of North America* 2 (1979): 527–54.

18. Robert Howland and Michael Thase, "A Comprehensive Review of Cyclothymic Disorder," *Journal of Nervous and Mental Disease* 181 (1993): 485–93.

19. Akiskal, "Prevalent Clinical Spectrum of Bipolar Disorders."

20. Howland and Thase, "Comprehensive Review of Cyclothymic Disorder."

21. Kraepelin, *Manic-Depressive Insanity,* 2.

22. Hagop Akiskal and Gopinath Mallya, "Criteria for 'Soft' Bipolar Spectrum: Treatment Implications," *Psychopharmacology Bulletin* 23, no. 1 (1987): 68–73.

23. Akiskal, "Prevalent Clinical Spectrum of Bipolar Disorders."

24. See Goodwin and Jamison, *Manic-Depressive Illness,* 136–38.

25. R. W. Cowdry, T. A. Wehr, A. Zis, and F. K. Goodwin, "Thyroid Abnormalities Associated with Rapid Cycling Bipolar Illness," *Archives of General Psychiatry* 40 (1983): 414–20; and T. A. Wehr and F. K. Goodwin, "Rapid Cycling in Manic-Depressives Induced by Tricyclic Antidepressants," *Archives of General Psychiatry* 36 (1979): 555–59.

26. A. Koukopoulos, B. Caliari, A. Tundo, G. Floris, D. Reginaldi, and L. Tondo, "Rapid Cyclers, Temperament, and Antidepressants," *Comprehensive Psychiatry* 24, no. 3 (1983): 249–58.

27. William Coryell, Jean Endicott, and Martin Keller, "Rapid Cycling Bipolar Disorder: Demographics, Diagnosis, Family History, and Course," *Archives of General Psychiatry* 49 (1992): 126–31.

CHAPTER 3. BIPOLAR DISORDER AND THE *DSM-5*

1. At the time, epilepsy was considered to be a mental illness.

2. Alfred Kinsey, Wardell Pomeroy, and Clyde Martin, *Sexual Behavior in the Human Male* (Philadelphia: W. B. Saunders, 1948), 678, 639.

CHAPTER 4. THE MOOD DISEASE

1. Quoted in Stanley W. Jackson, *Melancholia and Depression, from Hippocratic Times to Modern Times* (New Haven, CT: Yale University Press, 1986), 251 ("peevish," "complain[ed]," and "At the height"); and in Frederick K. Goodwin and Kay Redfield Jamison, *Manic-Depressive Illness* (New York: Oxford University Press, 1990), 58 ("In my opinion").

2. Quoted in Jackson, *Melancholia and Depression,* 253–54.

3. Quoted in ibid., 257.

4. See ibid., 262–63.

5. Emil Kraepelin, *Manic-Depressive Insanity and Paranoia,* trans. R. M. Barclay, ed. G. M. Robertson (1921; reprint, New York: Arno Press, 1976), 1.

6. Jackson, *Melancholia and Depression,* 272.

7. Henry J. Berkley, *A Treatise on Mental Disorders* (1900; reprint, New York: Arno Press, 1980), 179.

8. John F. J. Cade, "Lithium Salts in the Treatment of Psychotic Excitement," *Medical Journal of Australia* 36 (1949): 349–52.

9. Ibid., 350–51.

10. It turns out that John Cade was not the first psychiatrist to give lithium to patients with mood disorders. More than fifty years earlier, the Danish psychiatrist brothers Carl and Friedrich Lange had used lithium salts to treat patients with depression and had seen some success. The Lange brothers wrote about this discovery in a German psychiatric research journal, but their report did not garner much attention and was not translated into other languages. It had been essentially forgotten by the time Cade started his work.

11. For a superb account of this shameful story, see Götz Aly, Peter Chroust, and Christian Pross, *Cleansing the Fatherland: Nazi Medicine and Racial Hygiene* (Baltimore: Johns Hopkins University Press, 1994).

12. Ronald R. Fieve, *Moodswing: The Third Revolution in Psychiatry* (New York: Bantam Books, 1975), 3.

13. M. Schou, N. Juel-Nielsen, E. Strömgren, and H. Voldby, "The Treatment of Manic Psychoses by the Administration of Lithium Salts," *Journal of Neurology, Neurosurgery, and Psychiatry* 17 (1954): 250–60.

14. Roland Kuhn, "The Treatment of Depressive States with G 22355 (Imipramine Hydrochloride)," *American Journal of Psychiatry* 115 (1958): 459–64, at 461.

15. Schou, Juel-Nielsen, Strömgren, and Voldby, "Treatment of Manic Psychoses," 256. Emphasis added.

CHAPTER 5. THE PLASTIC BRAIN

1. Nancy C. Andreasen, *The Broken Brain: The Biological Revolution in Psychiatry* (New York: Harper and Row, 1985).

2. R. J. Schloesser, J. Huang, P. S. Klein, and H. K. Manji, "Cellular Plasticity Cascades in the Pathophysiology and Treatment of Bipolar Disorder," *Neuropsychopharmacology* 33 (2008): 110–33.

1. Anastase Georgotas and Samuel Gershon, "Historical Perspectives and Current Highlights on Lithium Treatment in Manic-Depressive Illness," *Journal of Clinical Psychopharmacology* 1, no. 1 (1981): 27–31.

2. Paul Baalstrup and Morgans Schou, "Lithium as a Prophylactic Agent: Its Effect against Recurrent Depressions and Manic-Depressive Psychosis," *Archives of General Psychiatry* 16, no. 2 (1967): 162–72.

3. B. Blackwell and M. Shephard, "Prophylactic Lithium: Another Therapeutic Myth?" *Lancet* 1 (1968): 968–71.

4. P. Baalstrup, J. Poulsen, M. Schou, K. Thomsen, and A. Amdisen, "Prophylactic Lithium: Double-Blind Discontinuation in Manic and Recurrent-Depressive Disorders," *Lancet* 2 (1970): 326–30.

5. American Psychiatric Association, "Practice Guidelines for the Treatment of Bipolar Disorder," *American Journal of Psychiatry* 151, suppl. (1994): 6.

6. To be more precise, the therapeutic index is the ratio of the largest dose producing no toxic symptoms to the smallest dose routinely producing the desired therapeutic effects.

7. Alan Gelenberg, John Kane, Martin Keller, Phillip Lavori, Jerrold Rosenbaum, Karyl Cole, and Janet Lavelle, "Comparison of Standard and Low Levels of Lithium for Maintenance Treatment of Bipolar Disorder," *New England Journal of Medicine* 321, no. 22 (1989): 1489–93.

8. Morgans Schou, "Forty Years of Lithium Treatment," *Archives of General Psychiatry* 54 (1997): 9–13.

9. Ibid., 11.

10. R. J. Knebel, N. Rosenlicht, and L. Collins, "Lithium Carbonate Maintenance Therapy in a Hemodialysis Patient with End-Stage Renal Disease," *American Journal of Psychiatry* 167, no. 11 (2010): 1409–10.

11. For an excellent review, see T. J. Raedler and K. Wiedermann, "Lithium-Induced Nephropathies," *Psychopharmacology Bulletin* 40, no. 2 (2007): 134–49.

12. American Psychiatric Association, "Practice Guidelines for the Treatment of Bipolar Disorder," 7.

13. Frederick K. Goodwin and Kay Redfield Jamison, *Manic-Depressive Illness* (New York: Oxford University Press, 1990), 707.

14. Jonathan Sporn and Gary Sachs, "The Anticonvulsant Lamotrigine in Treatment-Resistant Manic-Depressive Illness," *Journal of Clinical Psychopharmacology* 17, no. 3 (1997): 185–89.

15. Joseph R. Calabrese, S. Hossein Fatemi, and Mark J. Woyshville, "Antidepressant Effects of Lamotrigine in Rapid Cycling Bipolar Disorder," *American Journal of Psychiatry* 153, no. 9 (1996): 1236.

16. C. L. Bowden, J. R. Calabrese, G. Sachs, L. N. Yatham, S. A. Asghar, M. Hompland, P. Montgomery, N. Earl, T. M. Smoot, and J. DeVeaugh-Geiss (Lamictal 606 Study Group), "A Placebo-Controlled 18-Month Trial of Lamotrigine and Lithium Maintenance Treatment in Recently Manic or Hypomanic Patients with Bipolar

I Disorder," *Archives of General Psychiatry* 60, no. 4 (2003): 392; J. R. Calabrese, C. L. Bowden, G. Sachs, L. N. Yatham, K. Behnke, O. P. Mehtonen, P. Montgomery, J. Ascher, W. Paska, N. Earl, and J. DeVeaugh-Geiss (Lamictal 605 Study Group), "A Placebo-Controlled 18-Month Trial of Lamotrigine and Lithium Maintenance Treatment in Recently Depressed Patients with Bipolar I Disorder," *Journal of Clinical Psychiatry* 64, no. 9 (2003): 1013–24.

17. J. R. Calabrese, J. R. Sullivan, C. L. Bowden, T. Suppes, J. F. Goldberg, G. S. Sachs, M. D. Shelton, F. K. Goodwin, M. A. Frye, and V. Kusumakar, "Rash in Multi-Center Trials of Lamotrigine in Mood Disorders: Clinical Relevance and Management," *Journal of Clinical Psychiatry* 63, no. 11 (2002): 1012–19.

18. See Charles Bowden and Susan McElroy, "History of the Development of Valproate for the Treatment of Bipolar Disorder," *Journal of Clinical Psychiatry* 56, suppl. 3 (1995): 3–5.

19. Charles L. Bowden, "Predictors of Response to Divalproex and Lithium," *Journal of Clinical Psychiatry* 56, suppl. 3 (1995): 25–29.

20. D. J. Muzina, K. Gao, D. E. Kemp, S. Khalife, S. J. Ganocy, P. K. Chan, M. B. Seranno, C. M. Conroy, and J. R. Calabrese, "Acute Efficacy of Divalproex Sodium versus Placebo in Mood-Stabilizer-Naïve Bipolar I or Bipolar II Depression: A Double-Blind, Randomized, Placebo Controlled Trial," *Journal of Clinical Psychiatry* 72, no. 6 (2011): 813–19; C. L. Bowden, J. R. Calabrese, S. L. McElroy, L. Gyulai, A. Wassef, H. G. Pope, J. C. Chou, P. E. Keck, L. J. Rhodes, A. C. Swann, R. M. Hirshfeld, and P. J. Wozniak, "A Randomized, Placebo-Controlled 12-Month Trial of Divalproex and Lithium in the Treatment of Outpatients with Bipolar I Disorder: Divalproex Maintenance Study Group," *Archives of General Psychiatry* 57, no. 5 (2000): 481–89.

21. K. A. Macritchie, J. R. Geddes, J. Scott, D. R. Haslam, and G. M. Goodwin, "Valproic Acid, Valproate, and Divalproex in the Maintenance Phase of Bipolar Disorder," *Cochrane Database of Systematic Reviews* 3 (2001): Art. No. CD003196.

22. American Psychiatric Association, "Practice Guidelines for the Treatment of Bipolar Disorder," 10.

23. See Frederick Jacobsen, "Low-Dose Valproate: A New Treatment for Cyclothymia, Mild Rapid-Cycling Disorders, and Premenstrual Syndrome," *Journal of Clinical Psychiatry* 54, no. 6 (1993): 229–34. Also J. A. Delito, "The Effect of Valproate on Bipolar Spectrum Temperamental Disorders," *Journal of Clinical Psychiatry* 54, no. 8 (1993): 300–304.

24. Gary Sachs, "Bipolar Mood Disorder: Practical Strategies for Acute and Maintenance Phase Treatment," *Journal of Clinical Psychopharmacology* 16, no. 2, suppl. 1 (1996): 32S–47S.

25. J. C. Ballenger and R. M. Post, "Carbamazepine in Manic-Depressive Illness: A New Treatment," *American Journal of Psychiatry* 137, no. 7 (1980): 782–90.

26. B. Lerer, M. Moore, E. Meyendorff, S. R. Cho, and S. Gershon, "Carbamazepine versus Lithium in Mania: A Double-Blind Study," *Journal of Clinical Psychiatry* 48, no. 3 (1987): 89–93.

27. Robert Post, Thomas Uhde, James Ballenger, and Kathleen Squillace, "Pro-

phylactic Efficacy of Carbamazepine in Manic-Depressive Illness," *American Journal of Psychiatry* 140, no. 12 (1983): 1602–4.

28. Ibid.

29. R. H. Weisler, A. H. Kalali, and T. A. Ketter, "A Multicenter, Randomized, Double-Blind, Placebo-Controlled Trial of Extended-Release Carbamazepine Capsules as Monotherapy for Bipolar Disorder Patients with Manic or Mixed Episodes," *Journal of Clinical Psychiatry* 65, no. 4 (2004): 478–84.

30. F. Centorrino, M. J. Albert, J. M. Berry, J. P. Kelleher, V. Fellman, G. Line, A. E. Koukopoulos, J. E. Kidwell, K. V. Fogarty, and R. J. Baldessarini, "Oxcarbazepine: Clinical Experience with Hospitalized Psychiatric Patients," *Bipolar Disorders* 5, no. 5 (2003): 370–74.

31. Joseph F. Goldberg, Katherine E. Burdick, and Carrie J. Endick, "Preliminary Randomized, Double-Blind, Placebo-Controlled Trial of Pramipexole Added to Mood Stabilizers for Treatment-Resistant Bipolar Depression," *American Journal of Psychiatry* 161, no. 3 (2004): 564–66.

32. Michael Berk, David Copolov, Olivia Dean, Kristy Lu, Sue Jeavons, Ian Schapkaitz, Murray Anderson-Hunt, and Ashley Bush, "N-Acetyl Cysteine for Depressive Symptoms in Bipolar Disorder—A Double-Blind Randomized Placebo-Controlled Trial," *Biological Psychiatry* 64, No. 6 (2008): 468–75; M. Berk, O. Dean, S. Cotton, C. Gama, F. Kapczinski, B. Fernandes, K. Kohlmann, S. Jeavons, K. Hewett, C. Allwang, H. Cobb, A. Bush, I. Schapkaitz, S. Dodd, and G. Malhi, "The Efficacy of N-Acetylcysteine as an Adjunctive Treatment in Bipolar Depression: An Open Label Trial," *Journal of Affective Disorders* 135, nos. 1–3 (2011): 389–94.

33. C. A. Zarate Jr., J. A. Quiroz, J. B. Singh, K. D. Denicoff, G. De Jesus, D. A. Luckenbaugh, D. S. Charney, and H. K. Manji, "An Open-Label Trial of the Glutamate-Modulating Agent Riluzole in Combination with Lithium for the Treatment of Bipolar Depression," *Biological Psychiatry* 57, no. 4 (2005): 430–32.

34. A. Fan, A. Berg, C. Bresee, L. Glassman, and M. Rapaport, "Allopurinol Augmentation in the Outpatient Treatment of Bipolar Mania: A Pilot Study," *Bipolar Disorder* 14, no. 2 (2012): 206–10.

35. Maura L. Furey and Wayne C. Drevets, "Antidepressant Efficacy of the Antimuscarinic Drug Scopolamine: A Randomized, Placebo-Controlled Clinical Trial," *Archives of General Psychiatry* 63, no. 10 (2006): 1121–29.

36. Rodrigo Machado-Vieira and Carlos A. Zarate Jr., "Proof of Concept Trials in Bipolar Disorder and Major Depressive Disorder: A Translational Perspective in the Search for Improved Treatments," *Depression and Anxiety* 28, no. 4 (2011): 267–81.

CHAPTER 7. ANTIDEPRESSANT MEDICATIONS

1. H. S. Lee, D. H. Song, C. H. Kim, and H. K. Choi, "An Open Clinical Trial of Fluoxetine in the Treatment of Premature Ejaculation," *Journal of Clinical Psychopharmacology* 16, no. 5 (1996): 379–82.

2. G. S. Sachs, A. A. Nierenberg, J. R. Calabrese, L. B. Marangell, S. R. Wisniewski, L. Gyulai, E. S. Friedman, C. L. Bowden, M. D. Fossey, M. J. Ostacher, T. A. Ketter,

J. Patel, P. Hauser, D. Rappaport, and J. M. Martinez, "Effectiveness of Adjunctive Antidepressant Treatment for Bipolar Depression," *New England Journal of Medicine* 356, no. 17 (2007): 1711–22.

3. See ibid.; and R. S. El-Mallakh, S. N. Ghaemi, K. Sagduyu, M. E. Thase, S. R. Wisniewski, A. A. Nierenberg, H. W. Zhang, T. A. Pardo, and G. Sachs, STEP-BD Investigators, "Antidepressant-Associated Chronic Irritable Dysphoria (ACID) in STEP-BD Patients," *Journal of Affective Disorders* 111, nos. 2–3 (2008): 372–77.

CHAPTER 8. ANTIPSYCHOTIC MEDICATIONS

1. Jeffrey Lieberman, Allan Safferman, Simcha Pollack, Sally Szmanski, Celeste Johns, Alfreda Howard, Michael Kronig, Peter Bookstein, and John Kane, "Clinical Effects of Clozapine in Chronic Schizophrenia: Response to Treatment and Predictors of Outcome," *American Journal of Psychiatry* 151, no. 12 (1994): 1744–52.

2. In a study of 11,555 patients treated with clozapine, 73 developed agranulocytosis (of whom 2 died of the infectious complications of the condition). See Jose Alvir, Jeffrey Lieberman, Allan Safferman, Jeffrey Schwimmer, and John Schaaf, "Clozapine-Induced Agranulocytosis: Incidence and Risk Factors in the United States," *New England Journal of Medicine* 329 (1993): 162–67.

3. Joseph R. Calabrese, Herbert Y. Meltzer, and Paul J. Markovitz, "Clozapine Prophylaxis in Rapid Cycling Bipolar Disorder," *Journal of Clinical Psychopharmacology* 11, no. 6 (1991): 396–97.

4. Joseph Calabrese, Susan Kimmel, Mark Woyshville, Daniel Rapport, Carl Faust, Paul Thompson, and Herbert Meltzer, "Clozapine for Treatment-Refractory Mania," *American Journal of Psychiatry* 153, no. 6 (1996): 759–64.

5. Carlos Zarate Jr., Mauricio Tohen, Michael Banov, Michelle Weiss, and Jonathan Cole, "Is Clozapine a Mood Stabilizer?" *Journal of Clinical Psychiatry* 56, no. 3 (1995): 108–12.

6. G. Parker and G. Malhi, "Are the Atypical Antipsychotic Drugs Antidepressants?" *Journal of Clinical Psychopharmacology* 59, no. 3 (2002): 94–95.

7. T. Baptista, N. M. Kin, S. Beaulieu, and E. A. de Baptista, "Obesity and Related Metabolic Abnormalities during Antipsychotic Drug Administration: Mechanisms, Management, and Research Perspectives," *Pharmacopsychiatry* 35, no. 6 (2002): 205–19.

CHAPTER 9. MORE MEDICATIONS, HORMONES, AND DIETARY SUPPLEMENTS

1. For a discussion of these drugs to treat anxiety in bipolar disorder, see P. E. Keck, J. R. Strawn, and S. L. McElroy, "Pharmacologic Treatment Considerations in Co-occuring Bipolar and Anxiety Disorder," *Journal of Clinical Psychiatry* 67, suppl. 1 (2006): 8–15.

2. M. S. Bauer, P. C. Whybrow, and A. Winokur, "Rapid Cycling Bipolar Affective Disorder I: Association with Grade I Hypothyroidism," *Archives of General Psychiatry* 47, no. 5 (1990): 427–32.

3. H. A. Oomen, A. J. Schipperijn, and H. A. Drexhage, "The Prevalence of Af-

fective Disorder and in Particular of a Rapid Cycling of Bipolar Disorder in Patients with Abnormal Thyroid Function Tests," *Clinical Endocrinology* 45, no. 2 (1996): 215–23.

4. D. P. Cole, M. E. Thase, A. G. Mallinger, J. C. Soares, J. F. Luther, D. J. Kupfer, and E. Frank, "Slower Treatment Response in Bipolar Depression Predicted by Lower Pre-treatment Thyroid Function," *American Journal of Psychiatry* 159, no. 1 (2002): 116–21.

5. Joseph R. Calabrese and Mark J. Woyshville, "A Medication Algorithm for Treatment of Bipolar Rapid Cycling?" *Journal of Clinical Psychiatry* 56, suppl. 3 (1995): 11–18.

6. There have been controversies as to whether all thyroid hormone preparations made by different manufacturers are equivalent and interchangeable. Lawrence K. Altman, "Caution Urged over Switch in Thyroid Drug," *New York Times,* April 17, 1997. The problem can be avoided by making sure that you take the same preparation of levothyroxine, whether brand name or generic, all the time, and also by getting your thyroid hormone levels tested regularly.

7. J. Sarris, D. Mischoulon, and I. Schweitzer, "Omega-3 for Bipolar Disorder: Meta-analysis of Use in Mania and Bipolar Depression," *Journal of Clinical Psychiatry* 73, no. 1 (2012): 81–86.

8. M. Berk, D. Copoloc, O. Dean, K. Lu, S. Jeavons, I. Schapkaitz, M. Anderson-Hunt, and A. Bush, "N-Acetyl Cysteine for Depressive Symptoms in Bipolar Disorder—A Double-Blind Randomized Placebo-Controlled Trial," *Biological Psychiatry* 64, no. 6 (2008): 468–75; M. Berk, O. Dean, S. Cotton, C. Gama, F. Kapczinski, B. Fernandes, K. Kohlmann, S. Jeavons, K. Hewerr, C. Allwang, K. Cobb, A. Bush, I. Schapkaitz, S. Dodd, and G. Malhi, "The Efficacy of N-Acetylcysteine as an Adjunctive Treatment in Bipolar Depression: An Open Label Trial," *Journal of Affective Disorders* 135, nos. 1–3 (2011): 389–94.

9. K. Linde, G. Ramirez, C. D. Mulrow, A. Pauls, and W. Weidenhammer, "St. John's Wort for Depression—An Overview and Meta-analysis of Randomised Clinical Trials," *British Medical Journal* 313, no. 7052 (1996): 253–58.

10. R. C. Shelton, M. B. Keller, A. Gelenberg, D. L. Dunner, R. Hirschfeld, M. E. Thase, J. Russell, R. B. Lydiard, P. Crits-Christoph, R. Gallop, L. Todd, D. Hellerstein, P. Goodnick, G. Keitner, S. M. Stahl, and U. Halbreich, "Effectiveness of St. John's Wort in Major Depression: A Randomized Controlled Trial," *Journal of the American Medical Association* 285, no. 15 (2001): 1978–86.

11. A. J. Gelenberg, R. C. Shelton, P. Crits-Christoph, M. B. Keller, D. L. Dunner, R. M. Hirschfeld, M. E. Thase, J. M. Russell, R. B. Lydiard, R. J. Gallop, L. Todd, D. J. Hellerstein, P. J. Goodnick, G. I. Keitner, S. M. Stahl, U. Halbreich, and H. S. Hopkins, "The Effectiveness of St. John's Wort in Major Depressive Disorder: A Naturalistic Phase 2 Follow-Up in Which Nonresponders Were Provided Alternate Medication," *Journal of Clinical Psychiatry* 65, no. 8 (2004): 1114–19.

12. E. Moses and A. Mallinger, "St. John's Wort: Three Cases of Possible Mania Induction," *Journal of Clinical Psychopharmacology* 20, no. 1 (2000): 115–17.

1. Emil Kraepelin, *Manic-Depressive Insanity and Paranoia,* trans. R. M. Barclay, ed. G. M. Robertson (1921; reprint, New York: Arno Press, 1976), 97.

2. C. Freeman and R. E. Kendell, "ECT I: Patients' Experiences and Attitudes," *British Journal of Psychiatry* 137 (1980): 8–16.

3. M. Valance, "The Experience of Electro-Convulsive Therapy by a Practising Psychiatrist," *British Journal of Psychiatry* 111 (1965): 365–67.

4. Larry Squire, Pamela Slater, and Patricia Miller, "Retrograde Amnesia and Bilateral Electroconvulsive Therapy, Long Term Follow-up," *Archives of General Psychiatry* 38 (1981): 89–95.

5. Larry R. Squire and Pamela C. Slater, "Electroconvulsive Therapy and Complaints of Memory Dysfunction: A Prospective Three-Year Follow-up Study," *British Journal of Psychiatry* 142 (1983): 1–8.

6. E. Anderson and I. Reti, "ECT in Pregnancy: A Review of the Literature from 1941 to 2007," *Psychosomatic Medicine* 71, no. 2 (2009): 235–42.

7. Frederick K. Goodwin and Kay Redfield Jamison, *Manic-Depressive Illness,* 2nd ed. (New York: Oxford University Press, 2007), 782.

8. Sukdeb Mukherjee, Harold Sackeim, and David Schnur, "Electroconvulsive Therapy of Acute Manic Episodes: A Review of Fifty Years' Experience," *American Journal of Psychiatry* 151 (1994): 169–76.

9. S. Mukherjee, H. Sackeim, and C. Lee, "Unilateral ECT in the Treatment of Manic Episodes," *Convulsive Therapy* 4 (1988): 74–80.

10. Much of the work comparing the effectiveness of ECT with that of medication compares it with treatment with lithium. As studies comparing it with treatment using newer agents (such as the anticonvulsants) are done, statements about ECT's superiority to medical treatments for mania may need to be revised. However, given that the new mood stabilizers are perhaps *less* effective than lithium for depression, ECT's claims as a more predictably effective treatment for bipolar depression remain unchallenged.

11. See Mark S. George, Eric Wasserman, and Robert Post, "Transcranial Magnetic Stimulation: A Neuropsychiatric Tool for the Twenty-First Century," *Journal of Neuropsychiatry and Clinical Neurosciences* 8 (1996): 373–82.

12. Mark George, Eric Wasserman, Tim Kimbrell, John Little, Wendol Williams, Aimee Danielson, Benjamin Greenberg, Mark Hallett, and Robert Post, "Mood Improvement following Daily Left Prefrontal Repetitive Transcranial Magnetic Stimulation in Patients with Depression: A Placebo Controlled Crossover Trial," *American Journal of Psychiatry* 154 (1997): 1752–56.

13. A. Pascual-Leone, B. Rubio, F. Pallardo, and M. D. Catala, "Beneficial Effect of Rapid-Rate Transcranial Magnetic Stimulation of the Left Dorsolateral Prefrontal Cortex in Drug-Resistant Depression," *Lancet* 348 (1996): 233–37; and Charles Epstein, Gary Figiel, William McDonald, Jody Amazon-Leece, and Linda Figiel, "Rapid Rate Transcranial Magnetic Stimulation in Young and Middle-Aged Refractory Depressed Patients," *Psychiatric Annals* 28 (1998): 36–39.

14. A. J. Rush, M. S. George, H. A. Sackeim, L. B. Marangell, M. M. Husain, C. Giller, Z. Nahas, S. Haines, R. K. Simpson Jr., and R. Goodman, "Vagus Nerve Stimulation (VNS) for Treatment-Resistant Depressions: A Multicenter Study," *Biological Psychiatry* 47, no. 4 (2000): 276–86.

15. L. B. Marangell, A. J. Rush, M. S. George, H. A. Sackeim, C. R. Johnson, M. M. Husain, Z. Nahas, and S. H. Lisanby, "Vagus Nerve Stimulation (VNS) for Major Depressive Episodes: One Year Outcomes," *Biological Psychiatry* 51, no. 4 (2002): 280–87.

CHAPTER 11. COUNSELING AND PSYCHOTHERAPY

1. Jan Scott, "Psychotherapy for Bipolar Disorder," *British Journal of Psychiatry* 167 (1995): 581–88.

2. Nick Kanas, "Group Psychotherapy with Bipolar Patients: A Review and Synthesis," *International Journal of Group Psychotherapy* 43 (1993): 321–33.

3. L. E. Pollack, "Content Analysis of Groups for Inpatients with Bipolar Disorder," *Applied Nursing Research* 6 (1993): 19–27.

4. D. Miklowitz, J. Price, E. Holmes, J. Rendell, S. Bell, K. Budge, J. Christensen, J. Wallace, J. Simon, N. Armstrong, L. McPeake, G. Goodwin, and J. Geddes, "Facilitated Integrated Mood Management for Adults with Bipolar Disorder," *Bipolar Disorder* 14, no. 2 (2012): 185–97.

5. Beck originally called CBT simply "cognitive therapy." Psychologist Donald Meichenbaum, who has written extensively on Beck's cognitive therapy as well as on other types of therapy that use the techniques of behavioral psychology to help change thinking patterns (cognition), is perhaps most responsible for creating the broader category we now call "cognitive-behavioral therapy." See Donald Meichenbaum and Roy Cameron, "Cognitive-Behavior Therapy," in *Contemporary Behavior Therapy: Conceptional and Empirical Foundations,* ed. G. Terence Wilson and Cyril M. Franks (New York: Guilford Press, 1982), 310–37. Although some researchers and theoreticians will describe subtle differences between the terms *cognitive therapy* and *cognitive-behavioral therapy,* they now seem to be used interchangeably by most clinical psychologists and by researchers as well.

6. The area of comparison studies of psychotherapy and medication in the treatment of depression can be accurately described as a hornet's nest of controversy. It's not difficult to find a study to support any possible view: superiority of medication over psychotherapy, superiority of psychotherapy over medication, and equal efficacy for both. A nicely designed and well-executed study that found cognitive therapy to be as helpful as imipramine for 107 patients with major depressive disorder is Steven Hollon, Robert DeRubeis, Mark Evans, Marlin Wiemer, Michael Garvey, William Grove, and Vincente Tuason, "Cognitive Therapy and Pharmacotherapy for Depression, Singly and in Combination," *Archives of General Psychiatry* 49 (1992): 774–81. Readers who would like to jump into the hornet's nest feet first are referred to Jacqueline Persons, Michael Thase, and Paul Crits-Chistoph, "The Role of Psychotherapy in the Treatment of Depression: Review of Two Practice Guidelines," *Archives of General Psychiatry* 53 (1996): 283–90, and to the four (yes, four) accompanying rebuttal-commentary articles in the same issue of *Archives.*

7. A. T. Beck, A. J. Rush, B. F. Shaw, and G. Emory, *Cognitive Therapy of Depression* (New York: Guilford Press, 1979), 11.

8. The linguistic purist in me wants the plural of *schema* to be *schemata* or perhaps *schemae*. But *schemas* is the plural used in cognitive-therapy literature.

9. See Jan Scott, "Cognitive Therapy of Affective Disorders: A Review," *Journal of Affective Disorders* 37 (1996): 1–11.

10. David J. Miklowitz, "Psychotherapy in Combination with Drug Treatment for Bipolar Disorder," *Journal of Clinical Psychopharmacology* 16, suppl. (1996): 56S–66S.

11. E. Frank, S. Hlastala, A. Ritenour, P. Houck, X. M. Tu, T. H. Monk, A. G. Mallinger, and D. J. Kupfer, "Inducing Lifestyle Regularity in Recovering Bipolar Disorder Patients: Results from the Maintenance Therapies in Bipolar Disorder Protocol," *Biological Psychiatry* 15 (1997): 1165–73.

12. Kay Redfield Jamison, *An Unquiet Mind: A Memoir of Moods and Madness* (New York: Vintage Books, 1996), 88–89.

CHAPTER 12. TREATMENT APPROACHES IN BIPOLAR DISORDER

1. The word *empirical* is derived from the Greek word *empeirikos,* which means "a doctor relying on experience alone."

2. C. Bowden, R. Perlis, M. Thase, T. Ketter, M. Ostacher, J. Calabrese, N. Reilly-Harrington, J. Gonzaliz, V. Singh, A. Neirenberg, and G. Sachs, "Aims and Results of the NIMH Systematic Treatment Enhancement Program for Bipolar Disorder (STEP-BD)," *CNS Neuroscience and Therapeutics* 18, no. 3 (2012): 243–49.

CHAPTER 13. BIPOLAR DISORDER IN CHILDREN AND ADOLESCENTS

1. Barbara Geller, Kai Sun, Betsy Zimerman, Joan Luby, Jeanne Frazier, and Marlene Williams, "Complex and Rapid-Cycling in Bipolar Children and Adolescents: A Preliminary Study," *Journal of Affective Disorders* 34 (1995): 259–68.

2. Roselind Neuman, Barbara Geller, John Rice, and Richard Todd, "Increased Prevalence and Earlier Onset of Mood Disorders among Relatives of Prepubertal versus Adult Probands," *Journal of the American Academy of Child and Adolescent Psychiatry* 36 (1997): 466–73.

3. American Academy of Child and Adolescent Psychiatry, "Practice Parameters for the Assessment and Treatment of Children and Adolescents with Bipolar Disorder," *Journal of the American Academy of Child and Adolescent Psychiatry* 36 (1997): 138–57, studies cited on 140.

4. See Barbara Geller and Joan Luby, "Child and Adolescent Bipolar Disorder: Review of the Past Ten Years," *Journal of the American Academy of Child and Adolescent Psychiatry* 36 (1997): 1168–76.

5. Geller, Sun, Zimerman, Luby, Frazier, and Williams, "Complex and Rapid-Cycling in Bipolar Children and Adolescents."

6. M. Strober and G. Carlson, "Bipolar Illness in Adolescents with Major Depression: Clinical, Genetic, and Psychopharmacologic Predictors in a Three- to Four-Year Prospective Follow-up Investigation," *Archives of General Psychiatry* 39, no. 5 (1982): 549–55.

7. T. Spencer, J. Biederman, and T. Wilens, "Attention-Deficit/Hyperactivity Disorder and Comorbidity," *Pediatric Clinics of North America* 46, no. 5 (1999): 915–27.

8. J. Biederman, S. Faraone, E. Mick, J. Wozniac, L. Chen, C. Ouellette, A. Marrs, J. Garcia, D. Mennin, and E. Lelon, "Attention-Deficit Hyperactivity Disorder and Juvenile Mania: An Overlooked Comorbidity?" *Journal of the American Academy of Child and Adolescent Psychiatry* 35, no. 8 (1996): 997–1008.

9. S. V. Faraone, J. Biederman, D. Mennin, J. Wozniak, and T. Spencer, "Attention-Deficit Hyperactivity Disorder with Bipolar Disorder: A Familial Subtype?" *Journal of the American Academy of Child and Adolescent Psychiatry* 36, no. 10 (1997): 1378–87.

10. See American Academy of Child and Adolescent Psychiatry, "Practice Parameters for the Assessment and Treatment of Children and Adolescents."

11. M. Strober, M. DeAntonio, S. Schmidt-Lackner, R. Freeman, C. Lampert, and J. Diamond, "Early Childhood Attention Deficit Hyperactivity Disorder Predicts Poorer Response to Acute Lithium Therapy in Adolescent Mania," *Journal of Affective Disorders* 51, no. 2 (1998): 145–51.

12. T. A. Henderson, "Mania Induction Associated with Atomoxetine," *Journal of Clinical Psychopharmacology* 24, no. 5 (2004): 567–68.

13. T. Spencer and J. Biederman, "Non-Stimulant Treatment for Attention-Deficit/Hyperactivity Disorder," *Journal of Attention Disorders* 6, suppl. 1 (2002): S109–S119.

14. M. Strober, S. Schmidt-Lackner, R. Freeman, S. Bower, C. Lampert, and M. DeAntonio, "Recovery and Relapse in Adolescents with Bipolar Affective Illness: A Five-Year Naturalistic, Prospective Follow-up," *Journal of the American Academy of Child and Adolescent Psychiatry* 34 (1995): 724–31.

CHAPTER 14. WOMEN WITH BIPOLAR DISORDER

1. Ellen Leibenluft, "Women with Bipolar Illness: Clinical and Research Issues," *American Journal of Psychiatry* 153 (1996): 163–73.

2. Ibid., 164.

3. K. Yonkers, S. Vigod, and L. Ross, "Diagnosis, Pathophysiology, and Management of Mood Disorders in Pregnant and Postpartum Women," *Obstetrics and Gynecology* 117, no. 4 (2011): 961–77.

4. Ibid., 961

5. J. Payne, D. MacKinnon, F. Mondimore, M. McGinnis, B. Schweitzer, R. Zamoiski, F. McMahon, J. Nurnberger, J. Rice, W. Scheftner, W. Coryell, W. Berrittini, J. Kelsoe, W. Byerley, E. Gershon, J. DePaulo, and J. Potash, "Familial Aggregation of Postpartum Mood Symptoms in Bipolar Disorder Pedigrees," *Bipolar Disorder* 10, no. 1 (2008): 38–44.

6. K. Yonkers, K. Wisner, Z. Stowe, E. Leibenluft, L. Cohen, L. Miller, R. Manber, A. Viguera, and T. Suppes, "Management of Bipolar Disorder during Pregnancy and the Postpartum Period," *American Journal of Psychiatry* 60, no. 1 (2004): 608–20.

7. J. Moore, P. Aggarwal, "Lamotrigine Use in Pregnancy," *Expert Opinions in Pharmacotherapy* 13, no. 8 (2012): 1213–16; A. Einarson and R. Boskovic, "Use and

Safety of Antipsychotic Drugs during Pregnancy," *Journal of Psychiatric Practice* 15, no. 3 (2009): 183–92.

8. Douglas Maskall, Raymond Lam, Shala Misri, Lakshmi Yatham, and Athanasios Zis, "Seasonality of Symptoms in Women with Late Luteal Phase Dysphoric Disorder," *American Journal of Psychiatry* 154 (1997): 1436–41.

CHAPTER 15. ALCOHOLISM AND DRUG ABUSE

1. D. A. Reger, M. E. Farm, and D. S. Rae, "Comorbidity of Mental Disorders with Alcohol and Other Drug Abuse: Results from the Epidemiologic Catchment Area Study," *Journal of the American Medical Association* 264 (1990): 2511–18.

2. Results quoted in Kathleen Brady and Susan Sonne, "The Relationship between Substance Abuse and Bipolar Disorder," *Journal of Clinical Psychiatry* 56, suppl. 3 (1995): 19–24.

3. Susan Sonne, Kathleen Brady, and W. Alexander Morton, "Substance Abuse and Bipolar Affective Disorder," *Journal of Nervous and Mental Disease* 182 (1994): 349–52.

4. Markus Henriksson, Hillevi Aro, Mauri Marttunnen, Martti Heikkinen, Erkki Isometsä, Kimmo Kuoppasalmi, and Jouko Lönnqvist, "Mental Disorders and Comorbidity in Suicide," *American Journal of Psychiatry* 150 (1993): 935–40.

5. J. Prochaska and W. Velicer, "The Transtheoretical Model of Health Behavior Change," *American Journal of Health Promotion* 12, no. 1 (1997): 38–48.

CHAPTER 16. THE SCIENCE OF CYCLES

1. A. J. Lewy, H. A. Kern, N. E. Rosenthal, and T. A. Wehr, "Bright Artificial Light Treatment of a Manic-Depressive Patient with a Seasonal Mood Cycle," *American Journal of Psychiatry* 139 (1982): 1496–98.

2. Emil Kraepelin, *Manic-Depressive Insanity and Paranoia*, trans. R. M. Barclay, ed. G. M. Robertson (1921; reprint, New York: Arno Press, 1976), 139.

3. Norman E. Rosenthal, *Winter Blues: Seasonal Affective Disorder, What It Is and How to Overcome It* (New York: Guilford Press, 1993), 6.

4. Ibid., 9.

5. Diane Boivin, Charles Czeisler, Derk-Jan Dijk, Jeanne Duffy, Simon Folkard, David Minors, Peter Totterdell, and James Waterhouse, "Complex Interaction of the Sleep-Wake Cycle and Circadian Phase Modulates Mood in Healthy Subjects," *Archives of General Psychiatry* 54 (1997): 145–52.

6. Michael Terman, Leora Amira, Jiuan Terman, and Donald Ross, "Predictors of Response and Non-response to Light Treatment for Winter Depression," *American Journal of Psychiatry* 153 (1996): 1423–29.

7. Alan O. Kogan and Patricia Guilford, "Side Effects of Short-Term 10,000-Lux Light Therapy," *American Journal of Psychiatry* 155 (1998): 293–94.

8. For an extensive discussion of circadian rhythms and bipolar disorder, see Frederick K. Goodwin and Kay Redfield Jamison, *Manic-Depressive Illness*, 2nd ed. (New York: Oxford University Press, 2007), chapter 16, "Sleep and Circadian Rhythms," 659–88.

9. F. Benedetti, B. Barbini, A. Lucca, E. Campori, C. Colombo, and E. Smeraldi, "Sleep Deprivation Hastens the Antidepressant Action of Fluoxetine," *European Archives of Psychiatry and Clinical Neuroscience* 247 (1997): 100–103.

10. T. Wehr, D. Sack, and N. Rosenthal, "Sleep Reduction as a Final Common Pathway in the Genesis of Mania," *American Journal of Psychiatry* 144 (1987): 201–4.

CHAPTER 17. THE GENETICS OF BIPOLAR DISORDER

1. Emil Kraepelin, *Manic-Depressive Insanity and Paranoia,* trans. R. M. Barclay, ed. G. M. Robertson (1921; reprint, New York: Arno Press, 1976), 165.

2. M. DelBello and B. Geller, "Review of Studies of Child and Adolescent Offspring of Bipolar Parents," *Bipolar Disorder* 3 (2001): 325–34.

CHAPTER 18. BIPOLAR BIOLOGY

1. Robert Sapolsky, *Why Zebras Don't Get Ulcers,* 3rd ed. (New York: Holt Paperbacks, 2004), 7.

2. C. J. Morales-Medina, F. Sanchez, G. Flores, Y. Dumont, and R. Quirion, "Morphological Reorganization after Repeated Corticosterone Administration in the Hippocampus, Nucleus Accumbens, and Amygdala," *Journal of Chemical Neuroanatomy* 38, no. 4 (2009): 266–72.

3. Lori Altshuler, John Curran, Peter Hauser, Jim Mintz, Kirk Denikoff, and Robert Post, "T2 Hyperintensities in Bipolar Disorder: Magnetic Resonance Imaging Comparison and Literature Meta-analysis," *American Journal of Psychiatry* 152 (1995): 1139–44.

4. M. J. Kempton, Z. Salvador, M. R. Munafò, J. R. Geddes, A. Simmons, S. Frangou, and S. C. Williams, "Structural Neuroimaging Studies in Major Depressive Disorder: Meta-analysis and Comparison with Bipolar Disorder," *Archives of General Psychiatry* 68 (2011): 675–90.

CHAPTER 19. BIPOLAR DISORDER AND CREATIVITY

1. Aristotle, attributed by Seneca in *Moral Essays,* "De tranquillitate animi" (On tranquility of mind), sec. 17, subsec. 10, quoted in *The Columbia Dictionary of Quotations* (New York: Columbia University Press, 1993; CD ROM ed., 1994).

2. Quoted in Kay Redfield Jamison, *Touched with Fire: Manic-Depressive Illness and the Artistic Temperament* (New York: Free Press, 1993), 203–5.

3. These studies are described and cited in ibid.

4. Emil Kraepelin, *Manic-Depressive Insanity and Paranoia,* trans. R. M. Barclay, ed. G. M. Robertson (1921; reprint, New York: Arno Press, 1976), 17.

5. Quoted in Jamison, *Touched with Fire,* 126.

6. Jean Cocteau, "Le coq et l'arlequin," in *Le rappel à l'ordre* (1926), quoted in *Columbia Dictionary of Quotations,* CD ROM ed.

7. These studies are cited and described in Frederick K. Goodwin and Kay Redfield Jamison, *Manic-Depressive Illness,* 2nd ed. (New York: Oxford University Press, 2007), 379–410.

CHAPTER 20. LIVING WITH BIPOLAR DISORDER

1. Emil Kraepelin, *Manic-Depressive Insanity and Paranoia,* trans. R. M. Barclay, ed. G. M. Robertson (1921; reprint, New York: Arno Press, 1976), 179–81.

2. For a complete discussion of these animal models of the kindling phenomenon, see Robert Post, "Transduction of Psychosocial Stress into the Neurobiology of Recurrent Affective Disorder," *American Journal of Psychiatry* 149 (1992): 999–1010.

3. Constance Hammen and Michael Gitlin, "Stress Reactivity in Bipolar Patients and Its Relation to Prior History of Disorder," *American Journal of Psychiatry* 154 (1997): 856–57.

4. T. Treuer and M. Tohen, "Predicting the Course and Outcome of Bipolar Disorder: A Review," *European Psychiatry* 25 (2010): 328–33.

5. K. R. Jamison, R. H. Gerner, and F. K. Goodwin, "Patient and Physician Attitudes toward Lithium: Relationship to Compliance," *Archives of General Psychiatry* 36 (1979): 866–69.

6. Mario Maj, Raffaele Pirozzi, and Lorenza Magliano, "Non-response to Reinstituted Lithium Prophylaxis in Previously Responsive Bipolar Patients: Prevalence and Predictors," *American Journal of Psychiatry* 152 (1995): 1810–11. A similar study concluded that "the efficacy of lithium did not differ significantly" when it was started a second time in patients who had stopped it. But almost 13 percent of these patients needed *another* medication added to the lithium to achieve remission the second time around. (This seems to me to indicate that the lithium was *not* as effective the second time around.) See Leonardo Tondo, Ross Baldessarini, Gianfranco Floris, and Nereida Rudas, "Effectiveness of Restarting Lithium Treatment after Its Discontinuation in Bipolar I and Bipolar II Patients," *American Journal of Psychiatry* 154 (1997): 548–50.

7. Erving Goffman, *Stigma: Notes on the Management of Spoiled Identity* (Englewood Cliffs, NJ: Prentice-Hall, 1963), 1, 2.

CHAPTER 21. PLANNING FOR EMERGENCIES

1. E. C. Harris and B. Barraclough, "Suicide as an Outcome for Mental Disorders: A Meta-analysis," *British Journal of Psychiatry* 170 (1997): 205–28.

2. See, for example, J. E. Bailey, A. L. Kellerman, G. W. Somes, J. G. Banton, F. Rivara, and N. Rushforth, "Risk Factors for Violent Death of Women in the Home," *Archives of Internal Medicine* 157 (1997): 777–82.

3. *American Heritage Dictionary of the English Language,* 3rd ed. (New York: Houghton Mifflin, 1992).

CHAPTER 22. THE ROLE OF THE FAMILY

1. Kay Redfield Jamison, *An Unquiet Mind: A Memoir of Moods and Madness* (New York: Vintage Books, 1996), 120.

2. Stephen Strakowski, Susan McElroy, Paul Keck, and Scott West, "Suicidality among Patients with Mixed and Manic Bipolar Disorder," *American Journal of Psychiatry* 153 (1996): 674–76.

1. DISC I is the name of a gene discovered in 1970 that is now known to code for a protein important for the growth and development of neurons. Among other things, this protein is essential for the growth of axons and dendrites, the fibers that connect one neuron to others in the nervous system. An abnormal variation (mutation) of the gene was first identified in a family whose members had an unusually high risk of mental illness. Almost half of the family members with the mutation had schizophrenia, bipolar disorder, major depression, or another psychiatric problem. The gene's name comes from "**D**isrupted **I**n **S**chizophrenia" because schizophrenia was the most common illness in affected family members. Subsequent research has indicated that DISC I may be important in bipolar disorder as well.

Index

Page numbers in *italics* indicate tables or figures.

antidepressants (*continued*)
74–75, 99; in treatment of bipolar disorder, 104–6, 150, 157–58; tricyclic, 98–100, *99. See also specific drugs and classes*

antioxidants, 96, 120–21

antipsychotic medications, 107–14, 125, 150, 153; atypical, 108, 110–14, *111, 113*; side effects of, 109–10, 113–14; typical, 108–10, *109. See also specific drugs*

anxiety, 26, *26*, 57, 117; medications for, 115–17, *116*

appetite changes, 6; in depression, *18*, 22, *40*, 188; drug-induced, 91, 113; in mania, *10*, 12

Aremis. *See* sertraline

Aricept. *See* donepezil

aripiprazole, *111, 113*

Aropax. *See* paroxetine

artistic accomplishment, xi, 207–13, *208, 210, 211*

ascertainment bias, 167

asenapine, *111*

Asendin. *See* amoxapine

Ativan. *See* lorazepam

atomoxetine, 166

attention-deficit hyperactivity disorder (ADHD), 57, 156, 163, 164–65; links between bipolar disorder and, 164–65; symptoms of, 156, 163, 164; treatment of, 156, 166–67

AZD6765, 97

Azona. *See* trazodone

Baalstrup, Paul Christian, 78–80, *79*

Baillarger, Jules, 59–60

Beck, Aaron, 139

Beers, Clifford, 51–52

behavioral family management for bipolar disorder, 143

benzodiazepines, 115–17, *116*

Besitran. *See* sertraline

beta blockers, for tremor, 85, 91

Bini, Lucio, 125

biological clock, 159, 184, 186–87, 192. *See also* chronobiology

biological psychiatry, 29, 71, 136; historical perspectives on, 62, 63, 64, 66, 135; medications and, 96–97, 136. *See also* brain

biology of bipolar disorder, 198–206; brain functioning, 203–6; hormones, 117–18, 202–3; stress response, 117–18, 198–202, *200, 201*

bipolar disorder: biology of, 198–206; chronobiology and, 22, 159–60, 184–92; course of, 2, 9, 12, 14–15, *34*, 34–37, *36*, 217, 221; creativity and, 160, 207–13; depressive episodes in, 2, 9,

17–25; diagnosis of, xii, 1, 28–53, 149–50; different forms of, 2, 9, 17; in *DSM-5*, 2, 44, 57; family of patient with, 215–16, 239–49; future perspectives on, 216, 250–53; gender and, 50; genetics of, 40, 160, 193–97; historical perspectives on, 58–68; living with, 215, 217–30; manic episodes in, 2, 9–15; mixed mood states in, 2, 9, 25–27; not elsewhere classified, 44, 57; pediatric, 159, 161–68; planning for emergencies in, 215, 231–38; prevalence of, xi, 52; rapid-cycling, 26–27, 49–50; relapse of, xi–xii, 34, 35, 37, 221–22 (*see also* relapse(s)); remission of, 34, 35, 78, 150, 162, 222; with seasonal pattern, 41, 185, 186–89; "soft" forms of, xii, 46–47, *47*, 52, 57, 91, 154; stages of, 14–15, 37; substance abuse and, 159; support groups for, 136–37, 227–28, 248; symptoms of, 1–2, 6, 8–27, 217, 218; treatment of, 69–158 (*see also* treatment(s)); in women, 50, 159, 169–73

bipolar I, 30–37, *37*; age at onset of, 32, *33*; development of, 32–34; mood changes in, 30–32, *32*; natural history of, *34*, 34–37, *36*; relapse of, xi–xii, 34, 35, 221–22; time line for treatment of, 152

bipolar II, 37–41, *40*; compared with bipolar I, 40–41; course of, 40, 41; mood changes in, 36–39, *39*; prevalence of, 39; seasonal variations in, 41

bipolar III, 46–49, *48*

bipolar spectrum disorders, 44–49

birth defects, drug-induced, 85, 92, 171

bizarre thinking/behavior, 8, 13, 15, 23, 50–51, 52, 107–8

bodily response to stress, 198–202, *200, 201*

bodily rhythms, 22, 143, 173, 184, 191, 192. *See also* chronobiology

bodily symptoms, *10, 18*, 22–23

botanicals, 119

brain, 71–76; bipolar disorder and functioning of, 203–6; drug stimulation of reward centers in, 178–79; gender differences in organization of, 170; imaging of, 204–5, 251; limbic system of, 205; medication effects on, 74–75; mind and, 135–37; mood regulation by, 5, 8, 199, 251; neurotransmitters in, *72*, 73–75; plasticity of, 73–76; stress effects on, *200*, 200–202, *201*

brain research, 62, 250–53

brain-stimulation treatments, 124–33, 151, 251; deep brain stimulation, 133; electroconvulsive therapy, 25, 124–30, 151, 156–57;

transcranial direct current stimulation, 133; transcranial magnetic stimulation, 130–32, 151, 205, 251, 252; vagal nerve stimulation, 132

breast-feeding, 85, 169, 172

The Broken Brain (Andreasen), 71

bupropion, 102, *102*, 105, 157

Cade, John F. J., *64*, 64–66, 77, 78

carbamazepine, 92–94; in pregnancy, 171; side effects of, 94; therapeutic profile of, 92–94, *94*

Catapres. *See* clonidine

catatonia, *18*, 25, 125

Celexa. *See* citalopram

Cerletti, Ugo, 125

chemical imbalance, 69–70, 74, 136, 146

children. *See* pediatric bipolar disorder

chlordiazepoxide, *116*

chlorpromazine, 107–8, *109*, 111, 136

cholesterol elevation, 113–14

chromosomes, 165, 178, 193, 194, 196, 251

chronobiology, 22, 159–60, 184–92; circadian rhythms, 186–87; seasonal affective disorder, 117, 173, 188–89; sleep-wake cycle, 22, 187, 189–91, *190*, 224

Churchill, Winston, xi

Cipralex. *See* escitalopram

Cipramil. *See* citalopram

circadian rhythms, 186–87; seasonal affective disorder and, 188–89; sleep-wake cycle, 22, 187, 189–91, 224

citalopram, *101*

clomipramine, *99*

clonazepam, 57, *116*

clonidine, 166

clorazepate, *116*

clozapine (Clozaril), 52, *111*, 111–12, 113, *113*

Cocteau, Jean, 213

Cognex. *See* tacrine

cognitive-behavioral therapy (CBT), 139

cognitive effects, 6; of depression, *18*, 20–21; of electroconvulsive therapy, 127–29; of lithium, 85; of mania, *10*

cognitive therapy, 139–42, 144

commitment, involuntary, 233, 244–46, 247

commitment to treatment, 218–19, 222–23, 248

conflict management, 142, 143, 144, 223–25

confronting illness, 217–19

contraception, 172–73

corticosteroids, 203

cortisol, 115, 186, 194, 199–200, 202, 203, 224, 225

counseling, 55, 56, 70, 134, 137, 142, 143, 151, 213, 230; benefits of, 146, 151, 158; for children, 167; for family, 142, 143, 249; professional training for, 147; situational supportive, 144; in split treatment, 147; for stress and conflict management, 223–25. *See also* psychotherapy

The Crackup (Fitzgerald), 21

creativity, 160, 207–13

Crick, Francis, 194

cyclothymic disorder, 41–44, *42*; mood, thinking, and behavior patterns in, *43*; mood changes in, *41*, 41–42; treatment of, 152

Cymbalta. *See* duloxetine

Davedax. *See* duloxetine

deep brain stimulation (DBS), 133

delirium after electroconvulsive therapy, 127

delusions, 37, 107; in bipolar I, *37*; in depression, *18*, 23, 24, 26, 51; grandiose, 10, 12–13; hypochondriacal, 23; in mania, *10*, 13, 15, *24*, 51; in mixed mood states, 26; mood-congruent, 50; in neurosyphilis, 61–62; paranoid, 23–24, 51; of persecution, 13; of poverty, 23; religious, 12–13; schizophrenic, 50–51, 52, 53

dementia praecox, 66

denial, 180, 218, 226, 229, 253

deoxyribonucleic acid (DNA), 194–96, 251, 252

Depakene; Depakote. *See* valproate

depression, 2, 9, 17–25, 247; ADHD and, 164–65; agitated, 2, 203; allopurinol for, 97; antidepressants for, 98–106, 139, 157–58; antipsychotics for, 108; atypical antipsychotics for, 112–13; in bipolar I, 31, 32, *32*, 36, 37; in bipolar II, 36–39, *39*, *40*, 40–41; in bipolar spectrum disorders, 44–49, *47*, *48*; cognitive theory of, 139–40; cognitive therapy for, 144; corticosteroid-induced, 203; in cyclothymic disorder, *41*, 41–42, *42*; diagnosis as basis of treatment for, 156; duration of episodes of, 35; electroconvulsive therapy for, 25, 129–30; individual therapy for, 139–42; lamotrigine for, 87; major (clinical), 18; mild, xii, *42*, 63; in mixed mood states, 25–26, *26*; "normal," 17–18, 19; in pediatric patients, 162, 163–64; postpartum, 171; pseudo-unipolar, 46; with psychotic features, *18*, 23, *24*, 26, 51, 164; seasonal, 185–86, 188–89; sleep deprivation for, 191–92; St. John's wort for, 122–23; substance abuse and, 179; switching between mania and, 36; symptoms of, 1, 17–25, *18*, 156; thyroid function and, 118; transcranial magnetic stimulation for, 131; unipolar, 40, *48*, 131, 171,

depression (*continued*)
188, 195, 205; vagal nerve stimulation for, 132; in women, 170, 171
Depression and Bipolar Support Alliance (DBSA), xii, 7, 235, 256
depressive stupor, 24
desipramine, *99*
desvenlafaxine, *102*
Desyrel. *See* trazodone
diabetes insipidus, 84
diabetes mellitus, antipsychotic-induced, 113–14
diagnosis, 28–53, 149–50; acceptance of, 217–20; of bipolar I, 30–37; of bipolar II, 37–41; of bipolar spectrum disorders, 44–49; classification system for, 28; of cyclothymic disorder, 41–44; development of tools for, 61–62; difficulty of, xii, 1; disclosure of, 226–27; psychiatric, 29–30; of rapid-cycling bipolar disorder, 49–50; of schizoaffective disorder, 50–53; traumatic impact of, 137; treatment based on, 155–56
Diagnostic and Statistical Manual of Mental Disorders (DSM), 54–57, 188–89; bipolar categories in *DSM-5*, 2, 44, 57; cyclothymic disorder in, 42, 57; history of, 54–55; uses and limitations of, 55–57
diazepam, 45, *116*
diet, 224; antipsychotic-induced weight gain and, 113–14; caffeine in, 224; MAOI interactions with, 103–4; nutritional supplements, 119–20
diffusion magnetic resonance imaging (dMRI), 205
disinhibition, 11, 13, 48, 177, 211, 237, 247
disorganized thinking and behavior, 13, 15, 16, 107, 108, 156, 212, 244
diurnal variation of mood, *18*, 21–22, 188, 191; reverse, 188, 189
doctor appointments, 218–19
donepezil, 166
dopamine, 251; medication effects on, 95, 102, 108–9, 111
double-blind, placebo-controlled studies, 79–80, 87
doxepin, *99*
drug interactions, 111; with lamotrigine, 87, 88; with MAOIs, 103
dry mouth, tricyclic antidepressant–induced, 100
duloxetine, 102, *102*
Dutonin. *See* nefazodone
dynamic psychology, 135–36

dysphoria, 20; antidepressant-associated chronic irritable, 105–6
dystonia, 110

Efexor; Efexor XR; Effexor; Effexor XR. *See* venlafaxine
Ehrlich, Paul, 61
Elavil. *See* amitriptyline
Eldepryl. *See* selegiline
electroconvulsive therapy (ECT), 124–30; for bipolar disorder, 25, 129–30, 151, 156–57; history of, 124–26; memory problems after, 127–29; procedure for, 126–27
electroencephalogram (EEG): for electroconvulsive therapy, 127; sleep, 190–91
emergency planning, 215, 231–38; insurance issues, 233–34, 235–37; safety issues and hospitalization, 237–38, 246–47; whom to call for help, 234–35
employment issues, 17, 138, 227
Emsam transdermal system. *See* selegiline
Endler, Norman, 16, 19, 21, 22, 23
energy level, 6; in bipolar III, 46, 47; in depression, 22–23; in mania, 10, 13, 16
Epitol; Equetro. *See* carbamazepine
Epival. *See* valproate
Erocap. *See* fluoxetine
erythema multiforme, 88, 94
escitalopram, 45, *101*
Eskalith; Eskalith CR. *See* lithium
essential fatty acids, 119, 120
euphoria, 9–15, *10*
EVT 101, 97
exercise, 22, 85, 114, 198, 224, 225
extrapyramidal symptoms (EPS), 109–11, 113

Facilitated Integrated Mood Management, 139
Falret, Jean-Pierre, 59–60
family, 239–49; bipolar disorder relapse and, 143, 243, 248; criticism of, 240, 243; education for patient and, 134–35, 138–39, 142–43; interventions for, 142, 143, 248–49; involuntary treatment and legal issues affecting, 244–46; safety issues and, 246–47; support for, 247–49; symptom recognition by, 239–42; whom to call for emergency help, 234–35
family history, 30, 31, *40*, 44, *47*, 50
Fanapt. *See* iloperidone
fatigue, 5, *18*, 22–23, 188, 191
fatty acids, 119, 120
Fieve, Ronald, 67
fight or flight response, 198–99

irritability (*continued*)
III, 46, 47; in cyclothymia, *43*; in mania, *10*,
13, 15, 16, 30, 152; in mixed mood states, *26*; in
pediatric patients, 164

James, Robert, 59
Jamison, Kay Redfield, 13, 25, 144, 209, 222, 246
jet lag, 152, 187

Keats, John, 212
kidney effects of lithium, 83, 84
Kinsey, Alfred, 57
Klonopin. *See* clonazepam
Kraepelin, Emil, 13, 14, 21, 23, 25, 26–27, 29,
35, 46, 62, 63, 66, 125, 150, 161, 185, 211, 221;
concept of cyclothymia, 41–43; concept of
manic-depressive insanity, 1, 12, 41, 60–61,
193
Kuhn, Roland, 67, 74, 99

lamotrigine (Lamictal), 44, 45, 86–89, 96; for
bipolar depression, 87; drug interactions
with, 87, *88*; mechanism of action of, 75,
86; in pregnancy, 171; side effects of, 88–89;
Stanford protocol for initiation of, 89, *89*;
therapeutic profile of, 87–88, *88*; time to
clinical effect of, 153–55
Latuda. *See* lurasidone
legal issues, 244–46
levothyroxine, 118
Lexapro. *See* escitalopram
Librium. *See* chlordiazepoxide
lifestyle regularization, 143, 192, 198, 221,
224–26
light therapy, 151, 185, 188–89
limbic system, 205
lithium (Lithobid; Lithonate; Lithotabs), xi, 14,
28, 30, 31, 77–85, 136, 152, 153; blood levels
of, 31, 81–82, *82*, 165–66, 218; for children,
165–66; compared with lamotrigine, 87;
compliance with, 219; discontinuation of,
80, 83, 222, 223, 248; effect on creativity, 213;
half-life of, 80–81, *81*; historical studies of,
64–68, 77–80, *79*; mechanism of action of,
75; during pregnancy and breast-feeding, 85,
86, 171; prevention of stress-induced brain
damage by, *201*, 201–2; prophylactic effect
of, 67, 78; psychotherapy and, 144; in rapid-
cycling bipolar disorder, 49; side effects of,
83–85, *84*; therapeutic profile of, 80–83, *81*;
toxicity of, 78, 81
living with bipolar disorder, 215, 217–30; building support system, 226–28; confronting and
accepting illness, 217–20; not becoming a
"bipolar victim," 228–30; practicing mood
hygiene, 220–26
lorazepam, 116, *116*
Lord Byron, xi, 207, *208*
Lovan. *See* fluoxetine
loxapine (Loxitane), *109*
Ludiomil. *See* maprotiline
lurasidone, *111*
Lustral. *See* sertraline
Luvox. *See* fluvoxamine
Lyrica. *See* pregabalin

magnetic resonance imaging (MRI), 204–5
major tranquilizers. *See* antipsychotic
medications
managed care, 235–37
mania, 2, 9–15; vs. ADHD, 163, 164; antipsychotics for, 108; in bipolar I, 30–31, 32,
32, 36, 37; creativity and, 212; delayed treatment for, 17; delirious, 14, 25; duration of
episodes of, 35; dysphoric, 15, 20, 25–26, 112,
247; electroconvulsive therapy for, 129–30;
vs. hypomania, 15–17; length of time before
hospitalization for, *17*; mixed, 25–26; mortality and, 14; in pediatric patients, 162, 163;
precipitated by ADHD medications, 166;
precipitated by antidepressants, *47*, 67, 68,
98, 105, 139, 157, 166; precipitated by sleep
deprivation, 192, 224; vs. schizophrenia, 14;
stages of, 14–15; switching between depression and, 36; symptoms of, 1–2, *10*, 10–14;
unpleasantness of, 14, 15
manic-depressive illness, 9, 17. *See also* bipolar
disorder
maprotiline, 99
marital relationship, 136, 142, 223
medical conditions, 160; Americans with Disabilities Act and, 227; painful, *18*, 22–23
medications: antidepressants, 98–106, 150,
157–58; antipsychotics, 107–14, 150, 153; for
anxiety and sleep disturbances, 115–17, *116*,
153, 155; compliance with, 218–19, 222–23;
contraceptive, 172–73; discontinuation of,
xi–xii, 80, 83, 171, 172, 222, 248; duration of
treatment with, 152–55, 222, 253; electroconvulsive therapy and, 129; insurance coverage
for, 236; management in split treatment, 147;
mood stabilizers, 44–45, 77–97; N-acetyl
cysteine, 96, 120–21; off-label prescribing of,
95–96, 113, 236; pharmacogenomics, 251–52;

during pregnancy and breast-feeding, 85,
86, 171–72; psychotherapy and, 136, 137, 144;
for relapse prevention, 67, 78, 112, 222, 223;
reminder systems for, 223; stimulants, 156,
166; therapeutic results as guide to use of,
148–51; time to clinical effect of, 152–55. *See
also specific drugs and classes*
Medscape, 257
melancholia, 38, 54, 58–60
melatonin, 117, 119–20, 186
Mellaril. *See* thioridazine
memory problems, 6, *18*, 21, 29; after electroconvulsive therapy, 127–29
Mendel, Emanuel, 15
Mendel, Gregor, 193–94
menstrually related mood fluctuations, 169,
172–73
mental status examination, 29
Miklowitz, David, 139
A Mind That Found Itself (Beers), 51
Mirapex. *See* pramipexole
mirtazapine, *102*
mixed mood states, 2, 9, 25–27, *47*
molindone (Moban), *109*
Molipaxin. *See* trazodone
monoamine oxidase (MAO-A and MAO-B),
102–4, 105
monoamine oxidase inhibitors (MAOIs), 98,
102–4, *103*
mood: affect and, 9; brain regulation of, 5, 8,
199, 251; creativity and, 212; definition of, 5,
9; diurnal variation of, *18*, 21–22, 188, 189,
191; good vs. low, 5–6; hormones and, 117–18;
menstrually related fluctuations of, 169,
172–73; reactivity of, *18*; seasonal changes in,
41, 117, 173, 185, 186–89
mood, abnormal, 2–3, 6–27; constricted mood,
18–19; depression, 17–25; hypomania, 15–17;
mania, 9–15; mixed states, 2, 9, 25–27; schizophrenia and, 52
mood chart, 143, 225
mood hygiene, 220–26
mood-stabilizing medications, 44–45, 77–97,
150, 153; carbamazepine, 92–94; for children,
165–66; effect on creativity, 213; on the horizon, 96–97, 150; lamotrigine, 86–89, 153–54;
lithium, 77–85; mechanisms of action of, 75;
N-acetyl cysteine, 96; oxcarbazepine, 94–95;
pramipexole, 95; during pregnancy and
breast-feeding, 85, 86, 171–72; riluzole, 96;
tiagabine, 96; valproate, 89–92; zonisamide,
96. *See also specific drugs*

N-acetyl cysteine (NAC), 96
Nardil. *See* phenelzine
National Alliance for the Mentally Ill (NAMI),
256
National Mental Health Association (NMH),
234–35, 257
natural history, *34*, 34–37, *36*
Navane. *See* thiothixene
nefazodone, *102*
neuroimaging, 204–5, 251
neuroleptics. *See* antipsychotic medications
neurons, *72*, 73–75; apoptosis of, 86;
hippocampal, 75, 199–201, *200*, *201*
Neurontin. *See* gabapentin
neuroplasticity, 73–76
neuroscience research, 62, 250–53
neurotransmitters, 70, *72*, 73–75; medication
effects on, 75, 99, 100, 102–3, 108
norepinephrine, 74; antidepressant effects on,
99, 100, 102, 103
Norpramin. *See* desipramine
nortriptyline, 99
nutritional supplements, 119–20

Occam's razor, 156
off-label prescribing, 95–96, 113, 236
olanzapine, *111*, 113
omega-3 fatty acids, 120
One Flew Over the Cuckoo's Nest, 125, 126
optimism, 5, 6, 46, *48*
organic illness, 135
orthostatic hypotension, MAOI-induced, 104
oxcarbazepine, 94–95
oxidative damage, 121

painful conditions, *18*, 22–23
paliperidone, *111*
Pamelor. *See* nortriptyline
panic attacks, 2, 13, 15, 57, 117, 136
Parnate. *See* tranylcypromine
paroxetine, *101*, 105
patient/family education, 134–35, 138–39,
142–43
Paxil; Paxil CR. *See* paroxetine
pediatric bipolar disorder, 159, 161–68; ADHD
and, 163, 164–65; age at onset of, 161; compared with adult bipolar disorder, 162, *162*;
course of, 161, 167; depression as first sign of,
162, 163–64; developmental effects of, 167;
future research in, 167–68; prognosis for, 167;
rapid-cycling, 161, 162, 165, 167; symptoms of,
163–64; treatment of, 161, 165–67

perphenazine, *109*
pessimism, 5, 6, 20, 139, 240
pharmacogenomics, 251–52
phenelzine, *103*
phenothiazines, 107. *See also* antipsychotic medications
photoperiod manipulation, 186, 188
phototherapy, 151, 185, 188–89
physical restraint of patient, 59, 63, 247
Plath, Sylvia, 212
Poe, Edgar Allan, xi
postpartum mood disorders, 117, 170–71
power of attorney, 246
pramipexole, 95
pregabalin, 117
pregnancy, 170–72; electroconvulsive therapy in, 129; medications during, 85, 86, 171–72
premenstrual syndromes, 172–73
pressured speech, 11, 15, 16, *26*
Pristiq. *See* desvenlafaxine
procrastination, 224–25
Prolixin. *See* fluphenazine
protriptyline, *99*
Prozac. *See* fluoxetine
pseudo-parkinsonism, 110
psychiatric care, 232–35
psychiatrist-psychotherapist, 147
psychoanalytic treatment, 63, 67
psycho-educational group therapy, 138–39
psychosis, 107; antipsychotics for, 107–14. *See also* delusions; hallucinations
psychotherapy, 70, 134–47, 151, 230; benefits in bipolar disorder, 137, 145, 146–47, 158; dynamic, 135–36, 144; for family, 142, 143, 249; group, 138–39; individual therapy for depression, 139–42; medications and, 136, 137, 144; new treatment models for, 142–43; professional training for, 145; in split treatment, 147; for stress and conflict management, 223–25; traditional individual, 144–46; types of, 136–37
PubMed, 257

quetiapine, *111, 113*

racing thoughts, *10*, 10–11, 13, 14, 15, 108, 152
rapid-cycling bipolar disorder, 49–50; antidepressants and, 49, 50, 98, 104, 105, 139, 157; in children, 161, 162, 165, 167; hypothyroidism and, 118; ultra-rapid–cycling, 26–27; in women, 50, 169–70
rapid eye movement (REM) sleep, *190*, 190–91

rash, drug-induced, 88–89, 94
relapse(s), 34, 35, *37*; after medication discontinuation, xi–xii, 80, 171, 172; antidepressants and, 157; family and, 143, 243, 248; lithium blood level and, 81, *82*; medications for prevention of, 112, 222, 223; in pediatric patients, 167; during pregnancy/postpartum, 171–72; psychotherapy and, 137, 138, 141, 142, 143, 144; in stages-of-change model, *181*, 182; stress and, 221–22, 243; suicidality and, 237, 238
relationship problems, 202, 218, 223, 225, 228, 248; with employers, 227; of pediatric patients, 167; psychotherapy for, 142–45
Remergil; Remeron. *See* mirtazapine
research, 250–53; genetic, 196–97, 251–53; neuroscience, 62, 250–53; in pediatric bipolar disorder, 167–68
resources, 255–57
riluzole (Rilutek), 96
risperidone (Risperdal), *111, 113*
Rosenthal, Norman, 185

sadness, 5, 6, 8, 14, 19, 20, 27, 42, 144, 145, 211
safety issues, 237–38, 246–47; electroconvulsive therapy, 126, 127, 151; involuntary treatment and, 244–46. *See also* suicidality
Saphris. *See* asenapine
Sapolsky, Robert, 199
Sarafem. *See* fluoxetine
schizoaffective disorder, 50–53
schizophrenia, 8, 15, 50–53, 60, 63; antipsychotics for, 107–8
Schou, Morgans, 67, 78–80, *79, 82*, 213
Schumann, Robert, 208–9, *210*
scopolamine, 97
Sealdin. *See* sertraline
seasonal affective disorder (SAD), 117, 173, 188–89
seasonal mood changes, 185–86
selective serotonin reuptake inhibitors (SSRIs), 100–101, *101*
selegiline, *103*, 104
Seroquel. *See* quetiapine
serotonin, 74, 251; medication effects on, 99, 102, 108, 111
serotonin and norepinephrine reuptake inhibitors (SNRIs), 102, *102*
Seroxat. *See* paroxetine
sertraline, *101*, 157
Serzone. *See* nefazodone
sexual behavior: in cyclothymia, *43*; in depression, *18*, 22; in hypomania, 16; in mania, *10*, 11, 12, 14; of pediatric patients, 163

sexual dysfunction, drug-induced, 101, 104
shame, 19, 38, 52, 145, 243
Sideril. *See* trazodone
Sinequan. *See* doxepin
skin effects of drugs: carbamazepine, 94; lamotrigine, 88–89; lithium, *84,* 85
sleep deprivation, 115, 143, 171, 189, 218, 225, 218;
mania precipitated by, 192, 224; therapeutic,
189, 191–92
sleep disturbances, 6; in cyclothymic disorder, 43; in depression, 21–22, *40,* 191–92; in
mania, *10,* 12; medications for, 115–17, *116,* 153,
155; in mixed mood states, *26;* in seasonal
affective disorder, 188, 189
sleep-wake cycle, 22, 187, 189–91, *190,* 224
slow-wave sleep (SWS), *190,* 190–91
social rhythm metric, 143
social withdrawal, *18, 203*
spending sprees, 11, 14, 30, *43*
split treatment, 147
stages-of-change model, 180–83, *181*
Stelazine. *See* trifluoperazine
Stevens-Johnson syndrome, 94
stigma, 229
stimulants, 156, 166
St. John's wort, 121–23
stocktaking, 224
Strattera. *See* atomoxetine
stress, 142–43, 218; bodily response to, 117–18,
198–202, *200, 201;* management of, 142, 143,
221, 223–24; neuroplasticity and, 76; relapse
and, 221–22, 243
stupor, depressive, 24
Styron, William, 19, 20, 22, 24
substance abuse/addiction, 11, 12, *43,* 45, 159,
174–83; bipolar binges and, 174–77; brain
effects of, 178–79; relationship between
bipolar disorder and, 178; stages-of-change
model and treatment of, 180–83, *181;* suicide
and, 179–80
suicidality, xii, *18,* 24, 26, 31, 41, 47, 61, 212, 246–47;
electroconvulsive therapy for, 129; hospitalization for, 237–38, 247; prevention of, 237; risk
factors for, 247; substance abuse and, 179–80
support groups, 136–37, 227–28, 230, 248
support system, 226–28; for family, 247–49
symptoms, 1–2, 6, 8–9, 217, 218; of depression,
17–25; family recognition of, 239–42; of
hypomania, 15–17; of mania, 1–2, 9–15, 152; in
pediatric patients, 163–64; remission of, 34,
35, 78, 150, 162, 222; seasonal variation in, 41,
117, 173, 185, 186–89; in women, 169–70

synapses, *72, 73*–74
Synthyroid. *See* levothyroxine
syphilis, 61–62, 125, 135
Systematic Treatment Enhancement Program
for Bipolar Disorder (STEP-BD), 104–5,
151–52, 157–58

tacrine, 166
"talking cure," 62, 67. *See also* psychotherapy
tardive dyskinesia (TD), 110
Tegretol. *See* carbamazepine
temperament, 42; bipolar spectrum disorders and, 46, *47;* cyclothymic, 41–42;
hyperthymic, *47, 48*
Tenex. *See* guanfacine
testosterone, 170, 194
thinking patterns: in cyclothymic disorder, *43;*
in depression, 18, 20–21; in mania, 10–14, 26
thioridazine, *109*
thiothixene, *109*
Thombran. *See* trazodone
Thorazine. *See* chlorpromazine
thyroid disorders, 49, 202–3, *203;* lithium-
induced, *84,* 85
thyroid hormones, 118, 202–3
tiagabine, 96
Tofranil. *See* imipramine
toxic epidermal necrosis, 88–89
transcranial direct current stimulation (tDCS),
133
transcranial magnetic stimulation (TMS),
130–32, 151, 205, 251, 252
Tranxene. *See* clorazepate
tranylcypromine, *103*
trazodone, *102*
treatment(s): algorithms for, 151; antidepressants, 98–106, 150; antipsychotic medications, 107–14, 150; for anxiety and sleep
disturbances, 115–17, *116;* brain-stimulation
techniques, 124–33, 151, 205, 251; counseling/
psychotherapy, 134–47, 151, 158; duration
of, 152–55, 222, 253; genetic research and,
196–97, 251–53; herbal preparations and
nutritional supplements, 119–20; historical,
63–68; involuntary, 17, 232–33, 244–46, 247;
mood-stabilizing medications, 44–45, 77–97,
150; omega-3 fatty acids and fish oil, 120;
patient commitment to, 218–19, 222–23, 248;
for pediatric patients, 161, 165–67; phototherapy, 151, 185, 188–89; refusal of, 248; sleep
deprivation, 189, 191–92; STEP-BD study of,
104–5, 151–52, 157–58; for substance abuse/